Symposium on clinical frontiers in reconstructive microsurgery

Volume twenty-four

Symposium on clinical frontiers in reconstructive microsurgery

Editors

HARRY J. BUNCKE, M.D.

*Clinical Professor of Surgery and Chief,
Division of Microsurgery,
Ralph K. Davies Medical Center,
University of California, San Francisco,
San Francisco, California*

DAVID W. FURNAS, M.D.

*Clinical Professor and Chief,
Division of Plastic Surgery,
University of California, Irvine,
Irvine, California*

Proceedings of the Symposium of the Plastic Surgery Educational Foundation
of the American Society of Plastic and Reconstructive Surgeons, Inc.,
held in Anaheim, California, June 25-28, 1981

with 782 illustrations

The C. V. Mosby Company

St. Louis   Toronto   1984

MOSBY

A TRADITION OF PUBLISHING EXCELLENCE

Editor: Karen Berger
Assistant editor: Terry Van Schaik, Sandra Gilfillan
Editing supervisor: Elaine Steinborn
Manuscript editor: Suzanne Blackledge
Design: Staff
Production: Carol O'Leary, Barbara Merritt

Volume one copyrighted 1969, Volume two copyrighted 1969,
Volume three copyrighted 1971, Volume four copyrighted 1972,
Volume five copyrighted 1973, Volume six copyrighted 1973,
Volume seven copyrighted 1973, Volume eight copyrighted 1974,
Volume nine copyrighted 1974, Volume ten copyrighted 1974,
Volume eleven copyrighted 1975, Volume twelve copyrighted 1976,
Volume thirteen copyrighted 1976, Volume fourteen copyrighted 1976,
Volume fifteen copyrighted 1976, Volume sixteen copyrighted 1978,
Volume seventeen copyrighted 1978, Volume eighteen copyrighted 1978,
Volume nineteen copyrighted 1978, Volume twenty copyrighted 1979,
Volume twenty-one copyrighted 1982, Volume twenty-two copyrighted 1983,
Volume twenty-three copyrighted 1984

Printed in the United States of America

The C.V. Mosby Company
11830 Westline Industrial Drive, St. Louis, Missouri 63146

Library of Congress Cataloging in Publication Data

Symposium on Clinical Frontiers in Reconstructive Micro-
    surgery (1981: Anaheim, Calif.)
Symposium on Clinical Frontiers in Reconstructive Microsurgery

    "Volume twenty-four."
    Bibliography: p.
    Includes index.
    1. Surgery, Plastic—Congresses.   2.   Microsurgery—
Congresses.   I.   Buncke, Harry J.   II.   Furnas,
David W.   III.   Plastic Surgery Educational
Foundation (American Society of Plastic and Reconstructive
Surgeons)   [DNLM: 1.   Microsurgery—Methods—Congresses.
2.   Surgery, Plastic—Methods—Congresses.   WO 600 S98845s
1981]
RD118.A2S92   1981   617'.05   83-19305
ISBN 0-8016-1714-6

AC/MV/MV   9 8 7 6 5 4 3 2 1   02/B/220

Contributors

Bruce M. Achauer, M.D., F.A.C.S.

Associate Professor, Division of Plastic Surgery, University of California, Irvine; Director, U.C.I. Burn Center, University of California, Irvine, Medical Center, Orange, California

Bernard S. Alpert, M.D.

Assistant Clinical Professor, Department of Plastic Surgery, University of California, San Francisco; Co-Director, Microsurgical Laboratories, Department of Plastic Surgery, Ralph K. Davies Medical Center, San Francisco, California

Dr. med. Edgar Biemer

Consultant for Plastic Surgery, Klinikum rechts der Isar, Technical University, Munich, Germany

Kirby S. Black, B.S.M.E., P.E.

Technical Director, Reconstructive Microsurgery Laboratories, Division of Plastic Surgery, University of California, Irvine; Irvine, California

Willi Boeckx, M.D., Ph.D.

Associate Professor, Department of Surgery, Catholic University of Leuven; Consultant Plastic Surgery, Department of Surgery, Leuven, Belgium

Kenneth L.B. Brown, B.Sc., M.D., F.R.C.S.(C)

Assistant Professor of Surgery, McGill University; Attending Orthopedic Surgeon, The Montreal Children's Hospital, Montreal, Quebec, Canada

Harry J. Buncke, M.D.

Clinical Professor of Surgery and Chief, Division of Microsurgery, Ralph K. Davies Medical Center, University of California, San Francisco; San Francisco, California

Hsu Hsi Cheng, M.D.

Associate Professor, Department of Orthopaedics, Peking Medical College; Chief of Microsurgery, Division of Microsurgery, Department of Orthopaedics, Chi Shui Tan Hospital, Peking, China

Shu Lan Chia, M.D.

Attending Doctor, Division of Microsurgery, Department of Orthopaedics, Chi Shui Tan Hospital, Peking, China

Richard L. Cruess, M.D.

Dean, Faculty of Medicine, and Professor of Surgery, McGill University, Montreal, Quebec, Canada

Rollin K. Daniel, M.D., F.R.C.S.(C), F.A.C.S.

Professor of Surgery, McGill University; Chief of Plastic Surgery and Director, Microsurgical Laboratories, Royal Victoria Hospital, Montreal, Quebec, Canada

Don R. DeFeo, M.D.

Assistant Clinical Professor, Division of Neurosurgery, University of California, Irvine; Irvine, California

Marcus Castro Ferreira, M.D.

Associate Professor, Plastic Surgery Division, University of São Paulo Medical School; Surgeon in Charge, Microsurgery Unit, Hospital Das Clinicas, University of São Paulo Medical Center, São Paulo, Brazil

Frederick Finseth, M.D.

Mountain View, California

John D. Franklin, M.D.

Associate Clinical Professor and Chairman, Department of Plastic Surgery, University of Tennessee-Chattanooga; Chattanooga, Tennessee

Roger Friedman, M.D.

Fellow in Microvascular and Hand Surgery, Ralph K. Davies Medical Center, San Francisco, California; Resident in Plastic and Reconstructive Surgery, University of Michigan, Ann Arbor, Michigan

Toyomi Fujino, M.D., D. Med. Sci., F.A.C.S.

Professor and Chairman, Department of Plastic and Reconstructive Surgery, Keio University School of Medicine; Consulting Plastic Surgeon, Department of Plastic and Reconstructive Surgery, National Tokyo Second Hospital, Tokyo, and Hiratsuka City Hospital, Kanagawaken, Japan

David W. Furnas, M.D.

Clinical Professor and Chief, Division of Plastic Surgery, University of California, Irvine; Irvine, California

Nicholas G. Georgiade, D.D.S., M.D., F.A.C.S.

Professor and Chairman, Department of Plastic, Maxillofacial, and Oral Surgery, Duke University Medical Center, Durham, North Carolina

Alain L. Gilbert, M.D.

Chief, Microsurgery Laboratories, Hospitals of Paris; Attending Hand Surgeon, American Hospital, Hôpital Trousseau, Paris, France

Marjorie Girling, B.Sc. (Hons), Ph.D.

Senior Physicist, Department of Physics, Mount Vernon Hospital, Northwood, Middlesex, England

Leonard Gordon, M.D.

Assistant Clinical Professor, Department of Orthopaedic Surgery/Chief Orthopedic Hand Surgery Service, University of California, San Francisco; Attending Surgeon, Microvascular Surgery Unit, Hand and Microvascular Surgery Unit, Ralph K. Davies Medical Center, San Francisco, California

Kiyonori Harii, M.D.

Associate Professor, Department of Plastic Surgery, Faculty of Medicine, University of Tokyo; Tokyo, Japan

Douglas H. Harrison, M.B., F.R.C.S.

Consultant Plastic Surgeon, Mount Vernon Hospital, Northwood, Middlesex, England; Consultant Plastic Surgeon, Plastic Surgery Departments, Barnet General Hospital, Barnet, Hertfordshire, Edgware General Hospital, Edgware, Middlesex, Northwick Park Hospital, Harrow, Middlesex, England

Eiji Hatano, M.D.

Orthopaedic Surgeon and Research Assistant, Department of Orthopaedic Surgery, Hiroshima University School of Medicine, Hiroshima, Japan

Philip M. Hendel, F.R.C.S.

Assistant Professor, Department of Plastic Surgery, Tulane University School of Medicine, New Orleans, Louisiana

Yoshikazu Ikuta, M.D.

Chief of Microsurgery Unit, Department of Orthopaedic Surgery, Hiroshima University School of Medicine; Lecturer, Department of Orthopaedic Surgery, Hiroshima University School of Medicine, Hiroshima, Japan

Harold E. Kleinert, M.D.

Clinical Professor of Surgery, University of Louisville School of Medicine; Director of Hand Surgery Services, University of Louisville Hospitals, Louisville, Kentucky

David G. Kline, M.D.

Professor and Chairman, Department of Neurosurgery, LSU Medical Center; Department of Neurosurgery, Charity (Visiting Staff), Oshsner Foundation (Academic Staff), Southern Baptist, Touro, and H. Dieu (Active), Consultant, New Orleans VA Hospital and Kessler Air Force Base Hospital, New Orleans, Louisiana

John A. Kusske, M.A., M.D.

Professor and Chief, Division of Neurosurgery, University of California, Irvine; Irvine, California

Carroll B. Lesesne, M.D.

Resident, Plastic Surgery, Cornell University, Cornell–New York Hospital, New York, New York

Disa Lidman, M.D., M.Sc.

Department of Plastic Surgery, Linköping University Hospital, Linköping, Sweden

Tadeusz Lyczakowski, M.D.

General Surgeon, Krakow, Poland; Former Research Fellow, Microvascular Laboratories, Royal Victoria Hospital, Montreal, Quebec, Canada

Ralph T. Manktelow, M.D., F.R.C.S.(C)

Associate Professor, Department of Surgery, University of Toronto; Head, Division of Plastic Surgery, Toronto General Hospital, Toronto, Ontario, Canada

Carl H. Manstein, M.D.

Philadelphia, Pennsylvania; Former Christine Kleinert Fellow in Hand Surgery, Department of Surgery, University of Louisville Medical School, Louisville, Kentucky

Pierre J. Marie, Ph.D.

Director of Research, Lariboisière Hospital, Paris, France; Former Assistant Professor of Experimental Surgery and Director, Bone Histomorphometry Section, Shriners Hospital for Crippled Children, Montreal, Quebec, Canada

Stephen J. Mathes, M.D., F.A.C.S.

Associate Professor of Surgery, Division of Plastic, Reconstructive and Hand Surgery, University of California, San Francisco; San Francisco, California

Brian J. Mayou, M.B., F.R.C.S.

Consultant Plastic Surgeon, St. Thomas's Hospital, London; Queen Victoria Hospital, East Grinstead, Sussex, England.

Prof. Dr. Hanno Millesi

Head, Department of Plastic and Reconstructive Surgery, First Surgical Clinic, Vienna; Head, Ludwig-Boltzmann Institute for Experimental Plastic Surgery, Vienna, Austria

Brian D.G. Morgan, M.B., F.R.C.S.

Consultant Plastic Surgeon, Plastic and Maxillofacial Unit, University College Hospital, London, England; Regional Plastic Jaw Surgery Centre, Mount Vernon Hospital, Northwood, Middlesex, England

Wayne A. Morrison, M.B.B.S., F.R.A.C.S.

Assistant Plastic Surgeon, Senior Research Officer, Microsurgery Unit, St. Vincent's Hospital, Melbourne, Victoria, Australia

Godfrey Mott, M.I.ELEC.I.E.

Chief Technician, Physics Department, Mount Vernon Hospital, Northwood, Middlesex, England

R. Yaeger Mullen, B.S. (MT [A.S.C.P.])

Supervisor, Plastic Surgery Research Laboratories, Division of Plastic Surgery, Duke University Medical Center, Durham, North Carolina

Tom R. Norris, M.D.

Director, Microsurgery Laboratory, Attending Physician in Hand and Orthopaedic Surgery, Department of Hand Surgery, Pacific Medical Center, Presbyterian Hospital, San Francisco, California

Bernard McC. O'Brien, B.Sc., M.D., M.S., F.R.C.S. (Eng.), F.R.A.C.S., F.A.C.S.

Professorial Associate, Department of Anatomy, University of Melbourne; Plastic Surgeon and Director, Microsurgery Research Unit, St. Vincent's Hospital, Melbourne, Victoria, Australia

Samuel W. Parry II, M.D.

Chief Resident, Department of Surgery, Division of Plastic Surgery, University of California, San Francisco; San Francisco, California

Norman K. Poppen, M.D.

Clinical Assistant Professor, Department of Orthopedics, University of California, Davis, School of Medicine, Davis, California; Consultant, Hand Surgery Service, Chief Shoulder and Elbow Clinic, Department of Orthopedics, University of California, Davis, Medical Center, Sacramento, California

Ronald Riefkohl, M.D.

Assistant Professor, Division of Plastic, Maxillofacial and Oral Surgery, Duke University Medical Center, Durham, North Carolina

Donald Serafin, M.D., F.A.C.S.

Professor, Division of Plastic, Maxillofacial and Oral Surgery, Duke University Medical Center, Durham, North Carolina

William W. Shaw, M.D., F.A.C.S.

Associate Professor of Surgery (Plastic Surgery), New York University School of Medicine; Chief, Plastic Surgery Service, Bellevue Hospital, Director, Microsurgery and Replantation Surgery Service, New York University/Bellevue Hospitals, Institute of Reconstructive Plastic Surgery, New York University Medical Center, New York, New York

Susumu Tamai, M.D.

Associate Professor, Department of Orthopaedic Surgery, Nara Medical University Hospital, Kashihara, Nara, Japan

G. Ian Taylor, M.B.B.S., F.R.C.S., F.R.A.C.S.

Hunterian Professor, Associate Plastic Surgeon, University of Melbourne; Consultant Plastic Surgeon, Royal Melbourne Hospital; Senior Consultant Plastic Surgeon, Preston and Northcote Hospital, Melbourne, Victoria, Australia

Ivan Thomas, M.D.

Los Angeles, California

Jack W. Tupper, B.S., M.D.

Clinical Professor, Orthopaedic Surgery, University of California, San Francisco, California; Attending Physician, Chief, Division of Hand Surgery, Department of Orthopedics, Samuel Merritt Hospital, Oakland, California; Director, Hand Clinic, Department of Orthopedics, Highland Alameda County Hospital, Oakland; Director, Hand Clinic, Department of Orthopedics, Children's Hospital of Northern California, Oakland, California

Vincent E. Voci, M.D.

Department of Surgery, Section of Plastic and Reconstructive Surgery, The Mason Clinic and Virginia Mason Medical Center, Seattle, Washington

Da Ching Yin, M.D.

Attending Doctor, Division of Microsurgery, Department of Orthopaedics, Chi Shui Tan Hospital, Peking, China

Kaoru Yoshioka, M.D.

Orthopaedic Surgeon and Research Assistant, Department of Orthopaedic Surgery, Hiroshima University School of Medicine, Hiroshima, Japan

Preface

Symposium on Clinical Frontiers in Reconstructive Microsurgery is a written version of the Symposium of the same name held at Disneyland in Anaheim, California, in June 1981. The book gives a picture of the field, updated to 1984, at a time when microsurgery has made great advances in solving reconstructive problems of all parts of the body. This volume is a "still shot" of microsurgery's "Frontierland," and in the background are hints of "Fantasyland" and "Tomorrowland."

Our contributing authors come from ten nations on four continents. They represent a majority of the leading microsurgery centers of the world.

The symposium took place 15 years after the first experimental digital replantation, 12 years after the first clinical digital replantation, 8 years after the first clinical free flap of omentum with skin graft, and 7 years after the first clinical free flap of skin and subcutaneous tissue. The field is still new enough that all of the pioneers who achieved these landmarks are on our roster of authors.

The term "reconstructive microsurgery" has come to distinguish the work of the microsurgeon who deals with the integument, the musculoskeletal system, and the peripheral neurovascular structures. Our authors come from backgrounds in plastic surgery, orthopedic surgery, general surgery, and neurosurgery. They guide us through innovative techniques, instruct us in monitoring, and warn us of potential pitfalls, covering reconstructive problems from head to toe.

If microsurgeons weren't such a gregarious group, one might say that never again will such a group of pioneers and world authorities assemble in a single place; but gregarious they are—and we hope that *Symposium on Clinical Frontiers in Reconstructive Microsurgery* will simply stand as a noteworthy and happy landmark in one of surgery's most exciting spheres of work.

This volume was made possible by the efficient editorial and copy work of Karen Berger, Senior Editor, Medical and Dental Division, The C.V. Mosby Co., and Janet E. Inkster, Administrative Assistant, Division of Plastic Surgery, University of California, Irvine.

Harry J. Buncke
David W. Furnas

Contents

Part I

Microsurgery in the field

Chapter 1

Microvascular free flaps: survival, donor sites, and application

William W. Shaw

Since the advent of microvascular free flap surgery, several questions have frequently been asked: How reliable are free flaps? How often are they used? What is their role in the future?

To answer some of these questions, we started a survey based on 1,240 flaps from twelve microsurgery centers (all participants in the Leeds Castle [U.K.] Microsurgery Conference, 1980) (Fig. 1-1). In 1981 our survey group was augmented with nine more centers, bringing the total number of flaps to 2,233. Representing the microsurgery centers were: United States—H. Buncke, D. Serafin, W. Shaw, D. Baker, R. Acland, J. Franklin, J. May, S. Mathes, A. VanBeek, and W. Merritt; France—A. Gilbert, C. LeQuang, J. Baudet, J. Michon, and G. Foucher; Australia—B. O'Brien, J. Morrison, I. Taylor; United Kingdom—B. Bailey and M. Webster; Canada—R. Daniel; Japan—K. Harii and K. Ohmori; and China—T.S. Chang and Y. Song. Additional data on success rates and donor sites were obtained from a separate survey of 1,033 flaps in China. The total number of flaps per center ranged from 17 to 368. The average number of flaps per center was 112; the median was 67.

RATE OF SUCCESS OF FREE FLAPS

"Success" was defined as survival of the flap (or at least the major part of the flap) with achievement of the original reconstructive goal. The overall success rate was 94% for all years, starting with the first clinical successes in 1972. The data suggested that from 1972 to 1979 the success rate was about 89% and that it increased to 94% thereafter.

Ninety percent of all the flaps achieved an immediate and enduring success without further surgry. Ten percent of the flaps required additional operative procedures because of vascular complications, and the salvage rate among these flaps was 40%, bringing the total success rate to 94% (Table 1-1).

RECIPIENT SITES (Table 1-2)

The lower extremity was the most common recipient site (approximately 40% of flaps), followed closely by the head and neck (approximately 35%), the upper extremities (15%), and the breast and trunk (10%). The pattern of donor site choices varied greatly from center to center, probably representing a bias in the type of clinical case load as well as different emphasis.

DONOR SITES (Table 1-3)

Where a specific vessel could supply any of several blocks of tissue, each block is considered a separate flap. For example, the *dorsalis pedis artery* sup-

Table 1-1. Free flap survival data

Total flaps	Success*	Failure
2,233	2,083 (93.3%)	150 (6.7%)

*Ninety flaps (4%) were salvaged by reexploration.

Table 1-2. Free flap recipient sites in four groups (selected randomly to illustrate differences)

Head/ neck (%)	Breast/ trunk (%)	Upper extremity (%)	Lower extremity (%)
30	15	15	40
56	4	16	24
23	17	18	40
43	3	13	42

```
Participant:_____

  I.  Free Flaps Survival
```

	No. of Flaps	Success	Salvaged by Re-exploration	Failure
All years				
Recent 12 mos.				

```
 II.  Donor Sites:
            Free Skin Flaps _____   Myocutaneous Free Flaps_____
               Groin          _____      Latissimus dorsi     _____
               Delto-Ped.     _____      Tensor fascialata    _____
               Dorsalis Ped._____         Gracilis             _____
               Others         _____      Gluteus max.         _____
                                               Others

            Free Muscle                     Bone
               Gracilis       _____      Fibula
               Pectoralis     _____      Rib                  _____
               Extensor Brevis_____        Deep Iliac           _____
               Others         _____      Others               _____

            Compound
               Toe (1st)      _____      Others               _____
                   (2nd)      _____                           _____
               Rib & Skin     _____                           _____
               Ilium & Skin   _____                           _____

III.  Recipient Sites:
            Head/Neck         _____   Upper Extremity         _____
            Breast/Trunk      _____   Lower Extremity         _____

 IV.  Current Anticoagulation Routine (+):
```

	Heparin 1000 /hr	Heparin 1000 /hr	Dextran	ASA	Persan-tine	Coum-arin	Others
Free Flaps							
Replants							

Fig. 1-1. Questionnaire sent to twenty-one microsurgery centers.

Table 1-3. Reported free flap donor sites

Donor site	Artery	Reference
Skin flaps		
Scalp	Superficial temporal	34
Scalp	Occipital	59
Retroauricular	Posterior auricular	28
Forehead	Anterior superficial temporal	53, 58
Neck	Transverse cervical	67
Thorocoacromial	Thoracoacromial	67
Deltopectoral	Internal mammary perforator	33
Lateral thoracic (axillary)	Lateral thoracic	8, 9
Scapula	Circumflex scapular	6, 29, 51, 55
Deltoid	Posterior humeral circumflex	26
Medial arm	Septal cutaneous	23, 68, 69
Lateral arm	Septal cutaneous	68
Forearm	Radial	69

Table 1-3, cont'd. Reported free flap donor sites

Donor site	Artery	Reference
Groin	Superficial inferior epigastric and superficial circumflex iliac	21, 32, 56
Saphenous	Saphenous	1
Medial thigh	Branch of superficial femoral	5
Lateral thigh	Branch of profundus femoris	5
Dorsal foot	Dorsalis pedis	22, 58, 63
First toe web	Dorsalis pedis	53, 54, 70
Partial great toe	Dorsalis pedis	25
Myocutaneous flaps		
Latissimus dorsi	Thoracodorsal	47
Upper rectus abdominis	Inferior epigastric	67
Lower rectus abdominis	Inferior epigastric	61
Gracilis	Medial femoral circumflex	32
Rectus femoris	Lateral femoral circumflex	64
Tensor fascia lata	Lateral femoral circumflex	14, 39
Medial gastrocnemius	Medial sural	16
Gluteus maximus	Superior gluteal	27
Gluteus maximus	Inferior gluteal	44
Muscle for motion or coverage		
Pectoralis major	Thoracoacromial	18, 40
Pectoralis minor	Thoracoacromial	76
Latissimus dorsi	Thoracoacromial	45
Serratus anterior	Thoracoacromial	12, 71
Gracilis	Medial femoral circumflex	35, 48
Medial gastrocnemius	Medial sural	16, 43
Rectus abdominis	Inferior epigastric	67
Extensor brevis of toes	Dorsalis pedis	50
Vascularized bone		
Rib	Posterior intercostal	65
Rib	Anterior intercostal via internal mammary	3
Iliac crest	Deep circumflex iliac	72, 75
Iliac crest	Superficial circumflex iliac via groin skin flap	57, 72, 75
Fibula	Peroneal	18, 74
Second metatarsal	Dorsalis pedis	56, 60
Visceral organs		
Omentum	Gastroepiploic	4, 11, 14, 36, 52
Omentum and stomach	Gastroepiploic	7
Jejunum	Superior mesenteric branch	17, 38, 42, 62
Ileum	Superior mesenteric branch	31
Colon	Inferior mesenteric branch	24
Appendix	Appendicular	16
Ovary	Ovarian	78
Fallopian tube	?	16
Testes	Testicular	41
Adrenal gland	Adrenal	16
Specialized parts		
Great toe	Dorsalis pedis	13, 19, 30
Second toe	Dorsalis pedis	18, 77
Second and third toe	Dorsalis pedis	77
Second metatarsophalangeal joint	Dorsalis pedis	46
Fillet of foot	Posterior tibial	20
Lateral thigh	Profoundus femoris	20
Thumb	Radial	20
Fingers	Digital	2
Forearm	Radial and ulnar	20
Part of palm	Radial	49
Temporalis fascia	Superficial temporal	10
Serratus muscle with bone	Thoracodorsal	37
Latissimus dorsi muscle with rib	Thoracodorsal	37
Ulnar nerve	Ulnar	73
Radial nerve	Radial	73

plies (1) a *skin flap of the dorsum of the foot,* (2) the *great toe,* (3) the *second toe,* (4) the *extensor brevis muscle,* and (5) the *metatarsal phalangeal joint;* each is considered a separate flap. Where distinct differences in tissue composition are present, we have also considered each pattern to be a separate flap: the thoracodorsal artery may carry the *latissimus dorsi muscle* alone, the *serratus anterior muscle* alone, or the *serratus anterior muscle with bone.* However, a latissimus dorsi flap composed of only the anterior third of the latissimus dorsi muscle would still be considered in the same category as a flap composed of the complete muscle. Our initial survey yielded fifty-two donor sites, and fifteen more were added.

CUTANEOUS AND MYOCUTANEOUS FLAPS (Fig. 1-2)

Head and neck. Flaps from the head and neck are (1) *scalp flaps* based on the superficial temporal arteries and the occipital arteries; (2) *retroauricular flaps* based on the posterior auricular artery; (3) a *forehead flap* based on the frontal branch of the superficial temporal artery; (4) a *transverse cervical flap* based on the transverse cervical arteries; and (5) a *temporoparietal fascial flap* based on the superficial temporal vessels.

Upper half of the trunk. Flaps from the upper regions of the trunk are (1) the *thoracoacromial flap,* based on the thoracoacromial vessels; (2) a *deltopectoral flap* based on perforators of the internal mammary artery; (3) the *lateral thoracic flap* or *axillary flap* based on the lateral thoracic arteries; (4) the *latissimus dorsi myodermal flap* based on the thoracodorsal vessels; and (5) the *transverse scapular flap* and *vertical scapular flap* based on the circumflex scapular vessels.

Upper extremity. The upper extremity has provided (1) the *deltoid flap* based on the posterior humeral circumflex vessel; (2) the *medial and lateral upper arm flaps* based on separate cutaneous perforators; and (3) the *forearm flap* based on the lower half of the radial artery.

Lower half of the trunk. The lower parts of the trunk supply (1) the *groin flap* supplied by the superficial circumflex iliac artery; (2) the *rectus abdominis myodermal flap* (superior epigastric or inferior epigastric vessels); and (3) the *gluteus maximus flap* (superior gluteal artery or inferior gluteal artery).

Lower extremity. The lower extremities give (1) the *tensor fascia lata myodermal flap* (lateral femoral circumflex artery); (2) the *gracilis myodermal flap* (first branch of the profundus femoris artery); (3)

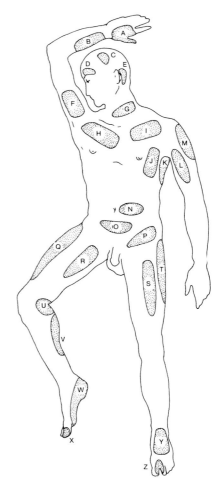

Fig. 1-2. Donor sites used for coverage. *A,* Part of palm, *B,* forearm, *C,* scalp, *D,* forehead, *E,* retroauricular skin, *F,* medial arm, *G,* neck skin, *H,* deltopectoral, *I,* thoracoacromial, *J,* lateral thoracic, *K,* latissimus dorsi myodermal flap, *L,* lateral arm skin, *M,* deltoid, *N,* abdominal skin with rectus muscle, *O,* lower abdominal skin with rectus muscle, *P,* groin flap, *Q,* lateral thigh skin and muscle flap, *R,* gracilis myodermal flap, *S,* rectus femoris myodermal flap, *T,* tensor flap, *U,* saphenous, *V,* medial gastrocnemius, *W,* sole skin myodermal flap, *X,* partial great toe, *Y,* dorsalis pedis, *Z,* first toe web space and sole of foot skin. Not included in the diagram are temporalis fascial flap, gluteus maximus myodermal flap, lateral thigh, and the entire forearm.

the *saphenous flap* (saphenous artery); (4) *medial and lateral thigh flaps* (skin perforators from deep vessels); (5) the *dorsalis pedis island flap* (dorsalis pedis artery); (6) *first toe web space flap* (first dorsal metatarsal artery); and (7) *partial great toe flaps.*

Amputated parts from accidental trauma. The skin of the palm, forearm, foot, and sole has been used for immediate microvascular repairs. Also, an amputated specimen consisting of the lateral half of the thigh with the tensor fascia lata muscle and

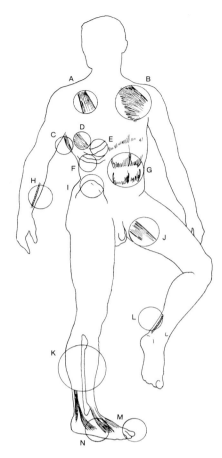

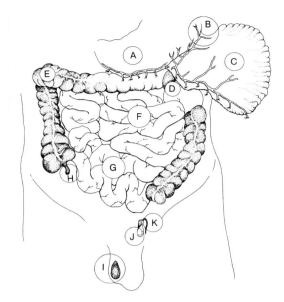

Fig. 1-3. Muscle, bone and nerve donor sites. *A,* pectoralis minor, *B,* pectoralis major, *C,* latissimus dorsi, *D,* serratus anterior, *E,* rib with anterior blood supply, *F,* rib with posterior blood supply, *G,* rectus abdominis muscle, *H,* radial nerve, *I,* iliac crest, *J,* gracilis muscle, *K,* fibula, *L,* sural nerve, *M,* great toe, second toe, and metatarsal phalangeal joint, *N,* extensor brevis muscle.

Fig. 1-4. Visceral donor sites. *A,* Part of stomach, *B,* part of stomach with omentum, *C,* omentum, *D,* adrenal gland, *E,* colon, *F,* jejunum, *G,* ileum, *H,* appendix, *I,* testis, *J,* ovary, *K,* fallopian tube.

the vastus lateralis muscle has been used for repairs to a lower limb stump.

Muscle, bone, and nerve (Fig. 1-3)

Muscle flaps. Muscle flaps were used as functioning muscles and included the *pectoralis major, pectoralis minor, latissimus dorsi, extensor hallucis brevis, medial head of the gastrocnemius,* and the *rectus abdominis muscle.*

Bone flaps. Vascular pedicles in these bone flaps supplied either the *periosteal surface* or the *endosteal surface,* or *both surfaces* of the bone. Flaps that have been transplanted include the *ribs* (posterior intercostal artery with its nutrient artery, or anterior intercostal artery with the attached internal mammary vessels); the *rib* with attached serratus anterior muscle; the *ilium* (as part of a groin

flap or as independent flaps supplied by deep circumflex iliac artery); the *fibula* (peroneal artery with both a nutrient artery and periosteal blood supply); the *metatarsal bone* and metatarsal phalangeal joint (dorsalis pedis artery); the *great toe, second, and third toes;* and *bones from amputated fingers and thumbs.*

Nerve transplants. The *radial, ulnar,* and *sural nerves* were transplanted by microvascular anastomosis a few times.

Visceral transplants (Fig. 1-4)

Omental flaps and gastrointestinal viscus flaps. The *omentum, omentum with attached stomach, jejunum, ileum, colon,* and even *appendix* have all been transplanted on their mesenteric blood supplies.

Genital transplants. The *testes* have been transplanted from the abdomen into the scrotum in cases of cryptorchidism. The *ovary fallopian tube* has been transplanted from one side to the other to match a functioning fallopian tube, and the *fallopian tube* has been transplanted to the opposite side to match a functioning ovary.

Endocrine transplants. *Adrenal gland* and *parathyroid transplants* have been reported in China.

DISCUSSION

We have made the following observations from this survey and a review of the literature.[1-78]

Free flaps are a reliable surgical technique with a high immediate success rate. A success rate of about 94% was achieved among the teams in this series. This figure for "success" gives a good general guide for the work of a center. However, it does not apply to the individual case with such factors as design constraints, patient's health, skill of the surgeon, or "point on the learning curve" of the surgeon.

Major vascular complications necessitate reoperations in about 10% of cases. A 10% rate of major vascular complications was seen fairly consistently from center to center. Even further reduction of major complications would increase the attractiveness of the free flap for routine reconstructive problems. Current efforts at improving monitoring, pharmacologic treatment, and surgical techniques are yielding results in this area. Four percent of the flaps beset by major vascular complications were saved by reoperation; this indicates that current methods of monitoring, imperfect as they are, are making an impact.

Potential donor sites are virtually unlimited. Any block of tissue that has an identifiable blood supply and that can tolerate a brief period of ischemia is a potential free flap. Donor sites are limited only by the surgeon's knowledge and imagination. Any combination of tissues that shares a common blood supply can be included in the design of a flap. Sometimes alternate vessels are available for supporting a specific flap: an iliac bone graft can be included with a groin flap by protecting the perforators from the superficial circumflex iliac artery. An iliac bone flap can be developed independently on the deep circumflex iliac artery. Skin and myodermal flaps predominated in this series, reflecting the types of problems for which solutions were needed.

The free flap technique is applicable all over the body. Just as in other reconstructive methods, the types of free flaps used depended on the types of clinical problems treated at a center. These clinical problems were weighted toward the head and neck in some centers, whereas defects of the lower limb or the upper limb predominated elsewhere. The types of flaps used reflected the types of problems treated.

SUMMARY

The data from a survey of 2,233 free flaps performed at microsurgery centers on four continents indicate that the free flap is a reliable reconstructive tool with wide applications. A number of donor sites are available. Ten percent of the flaps had major vascular complications and 4% of these were saved by repeated operation. The free flap is no longer considered an innovation but has attained the position as a routine reconstructive resource for the plastic surgeon. In the future we can look forward to an even greater variety of donor sites and flaps. Innovations in flap design and increasingly complex composition of flaps will be major areas of progress. As further experience is gained, we can look forward to operations that are safer, easier, and faster.

REFERENCES

1. Acland, R., et al.: The saphenous neurovascular free flap, Plast. Reconstr. Surg. **67:**763, 1981.
2. Alpert, B., and Buncke, H.: Mutilating multidigital injuries: use of a free microvascular flap from a non-replantable part, J. Hand Surg. **3:**196, 1978.
3. Ariyan, S., and Finseth, F.: The anterior chest approach for obtaining free osteocutaneous rib grafts, Plast. Reconstr. Surg. **62:**676, 1978.
4. Arnold, P., and Iron, G.: The greater omentum: extensions in transposition and free transfer, Plast. Reconstr. Surg. **67:**169, 1981.
5. Baek, S.M.: Two new cutaneous free flaps: medial and lateral thigh flaps, Plast. Reconstr. Surg. **71:**354, 1983.
6. Barwick, W., Goodking, D., and Serafin, D.: The free scapular flap, Plast. Reconstr. Surg. **69:**779, 1982.
7. Baudet, J.: Reconstruction of the pharyngeal wall by free transfer of the greater omentum and stomach, Inter. J. Microsurg. **1:**53, 1979.
8. Baudet, J., Guimberteau, J., and Nascimento, E.: Successful clinical transfer of two free thoracodorsal axillary flaps, Plast. Reconstr. Surg. **58:**680, 1976.
9. Boeckx, W., de Coninck, A., and Vanderlinden, E.: Ten free flap transfers: use of intraarterial dye injection to outline a flap exactly, Plast. Reconstr. Surg. **57:**716, 1976.
10. Brent, B.: Reconstruction of traumatic ear deformities, Clin. Plast. Surg. **5:**437, 1978.
11. Brown, R., Nahai, F., and Silverton, J.: The omentum in facial reconstruction, Br. J. Plast. Surg. **31:**58, 1978.
12. Buncke, H.: Presentation at the American College of Surgeons Meeting, Chicago, 1982.
13. Buncke, H., et al.: Thumb replacement—great toe transplantation by microvascular anastomosis, Br. J. Plast. Surg. **26:**194, 1973.
14. Caffee, H., and Asokan, R.: Tensor fascia lata myocutaneous free flaps, Plast. Reconstr. Surg. **68:**195, 1981.
15. Chang, T.S.: Experience in microsurgery in the People's Republic of China, J. Microsurg. **2:**83, 1980.
16. Chang, T.S.: Personal communication, 1981.
17. Chang, T.S., Hwang, O.L., and Wang, W.: Reconstruction of esophageal defects with microsurgically revascularized jejunal segments: a report of 13 cases, J. Microsurg. **2:**83, 1980.
18. Chen, Z.W., Yang, D.Y., Chang, D.S.: Microsurgery, New York, 1982, Springer-Verlag.

19. Cobbett, J.R.: Free digital transfer—report of a case of transfer of a great toe to replace an amputated thumb, J. Bone Joint Surg. **51B:**677, 1969.
20. Colen, S., Godfrey, N., Romita, M., and Shaw, W.: Salvage replantation, Clin, Plast. Surg. **10:**125, 1983.
21. Daniel, R., and Taylor, G.I.: Distant transfer of an island flap by microvascular anastomosis, Plast. Reconstr. Surg. **52:**111, 1973.
22. Daniel, R., Terzis, J., and Midgley, R.: Restoration of sensation to an anesthetic hand by a free neurovascular flap from the foot, Plast. Reconstr. Surg. **57:**275, 1976.
23. Dolmans, S., Guimberteau, J., and Baudet, J.: The upper arm flap. In Lie, T.S., editor: Microsurgery, Oxford, 1979, Excerpta Medica.
24. Flynn, M., and Acland, R.: Free intestinal autografts for reconstruction following pharyngoesophagectomy, Surg. Gynecol. Obst. **149:**858, 1979.
25. Foucher, G., Merle, M., Maneaud, M., and Michon, J.: Microsurgical free partial toe transfer in hand reconstruction: a report of 12 cases, Plast. Reconstr. Surg. **65:**616, 1980.
26. Franklin, J.: Deltoid free flap, Personal communication, 1982.
27. Fujino, T., Harashina, T., and Aoyagi, F.: Reconstruction for aplasia of the breast and pectoral region by microvascular transfer of a free flap from the buttock, Plast. Reconstr. Surg. **56:**178, 1975.
28. Fujino, T., Harashina, T., and Nakajima, T.: Free skin flap from the retroauricular region to the nose, Plast. Reconstr. Surg. **57:**338, 1976.
29. Gilbert, A., and Teot, L.: The free scapular flap, Plast. Reconstr. Surg. **69:**601, 1982.
30. Hamilton, R., and Morrison, W.: Microvascular segmental thumb reconstruction: a case report, Br. J. Plast. Surg. **33:**64, 1980.
31. Harashina, T., et al.: Secondary reconstruction of the esophagus with revascularized ileal transfer, Br. J. Plast. Surg. **34:**17, 1981.
32. Harii, K.: Microvascular free flaps for skin coverage, Clin. Plast. Surg. **10:**37, 1983.
33. Harii, K., Ohmori, K., and Ohmori, S.: Free deltopectoral skin flaps, Br. J. Plast. Surg. **27:**231, 1974.
34. Harii, K., Ohmori, K., and Ohmori, S.: Hair transplantation with free scalp flaps, Plast. Reconstr. Surg. **53:**410, 1974.
35. Harii, K., Ohmori, K., and Torii, S.: Free gracilis muscle transplantation with microneurovascular anastomosis for the treatment of facial paralysis, Plast. Reconstr. Surg. **57:**133, 1976.
36. Harii, K., and Ohmori, S.: Use of the gastroepiploic vessels as recipient or donor vessels in the free transfer of composite flaps by microvascular anastomosis, Plast. Reconstr. Surg. **52:**541, 1973.
37. Harii, K., et al.: A free transfer of both latissimus dorsi and serratus anterior flaps with thoracodorsal vessel anastomosis, Plast. Reconstr. Surg. **70:**620, 1982.
38. Hester, T., et al.: Reconstruction of cervical esophagus, hypopharynx and oral cavity using jejunal transfer, Am. J. Surg. **140:**487, 1980.
39. Hill, H., Nahai, F., and Vasconez, L.: The tensor fascia lata myocutaneous free flap, Plast. Reconstr. Surg. **61:**517, 1978.
40. Ikuta, Y., Kubo, T., and Tsuge, K.: Free muscle transplantation by microsurgical technique to treat severe Volkmann's contracture, Plast. Reconstr. Surg. **58:**407, 1976.
41. Janecka, I., and Romas, N.: Microvascular free transfer of human testes, Plast. Reconstr. Surg. **63:**42, 1979.
42. Jurkiewicz, M.: Vascularized intestinal grafts for reconstruction of the cervical esophagus and pharynx, Plast. Reconstr. Surg. **36:**509, 1965.
43. Keller, A., Allen, R., and Shaw, W.: Unpublished data, 1982, Bellevue Hospital, New York.
44. LeQuang, C.: Microvascular tissue transfer in plastic surgery. In Lie, T.S., editor: Microsurgery, Oxford, 1979, Excerpta Medica.
45. Manktelow, R.: Free muscle flaps. In Green, D.P., editor: Operative hand surgery, New York, 1982, Churchill Livingstone.
46. Mathes, S., Buchanan, R., and Weeks, P.: Microvascular joint transplantation with peripheral growth, J. Hand Surg. **5:**586, 1980.
47. Maxwell, G., Stueber, K., and Hoopes, J.: A free latissimus dorsi myocutaneous flap, Plast. Reconstr. Surg. **62:**462, 1978.
48. May, J., Gallico, G., and Lukash, F.: Microvascular transfer of free tissue for coverage of bone wounds of the distal lower extremity, N. Engl. J. Med. **306:**253, 1982.
49. May, J., and Gordon, L.: Palm of hand free flap for forearm length preservation in non-replantable forearm amputation: a case report, J. Hand Surg. **5:**377, 1980.
50. Mayou, B., Watson, J., Harrison, D., and Parry, C.: Free microvascular and microneural transfer of the extensor digitorum brevis muscle for the treatment of unilateral facial palsy, Br. J. Plast. Surg. **34:**362, 1981.
51. Mayou, B., Whitby, D., and Jones, B.: The scapular flap—an anatomical and clinical study, Br. J. Plast. Surg. **35:**8, 1982.
52. McLean, D., and Buncke, H.: Autotransplant of omentum to a large scalp defect with microsurgical revascularization, Plast. Reconstr. Surg. **49:**268, 1972.
53. Morrison, W., O'Brien, B.M., and MacLeod, A.: Clinical experience in free flap transfer, Clin. Orthop. **133:**132, 1978.
54. Morrison, W., et al.: Neurovascular free flaps from the foot for innervation of the hand, J. Hand Surg. **3:**235, 1978.
55. Nassif, T., et al.: The parascapular flap: a new cutaneous microsurgical free flap, Plast. Reconstr. Surg. **69:**591, 1982.
56. O'Brien, B.M., Morrison, W.A., and Dooley, B.J.: Microvascular osteocutaneous transfer using the groin flap and iliac crest and the dorsalis pedis flap and second toe, Br. J. Plast. Surg. **32:**188, 1979.
57. O'Brien, B.M., et al.: Successful transfer of a large island flap from the groin to the foot by microvascular anastomosis, Plast. Reconstr. Surg. **52:**271, 1973.
58. O'Brien, B.M., et al.: Free flap transfers with microvascular anastomosis, Br. J. Plast. Surg. **27:**220, 1974.
59. Ohmori, K.: Free scalp flap, Plast. Reconstr. Surg. **65:**42, 1980.

60. Ohmori, K., Sekiguchi, J., and Ohmori, S.: Total rhinoplasty with a free osteocutaneous flap, Plast. Reconstr. Surg. **63:**387, 1979.

61. Pennington, D., and Pelly, A.: The rectus abdominis myocutaneous free flap, Br. J. Plast. Surg. **33:**277, 1980.

62. Peters, C., McKee, D., and Berry, B.: Pharyngo-esophageal reconstruction with revascularized jejunal transplants, Am. J. Surg. **121:**675, 1971.

63. Robinson, D.W.: Microsurgical transfer of the dorsalis pedis neurovascular island flap, Br. J. Plast. Surg. **29:**209, 1976.

64. Schenck, R.: Free muscle and composite skin transplantation by microvascular anastomosis, Orthop. Clin. North Am. **8:**367, 1977.

65. Serafin, D., Villarreal-Rios, A., and Georgiade, N.: A rib-containing free flap to reconstruct mandibular defects, Br. J. Plast. Surg. **30:**263, 1977.

66. Shaw, W.W.: Microvascular free flaps: the first decade, Clin. Plast. Surg. **10:**3, 1983.

67. Shaw, W.W.: Unpublished data, 1982, New York University Hospital, New York.

68. Song, R., Song, Y., Yu, Y., Song, Y.: The upper arm free flap, Clin. Plast. Surg. **9:**27, 1982.

69. Song, R., et al.: The forearm flap, Clin. Plast. Surg. **9:**21, 1982.

70. Strauch, B., and Shafiroff, B.: The foot: a versatile donor site. In Serafin, D., and Buncke, H., editors: Microvascular composite tissue transplantation, St. Louis, 1979, The C.V. Mosby Co.

71. Takayanagi, S., and Tsukii, T.: Free serratus anterior muscle and myocutaneous flaps, Ann. Plast. Surg. **8:**277, 1982.

72. Taylor, G.: Current status of free vascularized bone grafts, Clin. Plast. Surg. **10:**185, 1983.

73. Taylor, G., and Ham, F.: The free vascularized nerve graft, Plast. Reconstr. Surg. **57:**413, 1976.

74. Taylor, G., Miller, G., and Ham, F.: The free vascularized bone graft—a clinical extension of microvascular techniques, Plast. Reconstr. Surg. **55:**533, 1975.

75. Taylor, G., Townsend, P., and Corlett, R.: Superiority of the deep circumflex iliac vessels as the supply for free groin flaps, Plast. Reconstr. Surg. **64:**595, 1979.

76. Terzis, J.K.: Presentation at the Third Microsurgical Symposium, New Orleans, 1983.

77. Yoshimura, M., et al.: Toe-to-hand transfer: experience with 38 digits, Aust. N.Z. Surg. **50:**248, 1980.

78. Yu, K.: Personal communication, Canton, China, 1982.

Part II

Replantation

Chapter 2

The classic: successful replantation of a completely cut-off thumb

Susumu Tamai

Since 1959 Yutaka Onji, Yasuhiro Murai, and I have been interested in replantation of amputated extremities, and we have continued animal experiments. Our clinical and laboratory experience indicates that replantation of large parts of the body, such as an entire leg, endangers the life of the host because of replantation toxemia characterized by metabolic acidosis, hyperpotassemia, and extravasation of plasma into the replanted extremity. Consequently we believe that this kind of surgery should be limited to small parts of the body such as fingers and hands, at least until the problem of toxemia is clarified and methods of treatment are established. In 1964 we asked members of our local medical association to send all patients with accidentally amputated fingers to us; this has given us the frequent opportunity to try reunion of amputated fingers. This is a difficult task, but finally, on July 27, 1965, Shigeo Komatsu and I succeeded in replanting an amputated thumb to its original position.

CASE REPORT

A 28-year-old male accidentally cut off his left thumb while working with a steel cutting machine. He was sent to our hospital 30 minutes after the accident. On the way to the hospital the severed thumb was dropped on the ground once. The thumb was completely cut off at the metacarpophalangeal joint. The wound was contaminated by a black, oily substance, but it was relatively clean and tissue damage was minimal.

Using lidocaine, we anesthetized the left arm with a brachial plexus block and applied a pneumatic tourniquet on the upper arm. The thumb was washed with sterile saline solution, and both wounds were debrided. A digital artery was cannulated with a 0.5 mm polyethylene tube, and the thumb was flushed with heparin diluted in low molecular weight dextran (Fig. 2-1). Venous return from the dorsal veins was seen.

The cartilage of the metacarpophalangeal joint was removed, and the joint was fused in an abducted position. Using a surgical microscope, we sutured two volar digital arteries and two dorsal veins end to end with atraumatic 7-0 braided silk and 8-0 monofilament nylon. (At that time, 8-0 monofilament nylon sutures were the smallest ones available in the world. At the time of this operation we had only two 8-0 nylon sutures, which had been given as samples by Dr. Julius Jacobson to Dr. Onji, who had visited him in New York in 1964.)

Magnification ranged from 10× to 16×. The external diameter of these vessels was approximately 0.8 to 1.0 mm, and a row of eight interrupted stitches was placed. Immediately after the reestablishment of circulation the thumb became pink. Pulsation of the digital arteries was noted, and venous return was present. The digital nerve was located at the same site as the arterial repair. We felt that our arterial anastomosis might be jeopardized by any effort at nerve repair, and it was therefore postponed. The extensor tendon was sutured end to end. The flexor tendon was not repaired because it had been cut in "no-man's-land." The tendon graft was also postponed. The skin was closed with interrupted sutures, and an elastic bandage was applied. The period between the accident and the reestablishment of circulation was 3 hours.

Slight edema developed on the second postoperative day but subsided within a week. The patient was discharged on the fortieth postoperative day. Four months

This report was initially presented in Japanese by Shigeo Komatsu at the ninth meeting of the Japanese Society for Surgery of the Hand in March 1966 in Tokyo and in English by Susumu Tamai at the annual meeting of the American Society of Plastic and Reconstructive Surgeons in November 1967 in New York. Panelists for the 1967 presentation were H.J. Buncke, J. Cobbett, J.W. Smith, and S. Tamai; moderator was C.C. Snyder.

13

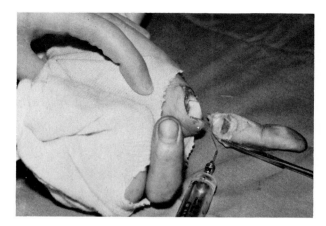

Fig. 2-1. Amputated left thumb is perfused with a diluted heparin solution before replantation. (From Komatsu, S., and Tamai, S.: Successful replantation of a completely cut-off thumb: case report, Plast. Reconstr. Surg. **42**:374, 1968.)

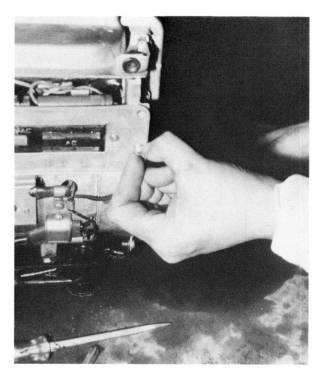

Fig. 2-3. Appearance of thumb 16 years after replantation. The patient still works at his original job.

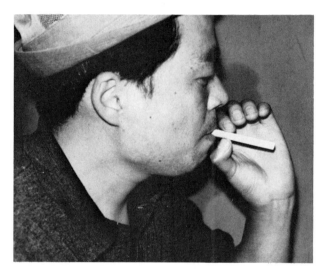

Fig. 2-2. At 2 years, 5 months after replantation, satisfactory functional result is demonstrated. (From Komatsu, S., and Tamai, S.: Successful replantation of a completely cut-off thumb: case report, Plast. Reconstr. Surg. **42**: 374, 1968.)

after the injury he returned to his original occupation. Although slight atrophy and loss of sensation was noticed, the patient had regained excellent pinch at 200 days postoperatively. We suggested that a neurovascular island flap be employed to improve sensation but the patient refused. According to another examiner, 2 years postoperatively the sensation had recovered surprisingly well on the ulnar side of the replanted thumb; a moderate flexion contracture was noted at the interphalangeal joint, but this position was satisfactory for the patient (Fig. 2-2).

An ancient Japanese legend states:

Amputated finger dropped on the ground once can never be replanted as a composite graft at its original site.

However, we have the exception that disproves this rule.

Microsurgical techniques are the key to the field of replantation surgery. This technique could be used to perform a one-stage Nicoladoni operation, using a toe to replace a thumb missing as a result of trauma or congenital causes. I hope we can now fulfill our patients' requests to have their amputated digits replaced.

Nineteen years have passed since this, the first successful replantation of a completely amputated thumb, and the patient is still working at his original job, using his replanted left thumb very well (Fig. 2-3). The interphalangeal joint is contracted to 60 degrees of flexion and the metacarpophalangeal joint is fused in a slightly abducted or extended position, but the power of the patient's pinch is almost normal. Protective sensation has returned to the entire thumb. The ulnar aspect of the pulp has the best sensation because of axonal regeneration in spite of the absence of a nerve repair.

Chapter 3

Replantation of digits

Harold E. Kleinert
Carl H. Manstein

The primary goal of replantation surgery is function; one cannot equate tissue survival alone with success.[1,3,6] Functional recovery of a finger necessitates adequate circulation, good sensibility, and restoration of a reasonable functional arc of motion. Motivation of the patient is also important; he must clearly have the desire and the capacity to participate in a long period of postoperative rehabilitation.

The amputated part is cooled to 2° to 4° C (Fig. 3-1), and cooling is maintained during surgical preparations. Larger amputated parts are cooled by irrigating the vascular system with cold heparinized saline solution or lactated Ringer's solution. Although we have replanted a digit after as long as 36 hours of cool ischemic time, the survival rate drops off sharply after 10 hours.

The ideal circumstance for replantation is a sharp, guillotine type of amputation that does not involve the joint and is located distal to the insertion of the flexor digitorum superficialis tendon. A single digit amputated at this level should be replanted, assuming that it is technically feasible and that the patient meets other qualifications. Digital replantation at the metacarpal level also usually results in good function. Good results are more difficult to achieve with digital replantation at the proximal phalanx level in the area of the A2 pulley.

Perhaps the most important factor in the success rate of replantation is case selection. Although the determination as to whether or not a digit is replantable is largely based on the surgeon's own experience, we have outlined some absolute and relative contraindications to replantation as guidelines. All of these contraindications must be tempered by the clinical situation and the surgeon's judgment.

Relative contraindications include:
1. Border finger amputation—except distal to insertion of flexor digitorum superficialis
2. Crushing or avulsion amputations
3. Double level injuries
4. Transarticular single digit amputation
5. Associated systemic disease
6. Patient more than 60 years old
7. Heavy soil contamination
8. A warm ischemic time of longer than 6 hours
9. Elderly patients (with certain exceptions)
10. Patients with preexisting major systemic diseases

Absolute contraindications include:
1. Extensive crush injury
2. Significant additional wounds of either the amputated part or the stump
3. Medical conditions that preclude a long operation

A basic goal in replantation is the restoration of the thumb, web space, and if possible, two other opposing digits. Digital transposition is often useful in multidigit amputations—the best digit is transferred to the most suitable stump and available parts are replanted to the best positions, regardless of their site of origin to obtain maximal function (Fig. 3-2).

Every effort is made to reattach a thumb at any level, even distal to the interphalangeal joint. Joint motion of the thumb is desirable, but even without its two joints this digit is the most crucial component of the hand.

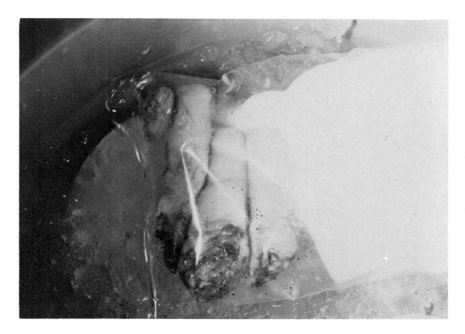

Fig. 3-1. Amputated parts sealed in plastic bag and placed in an iced, insulated chest for transport. (From Kleinert, H.E., et al.: Digital replantation—selection, technique, and results, Orthop. Clin. North Am. **8:** 309, 1977.)

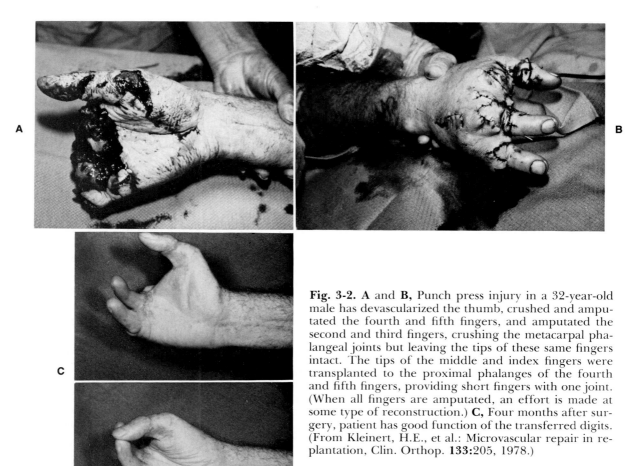

Fig. 3-2. A and **B,** Punch press injury in a 32-year-old male has devascularized the thumb, crushed and amputated the fourth and fifth fingers, and amputated the second and third fingers, crushing the metacarpal phalangeal joints but leaving the tips of these same fingers intact. The tips of the middle and index fingers were transplanted to the proximal phalanges of the fourth and fifth fingers, providing short fingers with one joint. (When all fingers are amputated, an effort is made at some type of reconstruction.) **C,** Four months after surgery, patient has good function of the transferred digits. (From Kleinert, H.E., et al.: Microvascular repair in replantation, Clin. Orthop. **133:**205, 1978.)

REPLANTATION TECHNIQUE

An orderly sequence is followed to achieve maximum success at surgery.

For most upper extremity replants we use an axillary block with bupivacaine HCl (Marcaine) 0.5% with epinephrine. A regional anesthetic is safer in these lengthy procedures, and it also provides a sympathetic blockade. Preoperative radiographs are made of the amputated part and the stump.

Low molecular weight dextran is given at the onset of surgery.

We proceed with cleansing, debridement, and repair. Crushed tissue is excised and the bone is shortened as indicated to aid tissue approximation without tension. The bone is usually shortened 0.5 cm beyond the soft tissue margin. Excessive bone shortening will interfere with dynamic balance of the hand (Fig. 3-3).

Firm, secure bone fixation is carried out with interosseous wires and Kirschner pins to decrease the likelihood of delayed union. The flexor and extensor tendons are then repaired, and vessel and nerve repairs are carried out under magnification.

Repairing the arteries before the veins allows quicker tissue perfusion and makes the identification of veins easier. Interposition vein grafts are needed for restoration of vessel length in half of the cases (Fig. 3-4). For each artery repair we repair two veins. The skin is closed loosely and skin grafts are applied as needed. Z-plasties are sometimes used to avoid constricting, circular scars.

In placing the dressings, we avoid tension, direct pressure, or constriction on the repaired structures. The dressing is designed to permit observation of the circulation of the replanted part and to facilitate elevation of the extremity (Fig. 3-5).

Postoperatively the patient is given dextran, 500 mg/day, for 3 days. Aspirin may also be used for its antiplatelet adhesive properties. In a replantation performed under suboptimal circumstances, heparin is given; one must watch for bleeding and

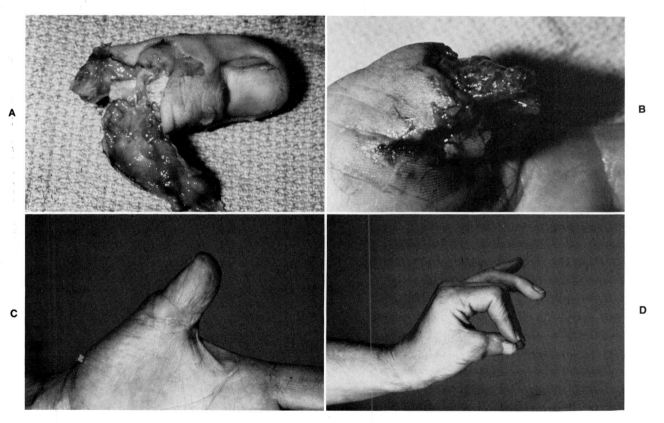

Fig. 3-3. A and **B,** Crush amputation of the thumb at the proximal phalanx from a forklift injury. (The thumb is always replanted if at all possible.) **C** and **D,** In spite of bone shortening, there is good function 4 months after surgery, with 30 degrees of flexion and full extension.

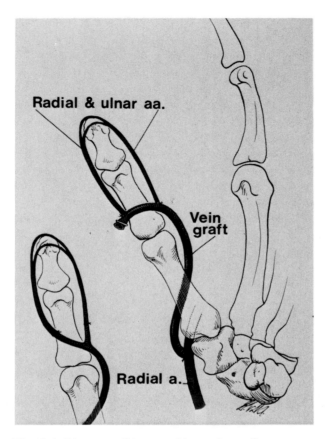

Fig. 3-4. Diagram of interposition vein graft to restore circulation to a crushed, replanted thumb. (From Kleinert, H.E., et al.: Replantation—an overview. Straub, L.R., and Wilson, P.D., editors: Clinical trends in orthopaedics, New York, 1982, Thieme-Stratton, Inc.)

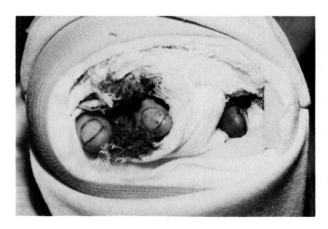

Fig. 3-5. Replantation dressing with fingertips exposed for monitoring circulation.

hematoma. Antibiotics are continued in the post operative period. The patient is discouraged from smoking.

Vessel thrombosis is the primary cause of failure of a replanted digit. Persistent bleeding necessitating reexploration is also an ominous complication.

Impending necrosis resulting from thrombosis can often be reversed by immediate reexploration, thrombectomy, and reanastomosis or vein grafts. A review of reexplorations that we carried out for circulatory embarrassment from 1976 to 1979 showed a salvage rate of 83%.[5] Fasciotomies may be needed for impending ischemia from swelling.

REHABILITATION

The postreplantation digit presents a rehabilitative challenge in which physical and occupational therapists play a key role. Most replant patients are well motivated, and psychologic problems are seldom an obstacle to long-term rehabilitation (Fig. 3-6).

Since both the flexor and extensor mechanisms are involved, early therapy should be based on active exercises, avoiding overly vigorous application of passive exercises. Regaining joint motion is as important as sensory return in the distal aspect of the replanted part. Splints are designed to provide stability yet allow for motion of the involved joints. Dynamic traction is instituted 3 weeks postoperatively to improve tendon gliding and range of motion.

Sensory feedback, touch desensitization, and a transcutaneous electrical nerve stimulator are used to deal with pain and cold intolerance.

RESULTS

To assess the results of replantation, we use a scheme of four grades of recovery.[2]

Grade I

- Ability to resume original work with a critical contribution from the reattached parts
- Collective range of joint motion exceeds 60% of normal, including the joint immediately proximal to the reattached part
- Recovery of sensibility to a high grade without excessive intolerance to cold
- Muscular power of 4 to 5 on a scale of 1 to 5

Grade II

- Ability to resume some gainful work but not original employment

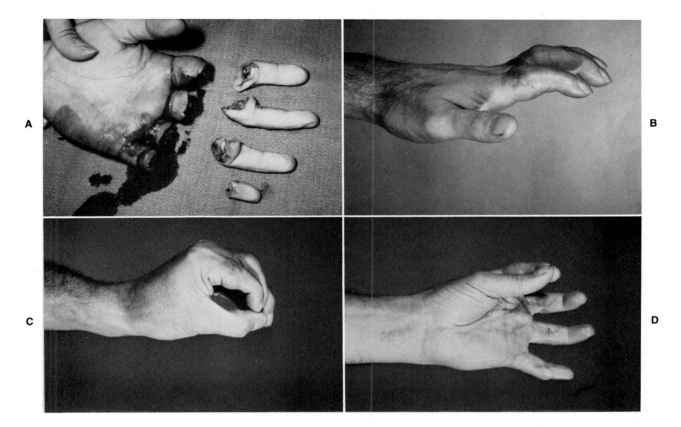

Fig. 3-6. A, Thirty-five-year-old male with saw amputation of all fingers of the left hand at proximal phalanges. **B** to **D,** Extension, opposition, and flexion at 10 months after surgery.

- Range of joint motion exceeds 40% of normal
- Recovery of near-normal sensibility in the median and ulnar nerve distributions without severe intolerance to cold
- Muscular power of grade 3 to 4 on a scale of 1 to 5

Grade III

- Independence in activities of daily living
- Range of motion of joints exceeds 30% of normal
- Poor but useful recovery of sensibility (for example, only median or ulnar recovery is good or quality is only protective in both median and ulnar areas)
- Muscular power of grade 3 on a scale of 1 to 5

Grade IV

- Tissue survival with no recovery of useful function

In surveys of our patients, nearly all said they would undergo the procedure again in preference to an amputation, whether their replantation was graded as successful or unsuccessful. Our recent overall survival rate for replanted digits exceeds 85%, approximating 100% in the "ideal" candidate.[4] Survival rates for crush amputations are much lower. The best results are achieved by primary repair of all structures. In our most recent series of digital and thumb replantations, 42% of the digits required secondary surgical procedures, including tenolysis, nerve graft, capsulectomy, tendon graft and/or transfer, pedicle flaps, and free flaps for soft tissue coverage.[5]

Return of sensation is better than one might expect, often better than for nerve repair alone. The motivation of the patient to regain function is undoubtedly important in the many cases regaining two-point discrimination of 7 mm or better.

Return to employment did not correlate with the mechanism of injury or the amputation level but depended largely on individual motivation. The average time for return to work for these patients was 6 months.

A 1980 survey of digital replantation in Louisville[2] revealed the following:

Grade of functional recovery	Thumb	Fingers proximal to PIP	Fingers distal to FDS	Total
I	3	6	16	25
II	9	23	16	48
III	11	42	16	69
IV	15	13	2	30
TOTALS	38	84	50	172
	32%	35%	65%	

Percent of total with grade I or II functional recovery

SUMMARY

Our survey shows that the ideal candidate for replantation is a young patient with a sharp, clean amputation distal to the insertion of the flexor digitorum superficialis tendon. A replantation center with a staff that is well trained in replantation surgery and rehabilitation techniques and that has adequate depth of personnel can achieve a worthwhile level of functional return in the majority of replantation patients. Careful case selection is the key to achieving a functional digit that is both cosmetically acceptable and of use to the patient.

REFERENCES

1. Chen, C.W., Chin, Y.C., and Pao, Y.S.: Further experience in the restoration of amputated limbs: report of two cases, Chin. Med. J. **84:**225, 1965.
2. Chen, Z.W., Meyer, V.E., Kleinert, H.E., and Beasley, R.W.: Present indications and contraindications for replantation as reflected by long-term functional results, Orthop. Clin. North Am. **12:**849, 1981.
3. Kleinert, H.E., Jablon, M., and Tsai, T.M.: An overview of replantation and results of 347 replants in 245 patients, J. Trauma **20:**390, 1980.
4. Kleinert, H.E., and Tsai, T.M.: Microvascular repair in replantation, Clin. Orthop. **133:**205, 1978.
5. Kleinert, H.E., Tsai, T.M., and Jupiter, J.B.: Replantation—an overview. In Straub, L.R., and Wilson, P.D., editors: Clinical trends in orthopaedics, New York, 1982, Thieme-Stratton, Inc.
6. Schlenker, J.D., Kleinert, H.E., and Tsai, T.M.: Methods and results of replantation following traumatic amputation of the thumb in 64 patients, J. Hand Surg. **5:**63, 1980.

Chapter 4

Digital replantation: indications and innovations

Roger Friedman
Leonard Gordon
Harry J. Buncke
Bernard S. Alpert

Technical refinements and clarification of the indications for digital replantation over the past decade have improved both digit survival and long-term function. We present in this chapter our current indications for digital replantation and discuss two new techniques—nail removal for treatment of venous congestion and dermal perfusion monitoring with fluorescein staining for assessment of digit viability. We believe that these techniques improve the success of replantation. The development of a transplantation team that works in centralized facilities is beneficial. In addition, the computerized recording of preoperative and postoperative data allows critical evaluation of the results of surgery and rehabilitation.

CENTRALIZATION OF FACILITIES

As more surgeons are trained in the indications for and techniques of replantation, the care of many patients will inevitably shift to extrametropolitan areas. The management of multiple digit trauma and complicated hand injuries should continue to be centralized in a regional microsurgical center where adequate numbers of personnel with expertise in operative and postoperative care are available. Such complex injuries require lengthy reconstructive procedures that should be instituted as soon after injury as possible. Emergency rooms over a wide geographic area should be in contact with a regional center where a replantation team is available around the clock. This team

should include surgeons, anesthesiologists, nurses, and assistants in sufficient numbers that work shifts do not exceed 4 to 6 hours. Since many of these patients have other severe injuries, additional surgical specialists should be readily available for consultation. In addition, transportation should be organized through a central system with staff members who know about weather conditions and available modes of ground and air transportation.

We are in the process of evaluating computerized information relating indications for surgery to functional results. Centralization facilitates such data collection.

INDICATIONS
General factors

The goal of replantation surgery has shifted in recent years from simple survival of the replanted part to attaining the optimal functional result. We emphasize individualization of the indications as our overriding philosophy. The decision to proceed with replantation requires consideration of several factors in addition to the mechanism of injury and the extent of damage. The age and functional requirements of the patient need to be evaluated, as well as the patient's general condition and the presence of chronic medical conditions.

Elderly patients may gain many years of function with replanted digits, despite the fact that nerve regeneration is not as efficient as in younger patients and that stiffness is often a serious prob-

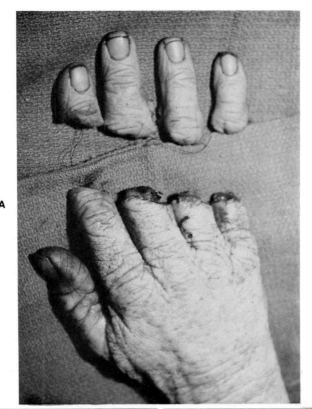

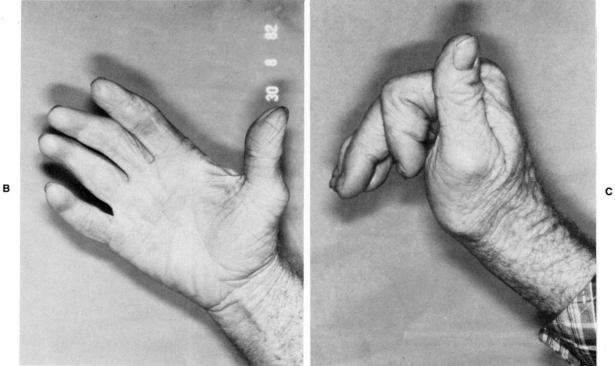

Fig. 4-1. A, Four-finger table saw amputation. Index finger level is distal to the superficialis tendon insertion. **B,** Seven months after replantation. **C,** Flexion from 0 to 90 degrees at proximal interphalangeal joint of the index finger. Other digits required tenolysis.

lem. Thus improved function must be weighed against the risks of lengthy anesthesia and prolonged rehabilitation in older patients.

The patient's emotional stability, adaptability, motivation, and occupational requirements must be evaluated; however, these factors are difficult to fully appreciate in the emergency situation. For this reason decisions regarding replantation cannot be based on these factors alone.

In patients with multiple trauma that jeopardizes survival, replantation may be precluded, although the amputated part may be cooled during treatment of the more severe injuries for possible replantation 24 hours or more later.[9]

Bone, vascular, and soft tissue damage in the amputated part must be carefully assessed. In many situations such damage may prevent viability or function. For example, even though the anastomoses are patent following replantation, extensive internal vascular damage may prevent perfusion of the digit.

If none of these factors contraindicate replantation, other details should be considered, such as the level of injury and the number and location of the involved digits.

Hand function

Two well-accepted indications for replantation are thumb and multiple digit amputations[2,11,12,16] (Fig. 4-1) because of the severe functional deficit that results. When more than one digit is amputated, the ulnar side of the hand should be reconstructed first to restore power grip and allow grasping of large objects. If the thumb is also amputated, it should be the first part replanted, but if the thumb is badly damaged, another digit should be transposed to the thumb position.

Single digit replantation

Amputation of one finger when accompanied by serious injury to other digits is sometimes referred to as a "single digit amputation" but actually constitutes "multiple finger injuries."

This affects prognosis, and such single digit amputations should be replanted. For example, in a patient with one digit amputated through the middle phalanx and an adjacent finger with a flexor tendon and nerve injury through the proximal phalanx (zone 2), the replanted digit may well have better long-term function than the other.

Digits replanted at the level of the dense pulley region close to the metacarpophalangeal joint tend to develop more scarring and regain less motion than those replanted distal to the flexor digitorum superficialis insertion. This is not surprising when one reviews the experience regarding the level of tendon repairs. For this reason a single digit amputation in zone 2, with no other injured digits, should not be replanted. In contrast, the functional results following single digit replantation in digits distal to the superficialis insertion are quite favorable (Fig. 4-2). Motion is of less importance at the level of the distal interphalangeal joint because digits fused or stiff at this level function quite adequately.[7] Similarly the functional results following single digit replantation in children are adequate to justify the procedure in most cases.[5,10] Nerves and arteries can be repaired a few millimeters proximal to the base of the nail.[15] If a vein is not available for repair at this level, we have used the technique of nail removal to provide a constant and slow venous egress from the small replanted part (see pp. 25 and 28).

The thumb has fewer demands for motion at the interphalangeal joint than fingers and plays a dominant functional role in the hand. For this reason all thumb amputations should be replanted, even with avulsive or crush injuries. In such cases nerve grafting may be performed at a later date to improve sensation (Fig. 4-3).

Crush and avulsive injuries

In many cases severe avulsive, crush, and multilevel injuries may preclude survival of the part after revascularization.[13] The liberal use of vein grafts[1] has allowed salvage of many such situations (Fig. 4-4). While a decreased average survival rate must be accepted if replantation is carried out in such circumstances, these efforts often result in greatly enhanced function. The individualized approach is particularly appropriate in such cases. In ring avulsion injuries the degloved part, which usually contains the distal phalanx, can often be replanted, resulting in good function and appearance (Fig. 4-5). Survival of an avulsed part is often difficult to achieve without the use of vein grafts. The decision to replant the digit depends largely on the personal attitudes of the patient and the experience of the replant surgeon.

TECHNICAL CONSIDERATIONS

The surgical technique used in replantation and the order of repair have become fairly standard.[1,4,6,8,12] Several aspects of our technique bear emphasis.

Whether osteosynthesis by Kirschner wires, interosseous wires, plates, or screws is used, a concerted effort should be made to leave joints mobile

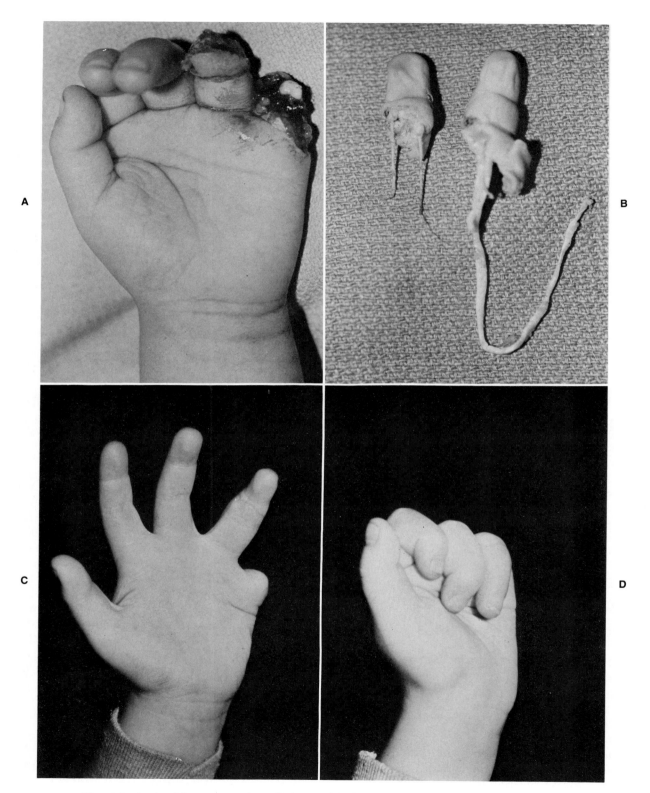

Fig. 4-2. A, Avulsive amputation of ring and little fingers in a 9-year-old. **B,** Exposed digital nerves of ring finger (left) secondary to avulsive injury. Little finger not replantable because of vascular injury. **C,** Successful replantation of ring finger distal to the superficialis insertion. **D,** Excellent flexion at proximal interphalangeal joint.

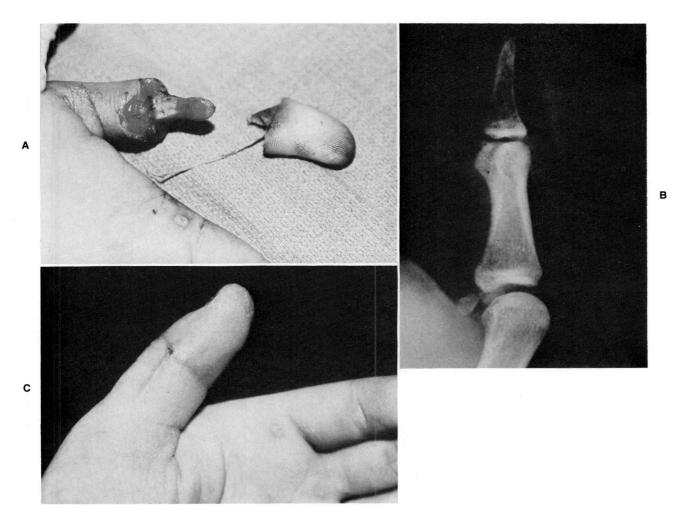

Fig. 4-3. A, Printing press avulsion of soft tissue of thumb at the interphalangeal joint level. **B,** Radiograph revealing intact bony structures. **C,** Successful replantation with vein graft interposed to reestablish arterial flow. Subsequent nerve grafting provided functional sensation.

for early motion. For this reason we prefer interosseous wiring for amputations close to joints. In patients with destruction of the metacarpophalangeal or proximal interphalangeal joints, a primary prosthesis can be used if the wound is clean and tissue destruction is limited.

The liberal use of vein grafts with removal of any damaged vessel segment cannot be overemphasized. We use the posterior wall-first suture technique for all anastomoses,[4] since it provides excellent exposure of the vessel lumen and avoids cumbersome stay sutures and clamp positioning in difficult situations. We emphasize placing extremely loose dressings; in many instances all dressings are removed in the recovery room when the patient is awake and cooperative. Antibiotic ointment

is placed on the wounds and the hand is positioned or a Kerlix roll and sterile towel, which avoids any pressure by blood-soaked dressings, especially if topical heparin sponges are being used.

POSTOPERATIVE CARE
Management of venous problems

Isolated instances occur during digital replantation in which venous congestion is a problem.[14] This may result from a distal level injury or crush and avulsive injuries in which no vein of adequate caliber is available in the amputated part. In other circumstances thrombosis of a venous anastomosis may occur that does not allow reexploration. In these cases we have had success in removing a portion of the nail plate in the replanted digit to pro-

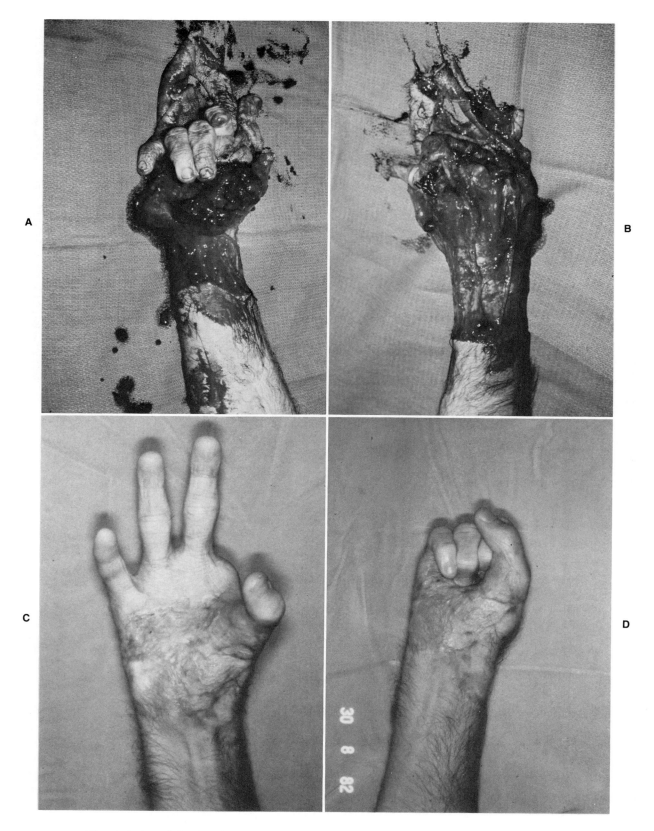

Fig. 4-4. A and **B,** Crushing and avulsive injury resulting in degloving from the distal forearm. Thumb sustained an avulsive amputation and all digits were devascularized. **C** and **D,** Five months after revascularization. Index finger was revascularized and subsequently failed. Reconstruction of superficial arch from ulnar artery did not provide adequate·flow to the index finger.

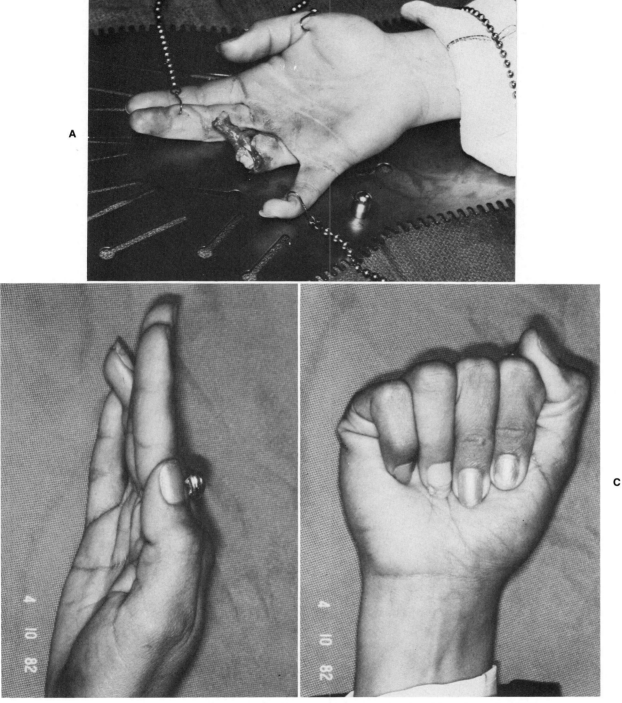

Fig. 4-5. A, Ring avulsion with intraarticular fracture through midportion of middle phalanx and open proximal interphalangeal joint. Amputated part includes distal phalanx and skin distal to the proximal interphalangeal joint. **B** and **C,** Six months after successful replantation, 0 to 100 degrees of flexion is present at the proximal interphalangeal joint, with a mallet finger deformity at the distal interphalangeal joint.

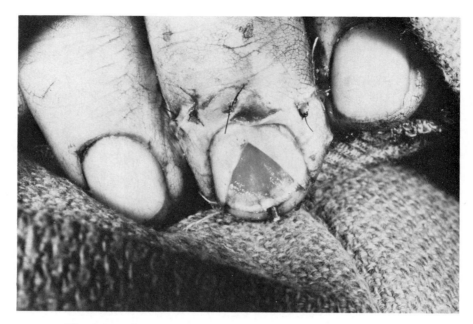

Fig. 4-6. Nail removal with preservation of the eponychial fold.

vide venous egress. This is performed preserving the eponychial fold (Fig. 4-6) and is combined with systemic heparinization and the application of topical heparin sponges (100 U heparin/1 ml saline solution) to the exposed nail bed for approximately 5 to 7 days. Constant, slow venous oozing from the nail bed limits congestion until newly developed venous channels can provide venous drainage.

Postoperative monitoring

Despite the plethora of monitoring devices currently being used or tested to provide postoperative evaluation of the adequacy of perfusion to replanted parts, none is ideal. The ideal device should provide a quantitative measurement and should be safe, noninvasive, and simple to use. Temperature probes, laser Doppler probes, skin and intraarterial thermocouples, and photoplethysmography are among the methods being used in various centers.

We are currently using a method that quantitates microscopic amounts of fluorescein in the dermis of a replanted part. This method has proved to be a reliable indicator of vascular perfusion. Sodium fluorescein (1.0 to 1.5 mg/kg) is administered intravenously every 2 hours for 36 to 48 hours beginning at the termination of surgery. Quantitative fluorescence readings of each injured digit are then obtained 10 minutes and 60 minutes after fluorescein injection and compared to uninjured (control) digits.[3] A ratio between the injured digit fluorescence and the control digit fluorescence may then be used for analysis. Viable digits demonstrate a significant increase in fluorescence 10 minutes after injection and a significant washout with return to the baseline values at 60 minutes (Fig. 4-7). By this method both arterial insufficiency (10-minute reading) and venous congestion (60-minute reading) can be detected and measured quantitatively, thereby alerting the surgeon to vascular problems before any clinical change can be detected. The test is performed by the nursing staff in the postoperative monitoring unit (Fig. 4-8).

We have reviewed data over a 1-year period, and such monitoring has proved valuable. Seventy-one patients underwent either replantation or revascularization of 111 fingers during 1981 and 1982. There were sixteen failed replants, for a survival rate of 86%. Eighteen replants were distal to the flexor digitorum superficialis tendon insertion, with one failure, for a survival rate of 95%. Monitoring led to early reexploration of sixteen digits, which resulted in salvage of ten digits.

Rehabilitation

The unique problem of upper extremity rehabilitation is that both flexor and extensor musculotendinous units must be protected and exercised simultaneously. Rigid internal fixation is necessary so that this may begin as soon as possible postop-

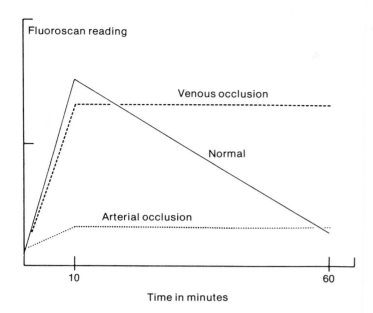

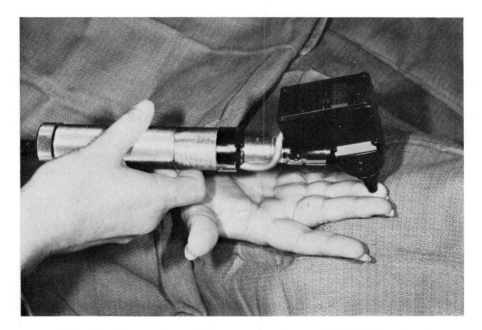

Fig. 4-7. Fluorescein index gives a reliable quantitative measure of digital blood flow. Normal (uninjured) and replanted digits display increased fluorescein at 10 minutes but return to the baseline by 60 minutes.

Fig. 4-8. Fluorescein perfusion monitor in use with digital readout.

eratively. The rehabilitation program after replantation consumes more time and effort than the original surgical procedure. Optimal functional results depend as much on a closely supervised program of postoperative hand therapy and splinting as on operative performance. Therapists should be well versed in conventional principles of hand surgery and therapy as well as in those problems unique to replantation. Our therapists make inpatient rounds with the medical staff on all replanta-

tion patients and, postoperatively, follow the patients independently and in conjunction with the medical staff.

Sensibility and the active motion of replanted parts are the two key variables that determine functional results postoperatively.

Sensibility is dealt with surgically in most patients by primary repair or occasionally by secondary nerve grafting or neurolysis. Restoration of active motion of replanted parts, however, depends both on surgical repair and attentive post-operative therapy. We have been discouraged in the past by the classic immobilization of replant patients for 3 weeks after surgery, followed by progressive institution of active and passive range-of-motion exercises. The resultant stiffness, especially in zone 2, has prompted us to introduce protocols with earlier gentle active and passive range-of-motion exercises as soon as pain and swelling permit. This may actually be toward the end of the first postoperative week and is almost always within the second week. Progressive motion is gradually added over the ensuing weeks, and dynamic splinting is begun. Static splinting and passive strengthening exercises are added as necessary in the later postoperative course. With a closely supervised protocol of this type, our results in the restoration of active tendon gliding have been better. A certain increased risk of tendon rupture may have to be accepted when using this approach; however, our encouraging results have stimulated us to continue this protocol.

SUMMARY

It has been approximately 19 years since the first digital replant, and finally a realistic approach to replantation is beginning to develop. The challenge ahead lies not in surgical technique but in the organization of facilities to take care of these patients and in the development of sound clinical judgment for patient selection. We still feel that the indications for digital replantation must be individualized.

The microsurgical team approach is helpful not only in allowing lengthy procedures but also in providing meticulous postoperative care. Recently two advances appear to have improved our survival rates: the dermal fluorescein monitor as an early detector of problems with arterial perfusion and venous congestion, and nail removal as a useful adjunct for treating venous congestion. Stiffness remains the dominant functional problem, but with early motion and assistance by competent hand therapists, a gratifying functional result can be achieved in most cases.

REFERENCES

1. Alpert, B.S., Buncke, H.J., and Brownstein, M.: Replacement of damaged arteries and veins with vein grafts when replanting crushed, amputated fingers, Plast. Reconstr. Surg. **61:**17, 1978.
2. Buncke, H.J., Alpert, B.S., and Johnson-Giebink, R.: Digital replantation, Surg. Clin. North Am. **61:**383, 1981.
3. Graham, B.H., et al.: Serial quantitative skin surface fluorescence: a new method for postoperative monitoring of vascular perfusion in replanted digits. Paper presented at the 1983 American Society for Surgery of the Hand meeting, Anaheim. (Submitted for publication.)
4. Harris, G.D., Finseth, F., and Buncke, H.J.: Posterior wall-first microvascular anastomotic technique, Br. J. Plast. Surg. **34:**47, 1981.
5. Jaeger, S.H., Tsai, T., and Kleinert, H.E.: Upper extremity replantation in children, Orthop. Clin. North Am. **12:**897, 1981.
6. Lister, G.: Intraosseous wiring of the digital skeleton, J. Hand Surg. **3:**427, 1978.
7. May, J.W., Toth, B.A., and Gardner, M.: Digital replantation distal to the proximal interphalangeal joint, J. Hand Surg. **7:**161, 1982.
8. Nissenbaum, M.: A surgical approach for replantation of complete digital amputations, J. Hand Surg. **5:**58, 1980.
9. O'Brien, B.M.: Replantation surgery, Clin. Plast. Surg. **1:**405, 1974.
10. O'Brien, B.M., Franklin, J., Morrison, W., and MacLeod, A.: Replantation and revascularization surgery in children, Hand **121:**12, 1980.
11. Tamai, S.: Twenty years' experience of limb replantation—review of 293 upper extremity replants, J. Hand Surg. **7:**549, 1982.
12. Urbaniak, J.R.: Replantation of amputated parts—technique, results, and indications. In American Academy of Orthopaedic Surgeons: Symposium on microsurgery: practical use in orthopaedics, St. Louis, 1979, The C.V. Mosby Co., p. 64.
13. VanBeek, A.L., Kutz, J.E., and Zook, E.G.: Importance of the ribbon sign, indicating unsuitability of the vessel in replanting a finger, Plast. Reconstr. Surg. **61:**32, 1978.
14. Weiland, A.J., et al.: Replantation of digits and hands—analysis of surgical techniques and functional results in 71 patients with 86 replantations, Clin. Orthop. **133:**195, 1978.
15. Wilgis, E.F.S., and Maxwell, G.P.: Distal digital nerve grafts: clinical and anatomical studies, J. Hand Surg. **4:**439, 1979.
16. Zei-Wen, C., Meyer, V.E., Kleinert, H.E., and Beasley, R.W.: Present indications and contraindications for replantation as reflected by long-term functional results, Orthop. Clin. North Am. **3:**849, 1981.

Chapter 5

Functional results in a selected series of replanted and revascularized digits, including a singular tale of an attempted digital replantation nine days after amputation

Jack W. Tupper

To characterize the level of return of function that can be anticipated when a replantation or revascularization is carried out under excellent conditions, we selected fifty-three patients (thirty-six replantations and seventeen revascularizations) from a larger series of 150 patients with amputated digits. We subjected these patients to a modified Tamai scheme of analysis, from which we could derive the level of function achieved from our repairs (Fig. 5-1). We then summarized some general observations gleaned from this selected series and also from our larger series of cases.

MODIFIED TAMAI ANALYSIS OF A SELECTED SERIES OF FIFTY-THREE PATIENTS
Patient selection

All patients were over 20 years of age; all were followed for at least 2 years; all patients had good natural motor coordination. Final evaluation was made only after completion of all reconstructive procedures.

Special problems in using the modified Tamai method of testing

1. The maximum score, 100, can be achieved with less than normal function.
2. The tests of activities of daily living (Part I [2]) are difficult to apply. Many uninjured people can do things with the normal major hand that

they cannot do with their minor hand, and many activities involve just certain fingers and not others.
3. Sensory (Part II): the British Sensory System used by Tamai is more applicable to high nerve injuries and is not sufficiently sensitive for fingers. Most replanted fingers score S3 or S4 (Table 5-1).

Table 5-1. Results in our series of fifty-three selected patients graded by modified Tamai score

Thumb	Number of digits	Tamai score
Thumb replants	10	88
Thumb revascularizations	5	83
Average		86
Multiple digits		
Multiple digit replants	18	84
Multiple digit revascularizations	3	86
Average		84
Single digits		
Single digit replants	6	90
Single digit revascularization	6	88
Average		89
Digital avulsions		
Ring avulsion replants	2	90
Ring avulsion revascularizations	3	93
Average		92
TOTAL REPLANTS	36	
TOTAL REVASCULARIZATIONS	17	
TOTAL CASES	53	

```
REPLANTATION SCORE SHEET (DR. SUSUMU TAMAI)


A CRITERIA FOR THE POSTOPERATIVE EVALUATION OF THE REPLANTED DIGIT & HAND


I.   MOTION ----- 40
     (1)  R.O.M. ----- 20
          THUMB:  Opposition ----- possible (10), difficult (5), impossible (0)
                  MPj  flex/ext =     /       IPj flex/ext =     /
                  ROM of (MPj + IPj) = more than ½ of normal --- (10)
                                       less than ½ of normal --- ( 5)
                                       stiff thumb           --- ( 0)

          FINGER:
```

	MPj	PIPj	DIPj	Sum of flex.	Lack of ext.	ROM
II flex/ext						
III						
IV						
V						

```
                              ROM:  more than 151° --- (20)
                                    111°       150° --- (15)
                                     71°       110° --- (10)
                                    less than  70° --- ( 5)
                                    stiff digit    --- ( 0)

     (2)  A.D.L. ----- 20
               1)  Pushing                11)  Washing face
               2)  Tapping                12)  Knotting
               3)  Hanging or drawing     13)  Buttoning
               4)  Grasp a soft material  14)  Writing
               5)  Grasp a hard material  15)  Scissoring
               6)  Power grasping         16)  Hammering
               7)  Pick up a coin         17)  Use a screw driver
               8)  Pick up a needle       18)  Use a clothes-pin
               9)  Wring a towel          19)  Fumble in pocket
              10)  Dip up water           20)  Show "scissors," "paper," & "stone"

              easy --- (1)   difficult --- (0.5)   impossible --- (0)

II.  SENSATION (by B.M.R.C.) ----- 20
          S₀    S₁    S₂    S₃    S₃₊    S₄
          (0)   (4)   (8)  (12)  (16)   (20)

III. SUBJECTIVE SYMPTOM ----- 10

          such as Pain (Rest pain or Motion pain).  Cold intolerance.  Numbness.
          Paresthesia, Tightness, etc.
                  severe --- (-3)   moderate --- (-2)   mild --- (-1)

IV.  COSMESIS ----- 10

          such as Atrophy, Scar, Colour changes, Deformities (Angulation, Rotation,
          Mallet, Swanneck, Button-hole, etc.), etc.
                  severe --- (-3)   moderate --- (-2)   mild --- (-1)

V.   PATIENT'S SATISFACTION ----- 20

          highly satisfied (20), fairly satisfied (15), satisfied (10)
          poorly satisfied (5), not satisfied (0)

          Job status:  same --- (0)   changed --- (-5)   can not work --- (-10)
```

Fig. 5-1. Score sheet for Tamai method of analysis. (Courtesy Dr. Susumu Tamai.)

A   B

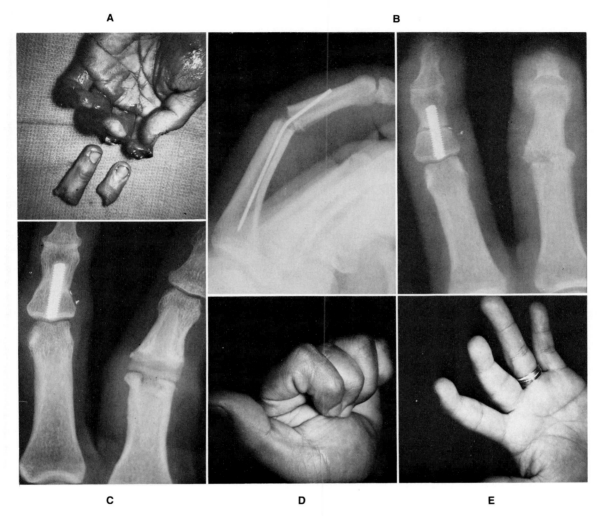

C   D   E

Fig. 5-2. A, Amputation of the index finger through the middle phalanx. Amputation of the long finger through the proximal interphalangeal (PIP) joint. **B,** (1) Temporary Kirschner wire fixation of the PIP joint will usually not result in fusion, but renders the finger immobile during the early rehabilitative phase. (2) Intramedullary screw fixation of the index finger. **C,** Swanson implant inserted in PIP joint of middle finger. Healing complete in index finger. **D,** Good flexion is present in both the index and middle fingers following flexor tenolysis. **E,** Good extension is also present. The patient returned to full-time work as a carpenter 1 year after the amputation.

GENERAL OBSERVATIONS FROM OUR REPLANTATION AND REVASCULARIZATION CASES

An amputated digit represents a complete division of all its tissues, and each tissue must be considered in the repair.

Skin. The problem of skin coverage is usually solved by resecting bone until primary skin closure may be obtained. Remaining defects in vessel length are handled with vein grafts. If there is a great loss of skin, replantation may not be warranted unless multiple digits have been lost.

Bone. Although the bone juncture should be fixed with dispatch, it should also be done with accuracy and security to allow early range of motion at 3 weeks when tendons are healed. If these points are observed, nonunion and malunion are uncommon.

Tendons. Restoration of tendon function is often a serious problem. Efforts at early motion are made under the supervision of the surgeon; a hand therapist is very helpful. The physical therapist is the most important person on the medical team at this stage. Secondary tenolyses for scarred or immobile tendons are commonly required.

Joints. Joint stiffness can occur either from direct damage to the joint or secondary contracture of capsular ligaments. High priority must be placed on gaining joint motion; otherwise the functional potential of a well-performed replantation may be nullified. If the original joint injury is so severe as to preclude the possibility of satisfactory function, an implant arthroplasty (Fig. 5-2) must be considered (either primarily or secondarily). A well-organized program of hand rehabilitation is essential.

Nerves. Restoration of nerve function is an elusive goal. No adult regains completely normal sensation after repair of a severed nerve. Success with the nerve repairs depends partly on the accuracy of the initial repair and partly on the adaptability of the patient. Although successful revascularization is the first criterion of success, return of nerve function to a useful level is equally important.

CHARACTERISTICS OF FAVORABLE AND UNFAVORABLE INJURIES

Digital injuries can be classified as either favorable or unfavorable for replantation or revascularization, and the ultimate functional result is closely related.

Characteristics of favorable injuries

1. *Limited zone of injury.* If the zone of injury is small, debridement of the damaged bone and tissues does not produce significant shortening and results will be better.
2. *Amputation distal to the superficialis insertion.* The vessels at this level are large enough for repair, sensory nerve regeneration is usually satisfactory, the proximal interphalangeal joint is unaffected, and mobilization is usually rapid.
3. *Amputation not through a joint.* If the joint is free of injury from the original trauma, a major obstacle to recovery is circumvented and prognosis is improved.

Characteristics of unfavorable injuries

1. *Wide zone of injury.* Complete debridement may bring about excessive shortening of the digit. Vessels may be damaged beyond repair. A single replantable finger that has a significant amount of damage to the bones, tendons, and nerves ordinarily should not be replanted. (The parts of this unreplantable finger may be useful for repairs elsewhere.)
2. *Avulsion amputation.* Avulsions often cause severe fascicular nerve damage at different levels, gravely diminishing the success of regeneration. Patients under 20 years of age recover more readily from this type of injury (Fig. 5-3).
3. *Excess warm ischemic time.* If the digit undergoes an excess period of warm ischemic time, not only are the chances of survival diminished, but also those digits that do survive may be compromised in their function.

SINGLE DIGIT VERSUS MULTIPLE DIGIT AMPUTATION

If replantation of a digit or digits is desirable as judged by all other criteria, we proceed with replantation whether the digit is single or one of several amputations (Fig. 5-4).

AGE

The young patient generally does better than the older patient, but there are many exceptions, and tissue age does not always correlate with chronologic age.

NATURAL MOTOR COORDINATION

Natural motor coordination is an important factor in regaining function. If properly motivated and properly supervised by a hand therapist or the surgeon, the patient with natural motor coordination will have the potential for a high level of adaptation and a high level of functional achievement. Apropos of this was one of our patients with four fingers amputated, all through the proximal phalanx, three of which were replanted. She learned

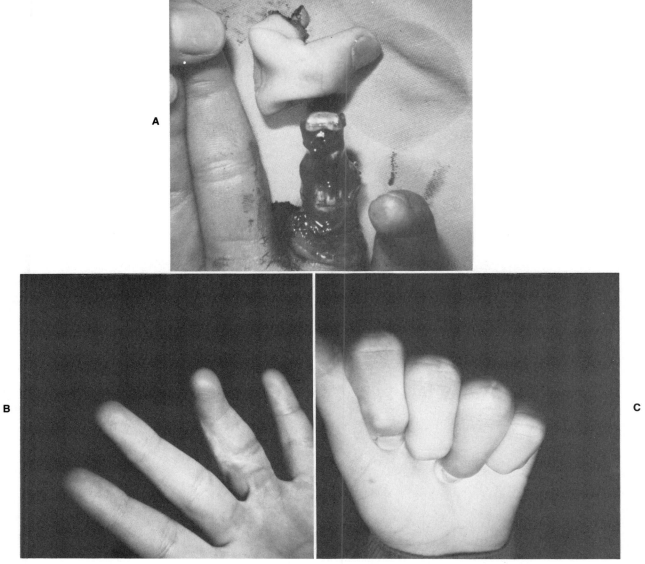

Fig. 5-3. A, Ring avulsion–amputation in a 12-year-old female. The distal phalanx remains with the amputated specimen. **B** and **C,** Postoperative appearance. Ring avulsion–amputations may be successful in teenagers, but have a lower rate of success in adults because of nerve damage.

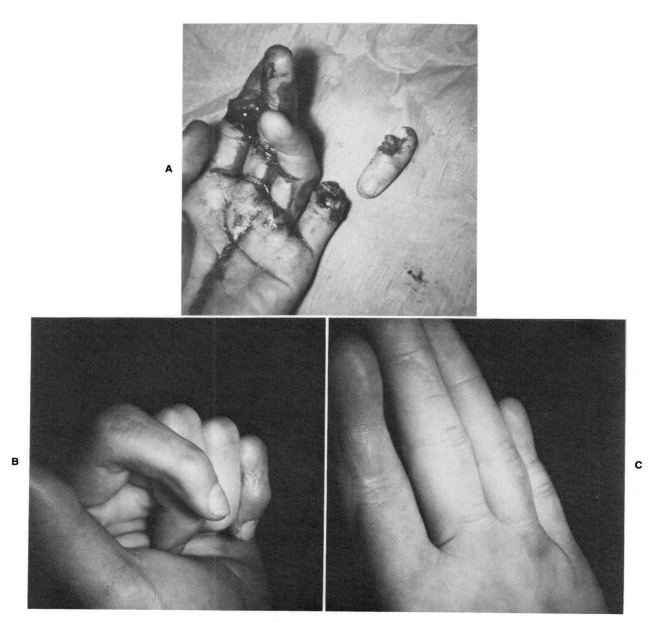

Fig. 5-4. A, Amputated left little finger at the base of the middle phalanx. The left index finger sustained a fracture of the proximal phalanx and lacerations of both digital nerves and flexor tendons. **B** and **C,** The replanted little finger functions better than the un-amputated but seriously injured index finger; replantation of a single amputated digit may be worthwhile.

to play the piano and type after the injury. Another patient with four replanted fingers plays golf again. Other patients with natural motor coordination are working as mechanics and have calluses on the replanted fingers as proof of active use.

COMMENTS

Replantation of amputated digits should be done by surgeons who are familiar with the general principles and techniques of hand surgery. The surgeon should be skilled in secondary surgical procedures, splinting, and hand rehabilitation. A close working relationship with a hand therapist is useful, if the therapist understands that the goal is motion, not strength. Strength may be easily obtained after motion is achieved; space-occupying materials (putty balls) or resistance gadgets should be avoided.

An amputated finger is not, per se, an indication for replantation; the overall function of the hand must be considered. In some occupations the patient can function very well without one or two fingers, and at times a prosthesis will serve the patient better. The financial and social impact should be considered and judgment must be used. However, under ideal conditions most finger or thumb replantations are worthwhile. When multiple digits are damaged, suboptimally functioning replanted digits may be better than no digits.

It should not be forgotten that repaired amputation stumps carry their own problems. An example of this is the 20% rate of recurrent, recalcitrant, painful neuromas, a problem rarely seen after replantation.

SUMMARY

Our results indicate that replantations and revascularizations under selected favorable conditions yield favorable functional results. Revascularizations in our series were indistinguishable from replantations in terms of functional results. Each type of tissue in the digit has its own problems that must be dealt with effectively to regain satisfactory function. Injuries of the favorable type in patients with natural motor coordination gave our best results.

A SINGULAR TALE OF AN ATTEMPTED DIGITAL REPLANTATION NINE DAYS AFTER AMPUTATION

A wealthy Arab from Mecca sustained a ring avulsion–amputation of his right ring finger, and for reasons that were unclear to me, he decided to come to Oakland, California, for replantation. Our

repeated cablegrams advised him to divert to nearer facilities, but to no avail. He boarded his private jet aircraft with his retinue and began his journey. Flying fatigued him, and about 4 PM each day he would stop in whatever country he was passing over and bed down for the night. The finger was meanwhile preserved, floating in a bottle of refrigerated intravenous solution.

Each morning, refreshed, he would continue his journey until the subsequent afternoon, when at 4 PM he would again stop for a night's sleep. Daily cablegrams gave assurances of his continued progress. Nine days after the amputation, he finally arrived at San Francisco Airport, his flight having taken him from the Middle East, across Europe, over the Atlantic Ocean, and across the North American continent. We were instructed to prepare for surgery. Soon the sirens of a police escort announced his passage as he made the transit of San Francisco, crossed the San Francisco–Oakland Bay Bridge, and arrived at Oakland's Merritt Hospital. After he had completed such an odyssey it seemed unthinkable to refuse him our best efforts at reuniting him with his well-traveled digit; we feared that the psychological consequences of making *no* effort would be worse than any untoward side effects of our surgical efforts.

The shrunken, gray member was retrieved from the IV bottle, and surgery began. The donor site was by now healed, and I suspected that the intima of the vessels was collapsed and sealed forever. However, I proceeded to obtain bone fixation, repair the tendons, and explore the vessels; I found to my surprise that one of the digital arteries could be repaired (at least it could be mechanically bridged) by means of a vein graft. I knew in my own mind, however, that there would be no return blood flow and that our vain effort would gracefully conclude. I removed the anastomosis clamps and witnessed an amazing sight: blood coursed through the vessels, the turgor of the finger reappeared, vigorous subdermal backbleeding began, and the color changed from gray to an astonishing brick red.

After retaining this brick red color for 2 days, the finger abruptly and rapidly mummified and we then amputated it. Probably any significant cellular function had ceased long before surgery, and what we were observing was the shell of a finger illuminating in silhouette the skeletal remains of the major vessels.

When does a finger die? Is there a way to rescue such structures when they are moribund? The value of these observations are difficult to assess!

Chapter 6

Replantation of the hand

Marcus Castro Ferreira

Replantation of amputated extremities has attracted the interest of surgeons for many years, but clinical application began only with the replantation of an arm in 1964 by Malt and McKhann.[4]

In the last two decades the development of microsurgical techniques and their application to replantation surgery has offered better prospects of success.

Our team has been performing replantation of extremities in São Paulo, Brazil, since 1965, and to this date a series of 125 cases of complete amputation has been carried out (forty arms and proximal forearms, twenty-six distal forearms and hands, and fifty-nine fingers). A survey of major limb replantations done before 1976 was reported elsewhere.[3]

We will deal here only with replantation at the level of the wrist and hand (Figs. 6-1 to 6-4), in which we had nineteen survivals of the replanted part in twenty-six cases (73%).

The amputation of a hand is a profound loss, so the indications for replantation are weighed with great care. Relative contraindications include (1) risk to the patient's life, (2) very severe crush or avulsive injuries, (3) multiple level amputations, (4) patient more than 50 years of age, (5) ischemic time longer than 12 hours, and (6) patient's mental status so poor that functional rehabilitation is precluded.

The overall care of the patient with a traumatic amputation has been extensively reviewed in the literature and we will not repeat it here. Only points peculiar to amputation at the level of the hand or related to our own experience on the subject will be mentioned.

The maximum ischemic time before replantation is still a matter of controversy; we fixed an empirical figure of 12 hours. Cooling should be provided as soon as possible. Perfusion of the vascular tree is no longer done.

BONE SHORTENING AND FIXATION

Bone shortening was done in our series only as needed to get good bone contact and was not done to lengthen the free vessel ends. Bone shortening was usually done by resecting one of the carpal rows, or the equivalent width of the radius and ulna if the level of injury was more proximal. In those cases in which the vessel stumps were short, vein grafts were used.

Fixation was obtained with Kirschner wires. Complications related to bone fixation were infrequent. Twice we observed nonunion at the wrist that needed revision and secondary arthrodesis.

VASCULAR ANASTOMOSES

Evaluation of the vascular stumps is carried out under the microscope. The arterial flow from the proximal stump should be strong and pulsatile. If any doubt persists, additional resection of the vessel is done and the flow reevaluated. If the resection is extensive, the gap is bridged with vein grafts taken from the foot or the forearm. In most cases of replantation of the hand, the ulnar artery is the main vascular supply for the superficial palmar arch and the circulation of the hand and digits; thus it should be repaired. In the wrist and at more proximal levels of amputation, the radial artery is present and should also be reanastomosed.

Venous drainage of the hand is usually provided by a superficial dorsal system. We always find at least two veins with good drainage in the subcutaneous tissues of the dorsal aspect of the hand.

Our policy has been to anastomose one artery

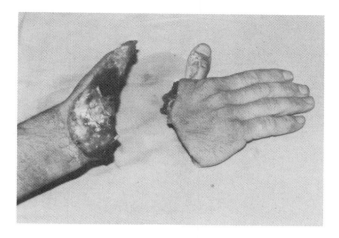

Fig. 6-1. Transmetacarpal amputation of the hand.

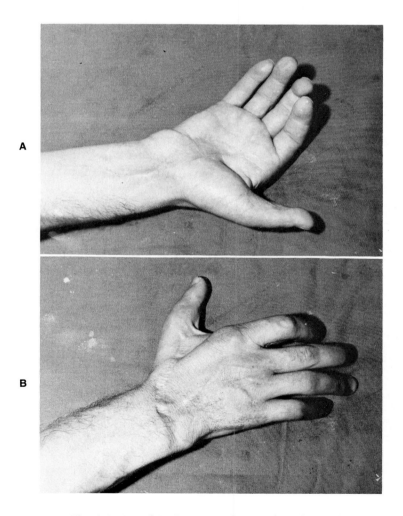

Fig. 6-2. A and **B,** Postoperative result at 8 months.

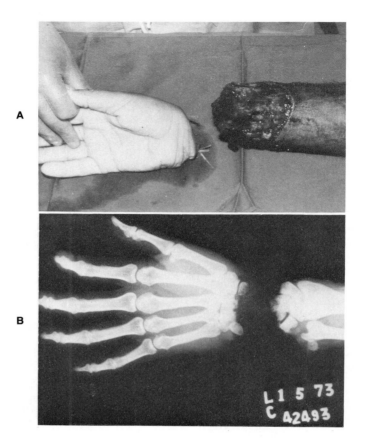

Fig. 6-3. A and **B,** Amputation of the hand at the carpal level.

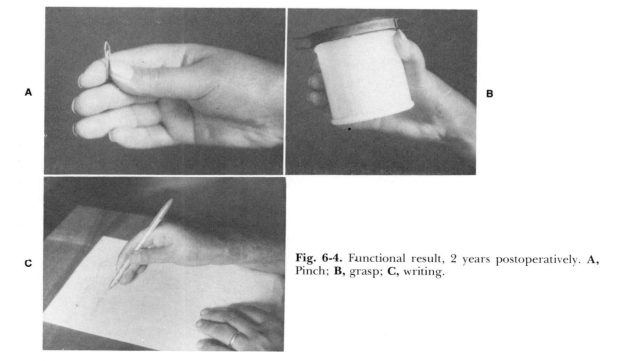

Fig. 6-4. Functional result, 2 years postoperatively. **A,** Pinch; **B,** grasp; **C,** writing.

and one vein before release of the arterial clamps. After circulation has been reestablished the other vascular structures are repaired.

No topical or systemic anticoagulant drug has been routinely used.

Satisfactory perfusion was achieved in almost every case, and technical problems did not seem to be responsible for the failures, which occurred 3 or 4 days postoperatively. The explanation probably lies in the status of the microcirculation and will be discussed later.

NERVE AND TENDON SUTURES

To achieve the best functional recovery, the repair of nerves and tendons should be done primarily. If for some reason it is not possible to do so primarily, they must be repaired secondarily, usually after 60 days. In these cases a marking suture is used to approximate the nerve stumps, preventing retraction of the nerve and thereby making the secondary operation easier. We favor use of the epiperineural suture for the primary repair of the median and ulnar nerves.

When feasible, and depending on the level of amputation, primary sutures were placed in the profundi flexor tendons, the flexor pollicis longus, the flexor carpi radialis, the flexor carpi ulnaris, the extensor digitorum communis, the extensor pollicis longus, the abductor pollicis longus, one extensor carpi radialis, and the extensor carpi ulnaris.

SKIN

The skin should be sutured loosely. Skin grafts and flaps are done as secondary procedures. One indication for a primary skin graft would be for the protection of exposed vascular structures, but we have never encountered such a problem in our series.

Fasciotomies were not done routinely. Only on rare occasions, when we faced massive edema with poor venous return, was such a procedure considered.

POSTOPERATIVE CARE

A bulky dressing and upper limb elevation were used; they were changed every 2 days.

Heparin and other anticoagulant drugs are no longer being used. We still favor the use of aspirin (1 g/day) and dextran-40, 500 ml/day, for 1 week. A vasodilator with ganglionic block action can be used intravenously to assure vasodilation of the extremity. In our country we have used naftidrofuril as a vasodilator in an intravenous drip for 1 week.

Gentle physical therapy is instituted as soon as possible, usually 2 weeks after the injury.

The patients were discharged in 10 days on the average, and the casts were removed in 45 to 60 days. Physical therapy can then be increased, with subsequent occupational therapy to help improve the functional result.

Results following replantation of the hand are difficult to assess and compare, since the cases are so dissimilar. The surgeon cannot influence the kind of injury, of course, but he can help affect the immediate success rate by decreasing the ischemic time for the extremities by disseminating an effective "limb replantation protocol" to all emergency rooms and hospitals likely to refer such patients. The surgeon should also establish a referral center for replantation surgery to attract a well-trained staff, to offer better care for the patients, and thereby to improve the success rate.[1,2,5]

The primary factor limiting success is the "no reflow phenomenon." It is not completely understood, but it seems to be related to the length of the ischemic time, the type of injury, and the level of the amputation. The measures we have today to prevent this phenomenon are totally empirical.

The results we have seen are comparable to those obtained in treating other major hand injuries. The main postoperative problems were related to joint stiffness and to impairment of the muscles (probably resulting from both denervation and ischemia of the intrinsic muscles).

A question has often arisen concerning the use of the replantation procedure in an attempt to provide a functional limb. This question is currently best answered by the results reported by the several replantation centers that have been established in many countries. In any event, the functional result of a replanted part should not be compared with the normal limb but with the best prosthesis currently available.

REFERENCES

1. American Replantation Mission to China: Replantation surgery in China, Plast. Reconstr. Surg. **52:**476, 1973.
2. Chen, C.W., Chien, Y.C., and Pav, Y.S.: Salvage of the forearm following complete traumatic amputation: report of a case, Clin. Med. J. **82:**632, 1963.
3. Ferreira, M.C., Marques, E.F., and Azze, R.J.: Limb replantation, Clin. Plast. Surg. **5:**211, 1978.
4. Malt, R.A., and McKhann, C.F.: Replantation of severed arms, JAMA **189:**716, 1964.
5. O'Brien, B.M.: Replantation surgery, Clin. Plast. Surg. **1:**405, 1974.

Chapter 7

Replantation of the upper arm and forearm

Susumu Tamai

Functional recovery of the replanted arm and forearm depends primarily on the operative indication. Even in a guillotine type of amputation near the elbow joint, it is generally difficult to obtain satisfactory function of the replanted extremity because of the anatomic characteristics of the distal arm and proximal forearm, where many motor branches from the three main nerves distribute into the extrinsic muscles of the hand. Also, sensory recovery may not be as satisfactory as that which can be obtained in replanted digits.

INDICATIONS

Replantation is indicated in patients in whom the following conditions are met:

1. The essential structures of the amputated part must be well preserved. Severe crush injuries or avulsive injuries in which important anatomic structures are missing are special problems and may obviate replantation. Patency of the major vessels in the severed part is the one absolute requirement for revascularization and replantation. If there are associated injuries in the distal part of the amputated limb, irrigation or angiography of the vessels may be needed for an accurate evaluation.

2. Warm ischemic time should preferably not exceed 6 hours. Although the "golden period" for the restoration of arterial flow to intact limbs is 6 to 8 hours (or a maximum of 12 hours), in complete or incomplete amputation ischemic changes in the tissues are greater, since collateral circulation is absent. Muscle tissue is the most vulnerable to ischemia, while skin and bone are probably the least vulnerable. To lower tissue metabolism, the amputated limb should be cooled in ice to 0° to 4° C immediately after the injury.

3. The patient must be in good general condition without any serious associated injuries or systemic diseases. The patient's age, sex, occupation, and desire for replantation are all given consideration in making the final decision.

PRIMARY CARE

Since an amputation injury to the upper extremity can be life threatening, resuscitation takes priority. The amputated part should be sealed in a polyethylene bag, without washing or sterilization, and should be cooled in ice to 0° to 4° C (Fig. 7-1, *A*). Bleeding from the proximal stump of the limb is controlled with sterile pressure dressings. Application of a pneumatic tourniquet on the upper arm may be indicated, depending on the level of amputation. In an incomplete amputation only the ischemic distal part should be surrounded by ice bags, while a compression bandage is applied to the wound itself (Fig. 7-1, *B*). If the replantation center is contacted before the patient's arrival, preparations for surgery can be made so that the procedure will go as smoothly as possible.

TRANSPORTATION

Most patients are brought directly to the replantation center by ambulance and are closely attended by a knowledgeable ambulance team. At the beginning of our series of replantations, there were few replantation centers in our country and patients were transported from distant locations by airplane or helicopter. However, with the increasing number of hospitals in Japan capable of replantation (now about 100), our case load in Nara is decreasing year by year. In a modern replanta-

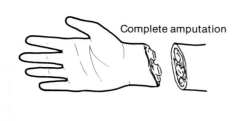

Complete amputation

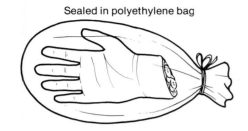

Sealed in polyethylene bag

A

Cooled in ice bag

Air tourniquet

Compression bandage

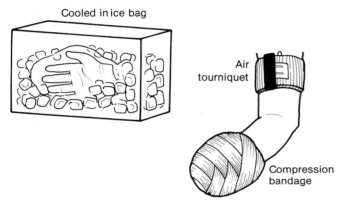

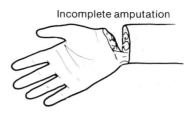

Incomplete amputation

B

Compression bandage

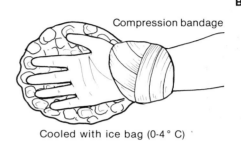

Cooled with ice bag (0-4° C)

Fig. 7-1. A and **B,** Schematic drawings showing primary care of the amputated part and the proximal stump of the extremity.

tion center a heliport on the roof or near the center is essential to receive patients with amputation injuries as quickly as possible.

PREOPERATIVE CARE AT THE CENTER OR UNIT

A history of the injury and an assessment of the patient's general condition are carried out, followed by a more detailed examination. A history of systemic diseases is obtained from the patient or relatives. Radiographs of the amputated limb and the proximal stump are taken, and then the injury is reassessed by the surgeon to determine whether or not replantation is possible. An extensively crushed or avulsed limb may not be acceptable for replantation. In an avulsion injury, when the major nerves are avulsed from proximal to distal, there is a good possibility of functional recovery. On the contrary, when the major nerves are avulsed from distal to proximal, especially around the elbow joint, no recovery in motor function can

be expected, since distal branches are pulled directly out of the muscles. Routine laboratory studies are performed when possible. An electrocardiogram and chest radiograph are also important to exclude heart and lung diseases. Intravenous infusions are started, and blood is typed and crossmatched if needed. Preoperative medications, antibiotics, and antitetanus and anticlostridial preparations are given.

In a complete amputation of the upper extremity, preparation of the amputated part and the proximal stump should be performed by two separate surgical teams. The wounds are washed with a chlorhexidine (Hibitane) solution and brush, and the nonviable tissues are thoroughly debrided. Manual milking or squeezing of the amputated part, going from distal to proximal, is an important maneuver (Fig. 7-2, *A*), since it helps to remove microthrombi or emboli lodged in the vascular lumen (Fig. 7-2, *B*). If revascularization is commenced without this maneuver, a thrombus may

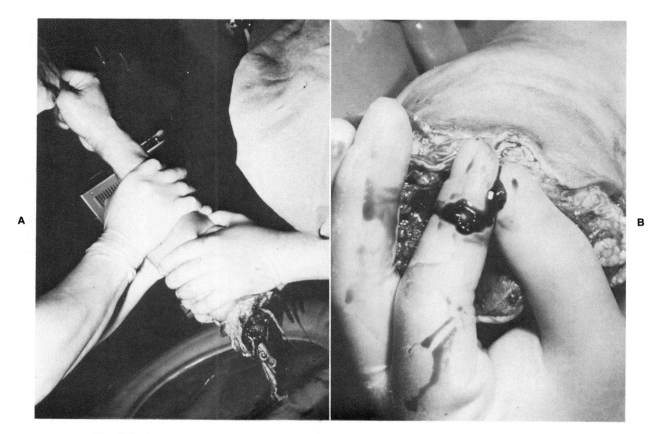

Fig. 7-2. A, Amputated upper extremity is squeezed manually. **B,** Large thrombus is squeezed out of the brachial artery.

be trapped in the distal artery and a critical circulatory problem will arise. Next a siliconized polyethylene catheter is carefully inserted into the arterial lumen; the amputated part is irrigated using heparin diluted in a low molecular weight dextran solution or saline solution, 10 U/ml; some replantation surgeons prefer to omit this step. Irrigation is stopped when the perfusate from the veins is clear, since prolonged perfusion is harmful and promotes edema in the severed part. Using this maneuver we not only thoroughly wash out the microclots and anaerobic metabolites but also assure the patency of the vascular channels in the amputated part. Failure to readily obtain venous return of the perfusate arouses suspicion that there are associated vascular injuries in the distal part. The less the return flow of perfusate, the greater the degree of obstruction or interstitial leakage that is suspected. In such an event, a preoperative angiogram of the amputated part may help define the problem. In every case we take color photographs of the dismembered part and the proximal stump from several views for the clinical records.

ANESTHESIA

In replanting an arm or forearm, we ordinarily use general anesthesia, but cervical epidural anesthesia with neuroleptoanalgesia is also employed in our center. Brachial block anesthesia such as bupivacaine (Marcaine) or lidocaine may be used for a forearm replantation but not for the upper arm.

REPLANTATION TECHNIQUE

A pneumatic tourniquet is used to control bleeding during a forearm replantation. To control bleeding during an upper arm replantation, the axillary artery can be exposed and occluded with an umbilical tape tourniquet. If ischemic time has been excessive, limb perfusion with oxygenated blood may aid in recovery. Continuous cooling of the limb during the operation, applying an ice bag or pillow until the circulation is reestablished, is used in most replantations.

The first step in replantation is shortening and fixation of the bone. After shortening the bone with an electric bone saw to a suitable length, averaging 2 to 5 cm to match the debridement of the soft tissues, we immobilize the bone firmly by any of a variety of methods of osteosynthesis. Intramedullary nailing is advisable at the level of the diaphysis. A compression plate may be used, but there is a risk of local swelling because of the bulk of the plate. In the metaphysis or epiphysis a bone screw or Kirschner wires are preferred. If the amputation involves a joint, primary arthrodesis in a functional position may be required.

After first suturing the periosteum and tissues around the bone as completely as possible, we perform the arterial anastomosis to revascularize the limb as soon as possible. The basic techniques of microvascular anastomosis are employed, using low-power magnification for the larger diameter vessels in the arm or forearm. When the clamps are released from the completed arterial repair, the skin turns pink and blood drips from the veins. The vein repairs follow after reinflation of the tourniquet to minimize blood loss. If the ischemic time permits, we sometimes do not release the clamps until both the arterial and venous anastomoses are complete. However, in replanting a major limb containing a large amount of muscular tissue, it may be preferable to use the former procedure to wash out the harmful anaerobic metabolites from the ischemic limb in an effort to avert replantation toxemia. One artery and two veins are repaired to gain a balanced circulation of the limb. Muscles and tendons are accurately repaired using 4-0 polypropylene (Prolene) or nylon sutures. From the standpoint of postoperative function, it is important to repair the minimum number of muscles or tendons required.

The nerve repairs are carried out primarily if possible, because secondary repairs are complicated by a widely scarred field and the need to do nerve grafts after neuroma resection.

We routinely use epineuroperineural sutures under low-power magnification. After making fasciotomies in several directions to prevent edema, we close the skin loosely. To avoid the development of constricting scars at the replantation site, we make relaxing incisions or Z-plasties at the suture line. The resultant skin defect is covered with an immediate split-thickness skin graft or by polyvinyl formaldehyde sponge (PVF sponge) followed by secondary skin grafting. PVF sponge has a special advantage because it drains wound exudates during the early postoperative period. In cases in which the skin defect exposes important deep structures, an immediate pedicle or free flap may be required for coverage. Finally, bulky dressings are applied with dorsal cast immobilization.

POSTOPERATIVE MANAGEMENT

The replanted part should be kept slightly higher than the heart, with the fingertips exposed for observation. Dressing changes are done daily. The patient's general condition must be maintained at an optimal level. Hourly observations of the replanted part are maintained. Skin color, temperature, capillary filling of the nail bed, and tension of the digital pulp are monitored. Pallor, coldness, and flattening of the digital pulp all indicate arterial problems. Timely reexploration and thrombectomy are indicated in the presence of such signs. On the contrary, darkness, turgidity, and abnormally brisk capillary return with excess tension of the pulp indicate venous problems. In the presence of these signs the hand is elevated higher than the heart; squeezing of the congested part is given a trial. If the signs persist, reexploration is done as quickly as possible. Venous congestion may cause significant edema of replanted major limbs, and additional relaxing skin incisions and fasciotomies might be needed.

Prevention of thrombosis at the site of the vascular anastomoses is of utmost importance, but in major limbs, systemic heparinization is generally not necessary and may even be harmful because of bleeding problems. Urokinase is effective for its fibrinolytic activity and is given when needed in an intravenous dose of 32,000 to 60,000 U/day in adults. Low molecular weight dextran, 500 ml/day, is also given intravenously for 3 to 5 days, during which time the patient is watched closely for any bleeding problems.

Prevention of bacterial infection is also important, since there is a greater exposure to the risk of infection in a major limb replantation than in a minor replantation. Massive doses of broad-spectrum antibiotics are given for 7 to 10 days. Factors considered in postoperative management are:

1. Good general condition
2. Observation of replant
3. Prevention of thrombosis
   Urokinase 32,000 to 60,000 U/day
   Low molecular weight dextran 500 ml/day
4. Prevention of infection
5. Rehabilitation (as early as possible) for prevention of joint stiffness and adhesion of muscle and tendon

Rehabilitation of the replanted limb starts on the first day, supervised by both the surgeon and the physical therapist. In an arm replant the passive range of motion exercises are carried out while awaiting regeneration of the motor nerves and return of power to the extrinsic muscles. The hand

and wrist joint are kept in a functional position throughout the postoperative period. On the tenth day, when all sutures are removed, moderate active motion exercise of the elbow joint is commenced. In a forearm replant, very mild active and passive motion of the proximal interphalangeal and distal interphalangeal joints is begun on the first day, while the metacarpophalangeal joints and the wrist are kept in a functional position. From the fifth to the tenth day, when the strength of the muscle-tendon suture lines is diminished, care is taken to avoid disruption. On the tenth day moderate active motion exercises in a warm bath are begun; after the fourth week active exercises using a dynamic splint are allowed. Until reinnervation has taken place, efforts are made to maintain muscular contractility and prevent denervation atrophy by the use of electrical stimulation to the paralyzed muscles.

RESULTS

As of December 1980, five cases of arm replantation (three complete and two incomplete) and twelve cases of forearm replantation (six complete and six incomplete) were performed in our hospital. Two forearms could not be salvaged because of arterial complications in the early postoperative period. In one forearm replant, significant edema developed postoperatively and has continued for approximately 1 year.

Table 7-1. Functional results of arm and forearm replantations

	*Excellent**	*Good*	*Fair*	*Poor*
Arm	0/5 (0%)	1/5 (20%)	3/5 (60%)	1/5 (20%)
Forearm	2/10 (20%)	3/10 (30%)	2/10 (20%)	3/10 (30%)
TOTAL	2/15 (13%)	4/15 (27%)	5/15 (33%)	4/15 (27%)

*Excellent, good, fair, and poor are equivalent to Grades I, II, III, and IV of Chen's criteria.

To obtain satisfactory function of the replanted limb, various secondary procedures were usually required (thirty-nine procedures in forearm replants and eight in arm replants). Capsulotomy of the metacarpophalangeal joint and musculotenolysis in the forearm were the most common procedures.

The best motor function was obtained after replantation of the distal forearm; the poorest results were obtained in replants at the level of the proximal third. Sensory recovery was limited in major limb replantations. Most patients regained protective sensation, but only in one case was there two-point discrimination of 10 mm at the fingertip. Our functional results, rated by Chen's criteria,[1] were fair or poor in 80% of the replanted arms and 50% of the forearms (Table 7-1).

CASE REPORT
Patient I

A 38-year-old male's right upper arm was amputated just above the elbow joint by a press machine. It looked somewhat like a guillotine-type amputation, but the median and ulnar nerves were avulsed distal to proximal for approximately 20 cm. Because of irreparable injuries to the motor branches of the nerves that innervated all the flexor muscles in the forearm, he seemed to be a poor candidate for replantation. The patient and his relatives, however, insisted on the procedure. After extensive bone shortening and fixation, one artery and three veins were repaired. An autogenous nerve graft taken from the proximal end of the avulsed ulnar nerve was transplanted to the defect in the median nerve as a bridge graft. None of the motor branches to the muscles could be repaired. The ulnar nerve also required an end-to-end repair of the main trunk. The extremity was successfully replanted. A skin defect caused by a relaxing skin incision was covered with a PVF sponge that in turn was replaced by a free skin graft later on.

Three years after the replantation sensation has returned to the palmar aspect of the fingers. His range of active motion at the elbow is 60 degrees (he misses full elbow extension by 60 degrees); he has 45 degrees of dorsiflexion of the wrist joint. He returned to his original job as a laborer 18 months following the replantation and performs his work surprisingly well (Fig. 7-3).

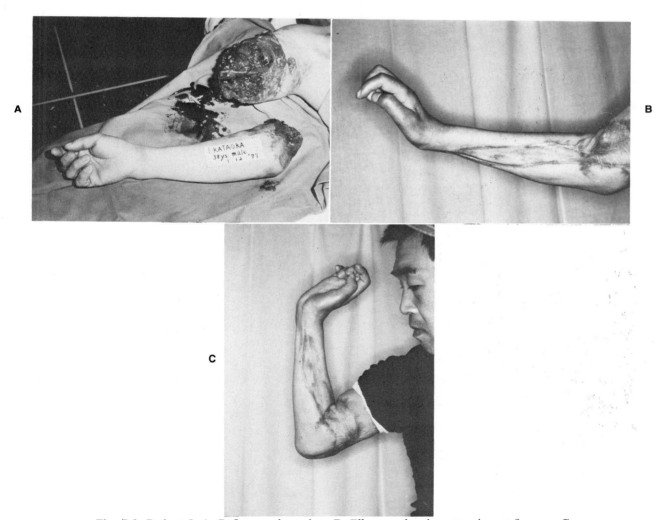

Fig. 7-3. Patient I. **A,** Before replantation. **B,** Elbow and wrist extension at 3 years. **C,** Elbow flexion.

Patient II

A 28-year-old male factory worker amputated his right forearm at the distal third in a cutting machine. He was transferred to our hospital with the amputated part cooled in ice. The operation started 4 hours after the injury; continuous cervical epidural anesthesia with 3% lidocaine (Xylocaine) was employed. The forearm bones were shortened approximately 2.5 cm. Fixation of the radius was obtained with a plate and a primary bone graft; the ulna was fixed with an intramedullary wire. Two arteries, five veins, and three nerves were repaired. The more important tendons and muscles were repaired with sutures. In long operations such as this, continuous cooling of the ischemic part with an ice bag or pillow helps to minimize ischemic changes. No systemic heparinization was used. Two units of blood and three units of intravenous fluid were given. Total operating time was 6 hours, and the extremity survived successfully. Since no bed was available in our hospital, the patient was transferred to a private hospital for postoperative care and rehabilitation under our supervision. Secondary procedures were not required, and 2 years postoperatively the functional recovery of the replanted hand was satisfactory, with recovery of intrinsic muscle function and a two-point discrimination of 20 mm on the pulp of the index finger (Fig. 7-4).

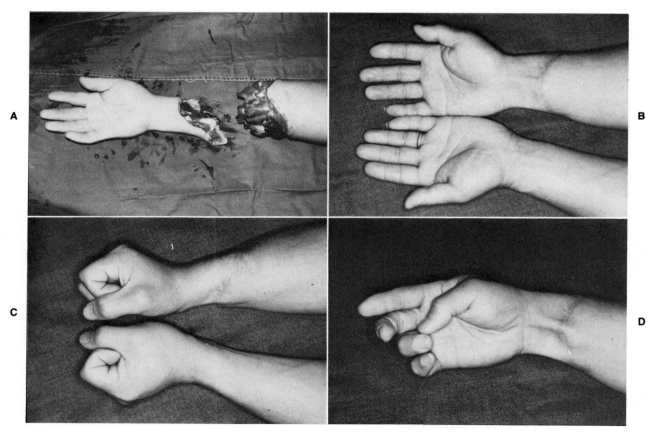

Fig. 7-4. Patient II. **A,** Before replantation. **B,** Appearance of both hands 2 years postoperatively. Muscle atrophy of the thenar and hypothenar regions has completely recovered, with good digital extension. **C,** Good flexion of digits. **D,** Thumb opposition is also recovering.

Patient III

A 17-year-old male sustained a moderately crushed amputation of his right forearm just proximal to the wrist from an electric saw. A general anesthesia was employed. Two arteries, five veins, and three nerves were repaired. The hand was successfully replanted, and 1 year after surgery extension and flexion of his digits was satisfactory, but function of the thenar muscles was very poor (Fig. 7-5). At 1 year and 6 months an opponensplasty was carried out, and function was much improved.

Since a number of factors influence the functional outcome of replanted extremities, final results vary. Primary factors include the level of amputation, the extent of tissue damage, the ischemic time before and during the operation, and the patient's age. Surgical technique is also an important factor. Circulatory problems, delayed nerve regeneration, tissue adhesions, and joint stiffness are secondary factors. The patient's cooperation throughout the treatment is essential for good results.[2]

REFERENCES

1. Chen, Z.W., et al.: Extremity replantation, World J. Surg. **2**:513, 1978.
2. Tamai, S., et al.: Major limb, hand, and digital replantation, World J. Surg. **3**:17, 1979.

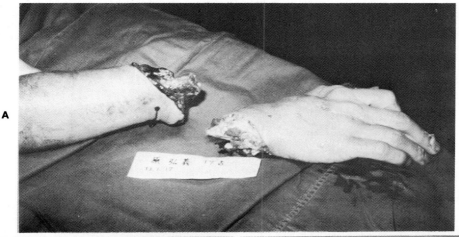

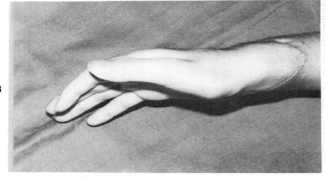 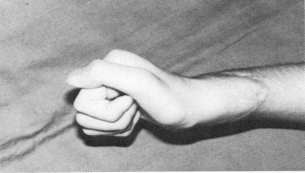

Fig. 7-5. Patient III. **A,** Before replantation. **B,** One year after replantation; although digital extension and flexion are satisfactory, opposition of the thumb is lacking.

Chapter 8

Replantation of other parts of the body

Edgar Biemer

Eleven surgeons are active on the replantation service of the Klinikum rechts der Isar. They have carried out replantation of nearly 1,000 amputated parts of the upper extremities and a great number of amputated parts from other areas of the body such as the scalp, ear, midface structures, toes, and feet.

INDICATIONS

Most of the patients have been transported to this center for replantation of parts that are virtually impossible to replant by other reconstructive procedures. Therefore the indications are very broad.

OPERATING TECHNIQUE

The details of operating technique for replantation of other parts of the body are similar to those employed in replantation of upper limb structures.[1] For replantation of the scalp, ear, midface, nose, and other such parts, the focus is chiefly on gaining successful microvascular anastomoses in unfavorable circumstances. The details of replantation of parts of the foot are essentially identical to the technique of replantation of amputated hand structures. Specific technical features are described in the following sections.

SCALP REPLANTATION

Accidental entanglement of long hair in the revolving parts of a machine is the most common cause of complete or partial avulsion of the scalp; vehicle accidents are another cause. In times past, coverage of the defect was furnished by means of split-thickness skin grafts or conventional pedicles. To be presentable in public, patients who underwent such grafts required wigs. These grafting methods have been superseded by microvascular

replantation whenever the procedure is feasible; only revascularization gives the possibility of *restitutio ad integrum*.[2]

Technique

The line of detachment varies from case to case and may even include an ear. The more proximal the level of detachment, the larger the diameter of the vessels, so if an ear has been included in the specimen, replantation is much easier. The best vessels for revascularization are the temporal or occipital arteries and veins.

If the level of vessel separation is more than 4 to 5 cm above the ear, suitable veins are extremely difficult to identify in the amputated part. In one case where the vessels were divided above this line, no suitable veins could be found and replantation was attempted with arterial anastomoses alone. In this case the scalp was well vascularized following the arterial repair, but because of massive loss of blood during the subsequent 2 postoperative days, the patient was taken back to surgery and the scalp was removed.

The plane of separation is usually between the galea aponeurotica and the periosteum; sometimes periosteum is included with the scalp. The hair is clipped and shaved in preparation for replantation. Arteries are identified by searching along the torn edge of the galea. The veins are embedded in the subcutaneous fat slightly superficial to the galea and are more difficult to identify. To facilitate identification of the veins, the arterial anastomoses are performed first, the vascular clamps are released, and then the veins are identified by their backflow. The blood perfusion requirement for the scalp will be fulfilled by a single temporal vascular anastomosis, plus a single occipital vascular anastomosis for either the artery or the vein. If the scalp tissues have been crushed in the accident, typical signs of trauma will become evident after the blood supply has been restored.

Cases

We have carried out replantation in three cases of total scalp avulsion in the past 5 years. Two avulsions resulted from accidents with revolving machines and one resulted from a car accident. The latter case was complicated by a fracture of the cervical spine. In two cases we achieved total survival of the scalp with normal hair growth as a result of our replantation. In the third case the line of separation ran 5 to 6 cm above the level of the ear, and suitable veins could not be found, even after two explorations during the subsequent 48 hours. Arterial anastomoses alone were performed, but because of massive blood loss and attendant transfusion coagulopathy, the viable scalp had to be removed and the bleeding vessels ligated.

EAR REPLANTATION

Total amputation of the ear is extremely rare. We have had only one case in 5 years.

CASE REPORT

A 46-year-old male lost his entire left ear when it was bitten off in an altercation. The amputated specimen was in good condition, and the divided ends of both the retroauricular artery and vein were identified. The diameter of each was about 1 mm. The corresponding vessel ends were identified at the site of detachment, and vascular anastomoses were successfully performed. The ear showed excellent perfusion on release of the vascular clamps; this continued for about 20 hours and then the onset of cyanosis was noted. A venous thrombosis was identified and a thrombectomy was attempted but was unsuccessful. Total necrosis of the ear resulted.

MIDFACE AMPUTATION

Our two cases of midface amputation occurred in children. One was caused by a dog bite and the other by a car accident.

CASE REPORT (Fig. 8-1)

A dog bit the face of a 4-year-old female, amputating her entire upper lip and the lower third of her nose. The specimen was taken from the dog's mouth immediately, and the patient and the specimen were sent directly to our replantation service.

On exploration of the specimen, we identified a side branch of the labial artery (diameter 0.4 mm). It was successfully anastomosed to its parent vessel with three sutures of 11-0 nylon. Excellent perfusion was seen when the clamps were removed. Two very tiny veins were then identified from their backflow. They were each anastomosed with three sutures of 11-0 nylon.

The postoperative course was marked by massive swelling of the entire face and extensive ecchymoses in both cheeks. This appeared to be associated with separation of the layers of the skin resulting from the tearing force of the dog's bite. After 5 days the swelling abruptly disappeared, and the facial structures survived completely. Two years after the surgery the upper lip has regained nearly normal function and the child is able to whistle.

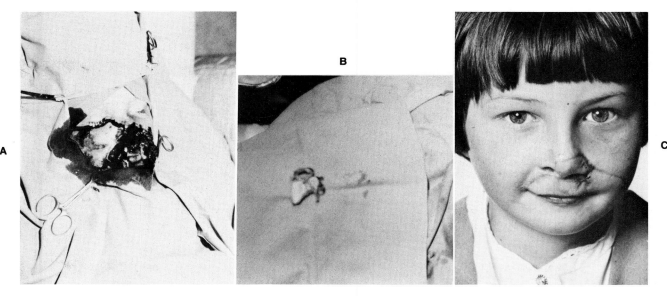

Fig. 8-1. A, Amputation of the upper lip and nose in a 4-year-old female as the result of a dog bite. **B,** Amputated specimen. **C,** Result 1 year after replantation.

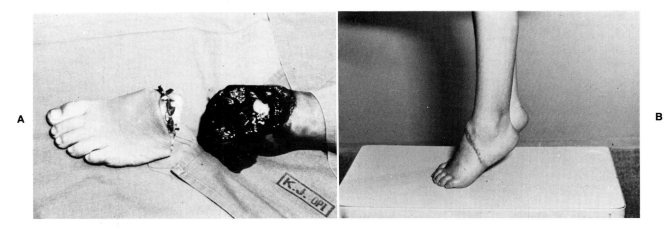

Fig. 8-2. A, Amputation of the midfoot in a 6-year-old female as the result of a harvesting machine accident. **B,** Normal function of the foot 8 months after replantation.

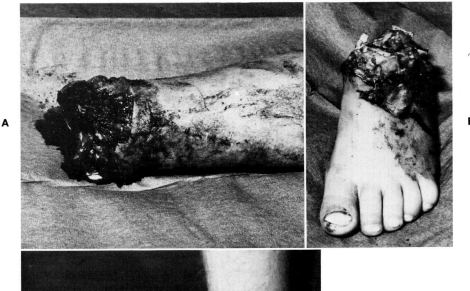

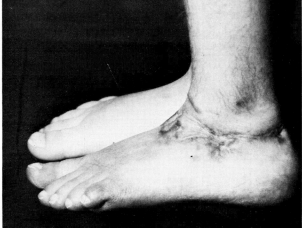

Fig. 8-3. A, Amputation of the entire foot through the ankle joint in a 7-year-old female as the result of a harvesting machine accident. **B,** Amputated specimen. **C,** Result 12 months after replantation.

TOE REPLANTATION

Only in very special circumstances are single toes replanted. Occasionally a cleanly amputated great toe has been replanted at the patient's request. The plantar arteries are the best candidates for anastomosis; because they are most easily found with the patient in prone position, the procedure is begun with the patient prone. The dorsal veins are the best veins for anastomosis. Therefore, once the arterial anastomoses are complete and the toes have been stabilized, the patient is turned over to a supine position. The replantation technique is in other respects identical to that used for fingers. Aesthetic and functional results have generally been excellent.

MIDFOOT REPLANTATION (Fig. 8-2)

If there is potential for replanting the amputated part without excessive shortening, replantation of amputations through the metatarsal area are clearly indicated.

Technique

The technique is identical to that employed in midhand replantations, except that the arterial connection is usually achieved by anastomosis of the dorsalis pedis artery. Every effort is made to gain successful repair of the nerves, particularly those to the sole of the foot. In a clean amputation, normal gait and the ability to wear ordinary shoes have been achieved.

TOTAL FOOT AMPUTATION

Whether or not a totally amputated foot should be replanted will depend on the type of injury. If a wide area of the foot is badly crushed, replantation will result in a short, crippled, poorly functioning foot. A good prosthesis is better for the patient than a badly functioning foot.

Technique

If possible one should carry out anastomoses on both the anterior and posterior tibial arteries, plus at least two veins. Repair of the sensory nerves is essential. Bone fixation is carried out with Kirschner wires or Rush pins.

CASE REPORT (Fig. 8-3)

In a harvesting machine accident a 7-year-old female sustained a sharp, guillotine-like amputation of the left foot at the level of the upper ankle. Because of the clean, sharp amputation, no shortening of the foot was needed. The divided ends of the anterior tibial artery were reunited with a single anastomosis. Two large veins were anastomosed. All sensory nerves were repaired. All extensor and flexor tendons, including the Achilles tendon, were repaired. The foot survived completely, and after 6 months the patient had a nearly normal gait. At first she wore special shoes because of a hallux valgus deformity, but this was corrected during the subsequent 2 years by conservative orthopedic measures. The patient regained full sensation and nearly normal ankle movements.

Table 8-1. Replantation of other parts of the body by microvascular anastomoses by the Department of Plastic Surgery, Klinikum rechts der Isar, Munich

Amputated part	Total	Subtotal	Success	Remarks
Scalp	4		3	No venous connection possible in one case
Ear	1		—	Venous thrombosis at the third day
Midface	2		1	
Toe	2	5	5	
Midfoot	3		2	
Foot	3		3	

DISCUSSION

In comparison to the number of amputations of parts of the upper limbs, amputations elsewhere on the body are rare. These amputations are of such special character that replacement by conventional reconstructive operations is not possible. This is particularly true for the scalp, ear, or midface (or male genitalia[3]). Therefore virtually no contraindication to replantation of these parts exists (Table 8-1).

In amputations of the foot the decision to carry out replantation must be made on the specific merits of each case. The main consideration is whether crushed tissues will deprive the foot of critical length.

SUMMARY

During the past 5 years our replantation team has replanted amputations of the scalp, midface, ear, toes, and foot. In the majority of cases the tissue that was replanted would have otherwise been irreplaceable. The aesthetic and functional results have been very promising.

REFERENCES

1. Biemer, D., and Duspiva, W.: Rekonstruktive mikrogefabchirurgie, Berlin, 1980, Springer-Verlag.
2. Miller, G.D.H., Anstee, E.J., and Suell, J.A.: Successful replantation of an avulsed scalp by microvascular anastomoses, Plast. Reconstr. Surg. **58:**133, 1976.
3. Tamai, S., Nakamura, Y., and Motomiya, Y.: Microsurgical replantation of a completely amputated penis and scrotum, Plast. Reconstr. Surg. **60:**187, 1977.

Part III

Pedicle design

Chapter 9

Free retroauricular flap

Toyomi Fujino

Excellent color match, inconspicuous donor scars, and a single-stage reconstruction are desired goals in facial resurfacing. The best color match is obtained from elsewhere on the face or forehead. A one-stage transfer of a forehead flap is feasible with a subcutaneous island flap[2] but leaves an unsightly scar. In our opinion the next best donor site for resurfacing part of the face is the retroauricular area, which leaves a hidden scar.

We will discuss a one-stage transfer of a retroauricular free flap by microvascular anastomosis.[4,5]

ANATOMY
Artery

The retroauricular artery usually arises from the external carotid artery (39/42 = 93%) and runs relatively deep, passing through the parotid gland (Figs. 9-1 and 9-2). It emerges in front of the anterior surface of the mastoid process behind the auricle.[6] Because this artery lies 3 cm beneath the skin near the mastoid process, one might anticipate problems when preparing it for transfer. However, inasmuch as the external diameter of this artery near the mastoid process is about 1.2 mm, we found that preparation was not difficult (Table 9-1). Furthermore, the retroauricular artery rises upward abruptly at the mastoid process to a position 1 cm below the skin surface in the central portion of the posterior aspect of the auricle. Therefore it is possible to expose this artery through careful dissection. It should be kept in mind that in three of forty-two cases studied (7%), the lower half of the retroauricular skin was nourished by a retroauricular artery from the external carotid artery, with the upper half fed by an artery branching from the occipital artery medial to the mastoid process (Figs. 9-2 and 9-3). In these latter specimens the retroauricular artery from the external

carotid artery penetrated through the auricular cartilage. The retroauricular artery runs lateral and slightly posterior to the trunk of the facial nerve. Thus, with care, injury to this nerve during preparation of the flap can be avoided. The relationship of the artery to the greater auricular nerve is not as uniform as the arrangement of the vessels and nerves in the intercostal space.

Table 9-1. Diameters (in millimeters) of vessels supplying the forty-two free flaps

	Right		Left	
Case	Artery	Vein	Artery	Vein
1	1.0	1.5	1.2	2.0
2	1.2	1.5	1.2	1.8
3	1.0	1.0	1.2	1.2
4	1.0	0.8	1.0	1.0
5	1.2	1.5	1.5	1.2
6	0.8	1.2	1.0	1.5
7	1.5	2.5	1.2	1.7
8	1.0	1.2	1.0	1.0
9	0.8	0.9	0.8	0.8
10	1.5	1.5	1.0	1.3
11	1.0	2.0	1.0	2.0
12	1.2	2.2	0.8	0.8
13	0.9	1.6	1.3	
14	1.0	1.0	0.6	
15	1.1	1.0		
16	1.0	1.0		
17	2.0		1.0	2.5
18	1.9		1.4	
19	1.4		1.5	
20			1.0	1.0
21			1.5	1.0
22			1.8	2.0
23			1.8	
24			1.1	
25			2.0	
Mean	1.1	1.4	1.2	1.4

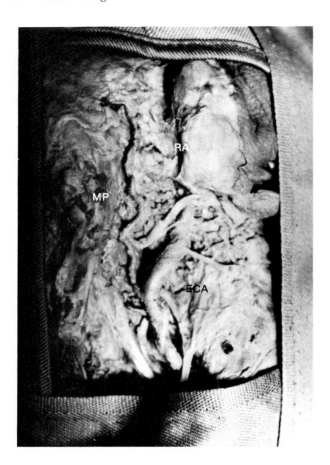

Fig. 9-1. Retroauricular artery originating from the external carotid artery in a right retroauricular flap. (*MP,* Mastoid process; *RA,* retroauricular artery; *ECA,* external carotid artery.)

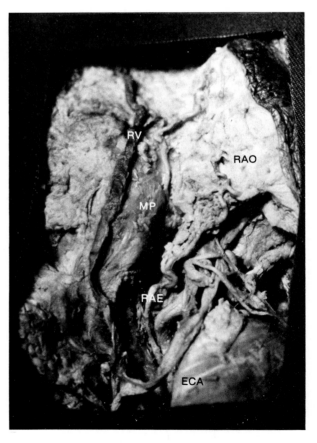

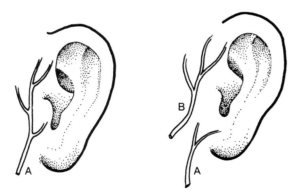

Fig. 9-2. Diagram of the types of retroauricular blood supply found in the flaps studied. On the left, the retroauricular artery *(A)* originates from the external carotid and supplies the entire flap region. On the right, the retroauricular artery *(A)* originates from the external carotid artery and supplies the lower portion of the flap; a second artery *(B)* originates from the occipital artery and supplies the upper portion of the flap area. (Adapted from Wada, M., and Fujino, T.: Anatomical description of the free retroauricular flap, J. Microsurg. **1:**108, 1979.)

Fig. 9-3. Retroauricular arteries arising from the external carotid artery and from the occipital artery. (*RAE,* retroauricular artery originating from the external carotid artery; *RAO,* retroauricular artery originating from the occipital artery; *ECA,* external carotid artery; *MP,* mastoid process; *RV,* retroauricular vein.)

Vein

The retroauricular vein does not always accompany the retroauricular artery. It courses in a more superficial zone, usually 1.5 cm below the surface of the mastoid region and 0.5 cm below the surface behind the auricle. The mean external diameter of the vein behind the auricle is 1.4 mm (Table 9-1); it tapers abruptly as it ascends above the auricle. The vein is situated in a posterosuperior position to the artery.

Size

The retroauricular artery gives off branches behind the auricle that are sufficient to support the flap area. From this area we can fashion a flap averaging 5 by 7 cm; the flap can be extended even more by taking advantage of the anastomoses between the retroauricular artery and the superficial temporal artery (Fig. 9-4).

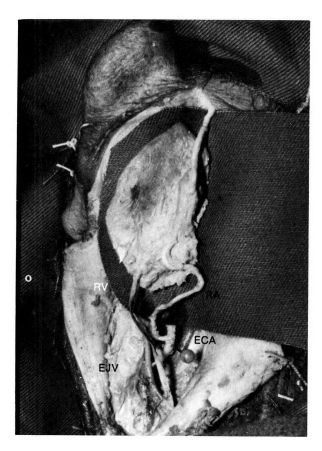

Fig. 9-4. Example of a free retroauricular skin flap. (*RA,* Retroauricular artery; *RV,* retroauricular vein; *ECA,* external carotid artery; *EJV,* external jugular vein.)

CASE REPORT

Our clinical experience with the free retroauricular flap is limited to one patient.

A 24-year-old male had had a cavernous hemangioma of the right upper and lower eyelids, the cheek, and the nose since birth. The hemangioma had been increasing in size, with occasional bleeding, proptosis, and a decrease in his vision (Fig. 9-5, *A*), for which the eye was removed. At this time the patient was admitted to the hospital for resurfacing of his nose (Fig. 9-5, *B*).

Before the microvascular surgery, the donor and recipient vessels were selected with the help of a Doppler probe.[1] For the recipient vessels we selected the left supratrochlear vessels. For the donor vessels we selected branches of the left postauricular vessels.

On May 14, 1974, the reconstruction was carried out with the patient under general anesthesia. A pigmented split-thickness skin graft on his nose was removed. The supratrochlear artery (0.7 mm in diameter) and the vein (1.0 mm in diameter) were identified and prepared as the recipient vessels. Next the trapezoid-shaped retroauricular skin flap (4 by 5 by 6 cm) was designed in an inverted position (Fig. 9-6, *A*). It was dissected superficial to the perichondrium; it contained one artery (0.7 mm in diameter) and four veins (the largest 1.0 mm, the next 0.5 mm in diameter).

The retroauricular flap was detached from its donor bed and was placed in a chilled normal saline solution containing heparin (10 IU/ml).

Under the operating microscope the adventitia of the donor and recipient vessels was removed. Then we did the microvascular anastomoses (Fig. 9-6, *B*).[3] The veins were 0.5 mm and 1.0 mm in diameter, and each required ten sutures of monofilament nylon; the arteries were each 0.7 mm in diameter, and each required six sutures. (The vein, which was the closest mate to the retroauricular artery, was not used because of a technical error in its preparation.)

Immediately after release of the arterial clamp the upper third of the flap turned pink; in about 15 minutes the entire flap was pink. After skin closure a white area was noted in the lower left part of the flap, so the sutures were removed to relieve tension.

On the following day the flap was pink-purple and edematous, although color return after finger pressure was immediate. However, the lower right part of the flap was dusky black; therefore all the flap sutures were immediately removed (Fig. 9-6, *C*).

Later the flap regained a normal color, and by the ninth day the edema had subsided. The flap was then resutured in place. No anticoagulants or dextran was used. The flap survived completely, and vessel patency has been consistently confirmed with a Doppler probe (Fig. 9-7).

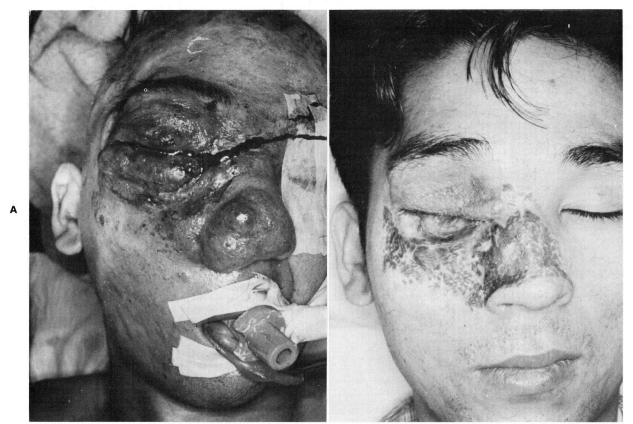

A   B

Fig. 9-5. A, Huge cavernous hemangioma with bleeding from the lower eyelid every other day and a progressive decrease in vision. The patient had received radiation therapy at 4 years of age. Bilateral carotid angiograms showed extensive involvement of the right orbit and maxillary sinus with some abnormal patterns in the left orbit and maxillary sinus. **B,** After radical excision of the main part of the lesion (including removal of the eye), the nose and cheek areas were resurfaced with a split skin graft. (From Fujino, T.: Free skin flap from the retroauricular region to the nose, Plast. Reconstr. Surg. **57:**338, 1976.)

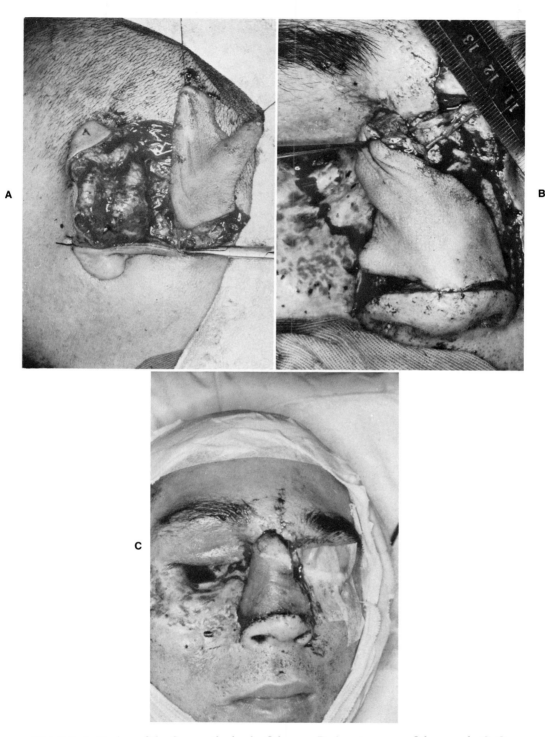

Fig. 9-6. A, Design of the flap on the back of the ear. **B,** Anastomoses of the vessels. **C,** On the first postoperative day it was necessary to remove all sutures from the flap edges; this was followed by satisfactory bleeding from all edges. (From Fujino, T.: Free skin flap from the retroauricular region to the nose, Plast. Reconstr. Surg. **57:**338, 1976.)

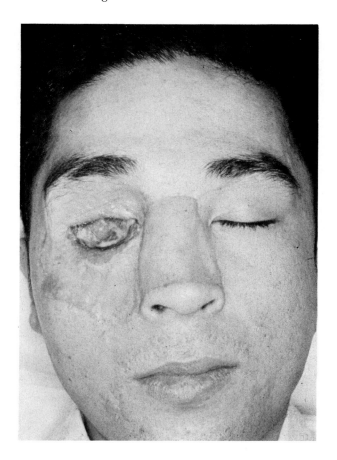

Fig. 9-7. Eleven months after the free flap to the nose and 10 months after the combined procedure on the cheek. (From Fujino, T.: Free skin flap from the retroauricular region to the nose, Plast. Reconstr. Surg. **57:** 338, 1976.)

DISCUSSION

For a one-stage resurfacing procedure, microvascular transfer of a free groin flap or free deltopectoral skin flap has been popular. However, these flaps are bulky and the flap must often be trimmed.

The free retroauricular skin flap is relatively thin and is suitable for resurfacing the nose, the upper part of the cheek, or the forehead. Our patient developed a good color match.

The postoperative course was marked by transient circulatory problems, possibly caused by insufficiency from a closed circuit of the anastomosed artery and vein in the flap. (The vein that was concomitant to the artery could not be used and a lesser choice was substituted.)

REFERENCES

1. Aoyagi, F., Fujino, T., and Ohshiro, T.: Detection of small vessels for microsurgery by a Doppler flowmeter, Plast. Reconstr. Surg. **55:**372, 1975.
2. Converse, J.M., and Wood-Smith, D.: Experiences with the forehead island flap with a subcutaneous pedicle, Plast. Reconstr. Surg. **31:**521, 1963.
3. Fujino, T., and Aoyagi, F.: A method of successive interrupted suturing in microvascular anastomoses, Plast. Reconstr. Surg. **55:**240, 1975.
4. Fujino, T., Harashina, T., and Nakajima, T.: Free skin flap from the retroauricular region to the nose, Plast. Reconstr. Surg. **57:**338, 1976.
5. Fujino, T., Ikuta, Y., and Harashina, T.: Technique of microsurgery, Tokyo, 1977, Igakushoin, pp. 72-76.
6. Warwick, R., and Williams, P.L.: Gray's anatomy, ed. 35, London, 1973, Longman Group, Ltd., p. 628.

Chapter 10

The deltoid flap: anatomy and clinical applications

John D. Franklin

During the wide excision of a melanoma in January 1980, we discovered a neurovascular pedicle supplying the skin over the deltoid muscle. After we made a circumferential incision around the melanoma, the tissue to be removed continued to bleed briskly despite fairly extensive undermining. On further examination and exploration, a neurovascular pedicle entering the flap was disclosed. It appeared beneath the deltoid muscle in the areolar tissue overlying the lateral head of the triceps. We further studied the anatomy of this pedicle in cadaver dissections and determined its cutaneous territory. Subsequently the flap was used clinically, and a preliminary report was presented in September of 1980.[1]

The deltoid flap is a fasciocutaneous, neurosensory free flap that is elevated primarily from above the deltoid muscle. Its blood supply is derived from a cutaneous branch of the posterior circumflex humeral artery, which emerges from beneath the deltoid muscle to vascularize the overlying skin. Sensation is supplied by a branch of the axillary nerve that is present in the pedicle. Advantages of the flap are that it is thin and pliable and that it may provide sensation to the reconstructed area. Primary applications of the flap have been in head and neck reconstruction and foot and ankle coverage.

From January 1980 to June 1982 free deltoid flaps were transferred in thirty-five patients. In this chapter we present the anatomy and elevation of the deltoid flap and examples of its clinical applications.

FLAP ANATOMY

The posterior circumflex humeral artery arises from the axillary artery and passes into the quadrilateral space, where its major branches supply the deltoid muscle. It anastomoses with the profunda brachii system and the anterior circumflex humeral artery. In addition, a cutaneous branch of the posterior circumflex humeral artery, about 1 mm in diameter at its origin, presents in the areolar tissue in the deltoid-triceps groove and vascularizes the skin over the deltoid muscle. The cutaneous artery lies between two veins that join the posterior circumflex humeral vein in the quadrilateral space.[2] The lateral brachial cutaneous nerve, originating from the inferior division of the axillary nerve, accompanies the cutaneous artery and veins laterally in the pedicle. This sensory nerve innervates the skin over the posterior inferior two thirds of the deltoid muscle and the upper portion of the triceps.[3]

An arteriogram demonstrates the large posterior circumflex humeral artery arising from the axillary artery. The cutaneous branch that supplies the deltoid flap is designated by the arrow in Fig. 10-1.

A vessel 2 to 4 mm in diameter is obtained by the division of the posterior circumflex humeral artery proximal to the origin of the cutaneous artery. The diameter of the accompanying posterior circumflex humeral vein is approximately twice that of the artery. The axillary nerve lies beneath and medial to the posterior circumflex humeral vessels. The neurovascular pedicle is 6 to 8 cm long.

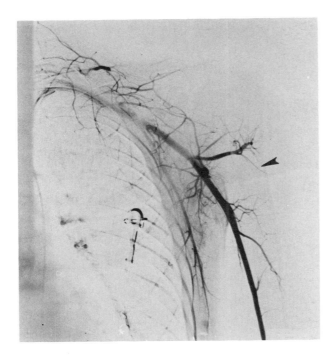

Fig. 10-1. Arteriogram of shoulder region. Arrow indicates cutaneous branch of posterior circumflex humeral artery.

FLAP DESIGN AND ELEVATION

In designing the deltoid flap, the surgeon must determine the approximate entry of the neurovascular bundle. One line is drawn from the acromion to the olecranon, while another line is drawn over the deltoid-triceps groove. The pedicle emerges from beneath the deltoid muscle, at a point 2 to 4 cm posterior to the intersection of the lines, along the deltoid-triceps groove (Fig. 10-2). More precise entry of the artery may be determined with a Doppler flowmeter. The flap is raised from over the deltoid muscle, with the neurovascular bundle entering along one edge. The flap may be centered over the vessels, if desired.

After the outline of the entire flap is drawn on the shoulder, a dome-shaped incision is made around the proposed flap. Usually no incision is made over the deltoid-triceps groove. Elevation is begun from the point most distal to the deltoid-triceps groove and continues until the inferior edge of the deltoid muscle is reached. The muscle fascia is raised sharply with the flap. In the process a pseudogroove in the deltoid muscle may be encountered and confused with the inferior edge of

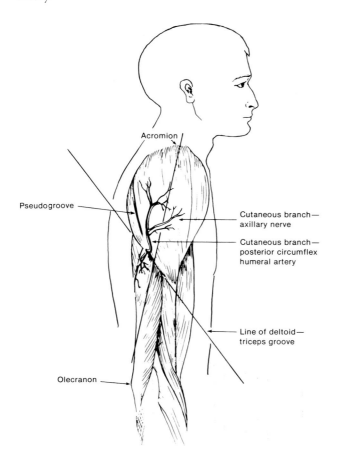

Acromion

Pseudogroove

Cutaneous branch—axillary nerve

Cutaneous branch—posterior circumflex humeral artery

Line of deltoid—triceps groove

Olecranon

Fig. 10-2. Diagram demonstrating anatomic location of the neurovascular pedicle.

the deltoid muscle. (In the pseudogroove all the muscle fibers are lying parallel to one another.) When the inferior edge of the deltoid is identified and elevated, the neurovascular bundle should be easily identifiable in the space between the deltoid and triceps muscles (Fig. 10-3).

The dissection of the vessels under the deltoid into the quadrilateral space is the most difficult part of the flap elevation. After the neurovascular bundle has been identified, the areolar tissue overlying the vessels is dissected and the vessels are traced into the quadrilateral space. The numerous arteries and veins that are associated primarily with the deltoid muscle are divided between vascular clips. The dissection is continued until 2 to 3 cm portions of the posterior circumflex humeral vein and artery have been freed. At this juncture an incision is made in the skin and subcutaneous tissue over the deltoid-triceps groove, and the flap is freed from the surrounding tissue. While the vessels are still intact, the viability of the flap is demonstrated by initiating bleeding from its edges. The artery and the vein are then divided, exposing the sensory nerve from the inferior division of the axillary nerve. The nerve is divided and the flap is removed.

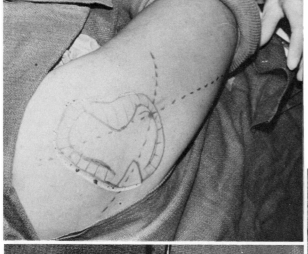

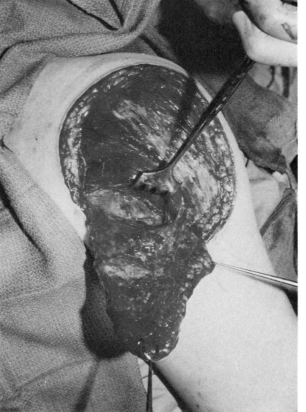

Fig. 10-3. Flap design and elevation. **A,** Outline of proposed flap and dome-shaped incision in the skin. **B,** Flap completely elevated excluding skin bridge inferiorly. **C,** Elevation of inferior edge of deltoid muscle demonstrating neurovascular pedicle.

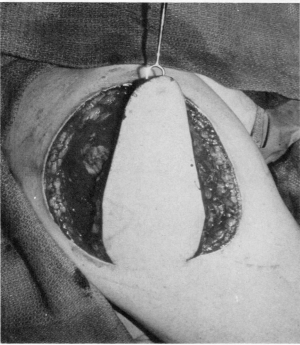

CASE REPORT

Between January 1980 and May 1982 a total of thirty-five patients received deltoid free flap transfers. The ages of these individuals (twenty-five males and ten females) ranged from 8 to 92 years. The largest flap measured 15 by 27 cm and the smallest 4 by 8 cm. Seventeen flaps were used in head and neck reconstruction, fifteen in foot and ankle reconstruction, and three for upper extremity coverage. The donor sites were closed primarily in twenty patients, and skin grafts were used in fifteen.

Head and neck reconstruction

The deltoid flap has been used in seventeen head and neck reconstructions. Two flaps were used for intraoral lining, two were deepithelialized to augment the tissue of the cheek, three were used to replace scalp defects, and ten were used for skin and soft tissue reconstruction of the cheek and neck. No flap failures or partial losses occurred in this group. Two examples of the use of this flap in the head and neck are given.

Patient I

A malignant parotid tumor had been removed from a 29-year-old female at age 2, and postoperative radiotherapy had been employed. The patient came to us desiring reconstruction of the atrophic, irradiated neck and parotid area and replacement of the thin skin over the carotid artery. The thin, atrophic skin over the carotid was removed and the adjacent tissue was undermined. The defect was filled with a 14 by 6 cm free deltoid flap. The edges of the flap were deepithelialized and feathered circumferentially to improve the contour of the neck and cheek. The inferior portion of the flap was further deepithelialized and placed low on the neck to reconstruct the defect resulting from the atrophy of the irradiated sternocleidomastoid muscle. The thyrocervical artery was used to vascularize the flap. The sensory nerve of the flap was anastomosed to one of the branches of the cervical plexus.

Fig. 10-4 shows the contouring and texture-color match of the flap with the surrounding tissues. The patient demonstrates no excess bulk of the flap. Within 3 months of the operation, response to light touch and two-point discrimination of 1.5 to 2 cm, almost identical to that of the skin of the opposite shoulder, was demonstrated. The donor site was closed primarily, and although the scar is thick because of its location on the posterior portion of the shoulder, it is easily concealed with clothing. This case is an example of a one-stage reconstruction for a significant defect.

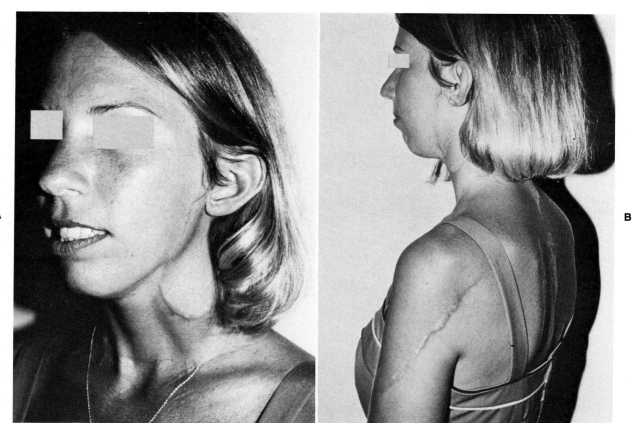

Fig. 10-4. Patient 1. **A,** Deltoid flap contouring left neck and cheek region. **B,** Posterior-lateral photograph of flap and donor site.

Patient II

A 73-year-old male sustained an electrical burn on the scalp 2 years before reconstruction. None of the numerous skin grafts and scalp flaps used to cover the defect were successful. The patient was initially seen with localized osteomyelitis in the temporal bone surrounded by thin skin grafts. The infected bone and the atrophic skin graft were removed. The defect was closed with a 6 by 15 cm free deltoid flap. The vessels of the flap were anastomosed to the superficial temporal artery and vein. In Fig. 10-5, 4 months postoperatively, the patient demonstrated good coverage from this one-stage procedure.

Foot and ankle reconstruction

Foot and ankle defects have been reconstructed with free deltoid flaps in fifteen patients. Six flaps have been placed on the weight-bearing portion of the foot and nine on non-weight-bearing portions of the foot or ankle. Only two failures of the thirty-five flaps occurred in this group. Venous thrombosis occurred in three flaps, but these were salvaged. Two examples of reconstruction about the foot and ankle are presented.

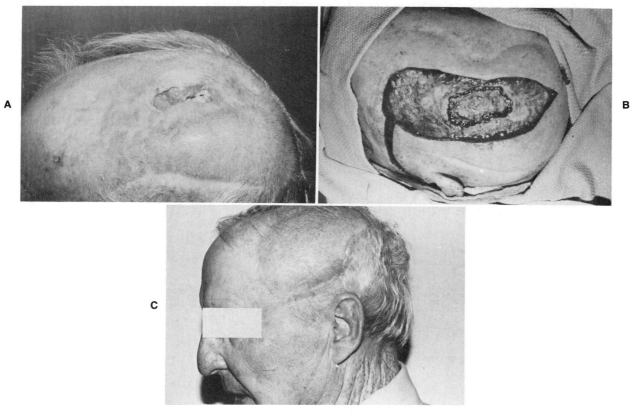

Fig. 10-5. Patient II. **A,** Exposed infected temporal bone surrounded by thin skin grafts. **B,** Excised skin graft and infected bone. **C,** Postoperative appearance at 4 months.

Patient III

A 17-year-old male sustained an avulsion injury of the heel 1 year before reconstruction. The area was closed with a skin graft, which became ulcerated, painful, and infected. Reconstruction was instituted with an 11 by 13 cm free deltoid flap. The posterior tibial artery was anastomosed to the posterior circumflex humeral artery end to side. Sensation was acquired in the heel by anastomosing the sensory nerve of the flap to one of the sensory branches of the posterior tibial nerve. The donor site was closed primarily and healed with a thick scar on the posterior aspect of the shoulder (Fig. 10-6). Two years after the procedure the patient continues to walk on the flap. He has good protective sensation and a two-point discrimination of 2 cm. Although he walks easily in a shoe, in his bare feet he bears little weight on the flap.

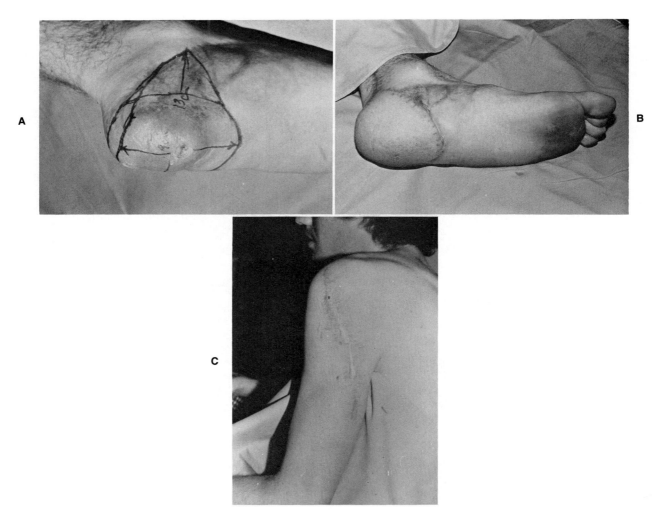

Fig. 10-6. Patient III. **A,** Preoperative appearance of heel. **B,** Postoperative appearance at 2 years. **C,** Donor site scar.

Patient IV

A 24-year-old male sustained a burn from a motorcycle exhaust on the medial aspect of the ankle. Six months later, after two local flaps had failed, the area was reconstructed with a 10 by 14 cm free deltoid flap. A venous thrombosis that developed during the postoperative period was corrected and the flap survived (Fig. 10-7).

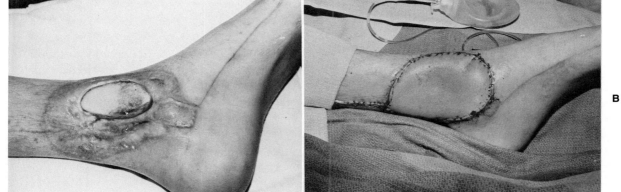

Fig. 10-7. Patient IV. **A,** Preoperative view of ankle defect. **B,** Appearance after reconstruction with deltoid flap.

DISCUSSION

Usable neurovascular pedicles are found in almost all deltoid elevations. There is some variation in the entry position of the neurovascular pedicle along the deltoid-triceps groove. Occasionally two pedicles enter the flap with a common origin from the posterior circumflex humeral vessels. Rarely the major vascular pedicle penetrates the lower portion of the deltoid muscle to enter the overlying skin.

In our experience the deltoid flap has proved of greatest use and advantage in reconstruction of the head and neck area, especially in females. Its low bulk and almost identical color and texture match to the cheek and neck make it ideal for reconstruction there. The deltoid flap has also proved quite useful as a one-stage foot and ankle reconstruction.

Sensation in the flap is easily obtained in the head and neck because there are many sensory nerves available for anastomosis in the neck. Good protective sensation has been obtained in foot and ankle reconstruction when the sensory nerve of this flap is anastomosed to sensory nerves in the recipient area.

Occasionally thinning of redundant tissue around the margins may be necessary, although bulkiness is minimal. The thinnest deltoid flaps are usually found on the most superior aspect of the shoulders of males. Deltoid flaps are usually thicker in females.

Coverage with a deltoid flap has proved less than ideal on weight-bearing portions of the foot. Barefooted patients bear minimal weight on the flap. Significant adherence of the flap tissue and dermis to the underlying bones and ligaments of the foot is lacking; consequently the flap tends to slide slightly when weight or stress is applied to it, giving the patient an unsteady feeling, especially while walking shoeless. Examinations indicate that weight is applied when shoes are worn, however. Breakdown of the flap has not been a problem on weight-bearing surfaces.

Most of the vascular problems encountered with the deltoid flap have occurred in the lower extremity as a result of poor arterial perfusion or venous obstruction. Three of the four flaps that developed venous obstruction were salvaged. In several individuals initially experiencing inadequate arterial blood flow, local vasodilation or stripping of the adventitia of the artery relieved the difficulty. The incidence of inadequate arterial profusion has decreased with the increased use of epidural anesthetics and better hydration.

The greatest objection to using the deltoid flap involves the donor site. The resulting scar on the shoulder tends to be thick and objectionable—often more so to the reconstructive surgeon than to his patient. In recent cases, skin grafts placed over the donor defects have filled in quite nicely and have produced more aesthetically pleasing scars.

Since the ages of patients in whom deltoid transfers have been performed have ranged from 8 to 92 years, we feel that extremes of age are no contraindication to this type of microvascular free tissue transfer.

SUMMARY

The deltoid flap is a relatively thin, pliable, fasciocutaneous flap that can provide sensation to the reconstructed area. It has provided an excellent color and texture match in head and neck reconstruction. Coverage of foot and ankle defects is possible, with little need for subsequent excision of redundant tissue or debulking.

The basic elevation of the flap is quite simple. Dissecting the neurovascular pedicle from beneath the deltoid muscle is tedious, however. With persistence a long pedicle with a large artery and vein can be obtained. The healing of the donor site with a thick scar is a distinct disadvantage in considering this flap for some reconstructive procedures. The deltoid flap has proved to be a useful resource to the reconstructive microsurgeon. It has been most ideal in reconstructing defects in the head and neck and contouring about the foot and ankle.

REFERENCES

1. Franklin, J.D., Rees, R.S., Madden, J.J., Jr., and Lynch, J.B.: The posterior circumflex humeral neurovascular free flap, Plast. Surg. Forum **3:**172, 1980.
2. Goss, C.M., editor: Gray's anatomy of the human body, ed. 29, Philadelphia, 1973, Lea & Febiger.

Chapter 11

The free groin flap

Bernard S. Alpert
Samuel W. Parry II
Harry J. Buncke
Leonard Gordon

HISTORY

The expansion of the number of free flap donor sites with longer vascular pedicles and larger vessel diameters has led to a decrease in the number of free groin flaps being performed. This flap, however, still leaves the most aesthetically pleasing donor site and will continue to have a place in the plastic surgeon's armamentarium.

The pedicled groin flap was first described in 1946 by Shaw and Payne,[10] but its popularity waned until 1972, when McGregor and Jackson extolled its dependability and worth.[5,11] It is an axial skin flap, similar in this sense to Bakamjian's deltopectoral flap.[1] The superficial circumflex iliac arteriovenous system provides the axial blood flow to the flap; however, frequent anatomic variations make use of this flap difficult.

Daniel and Taylor were the first to successfully perform and describe the free groin flap.[3] This followed the first free omental transplant by McLean and Buncke by 1 year and represented the first reported successful case of composite tissue transplantation by microvascular anastomoses.[6] Soon thereafter O'Brien reported a similar success,[7] and by 1976 the first series of free groin flaps appeared in the literature.[2,4,9] In 1978 Taylor and Watson introduced the vascularized osteocutaneous groin flap, which included iliac crest bone,[13] and subsequently Taylor beautifully demonstrated the experimental and clinical advantages of using the deep circumflex iliac vascular system as the blood supply for free groin skin and osteocutaneous flaps.[14,15]

ANATOMY

The vascular anatomy of the groin flap is the source of its primary disadvantages: (1) the vascular pedicle is very short, (2) the vessels exhibit considerable variability, and (3) the artery is usually small (approximately 1 mm in diameter) and occasionally too small for anastomosis. This is especially true in young women. Because of these shortcomings, Ohmori and Harii reported a 6% incidence of unsuitable donor vessels.[8]

Taylor and Daniel demonstrated the tremendous vascular variability of the groin flap in 100 cadaver dissections done bilaterally.[12] They found bilateral symmetry of the vascular pattern in only one third of the cases. They followed the origins and courses of the superficial circumflex iliac and superficial epigastric arteries in all cases and found (1) a common origin of both arteries in 48%, (2) a superficial circumflex iliac artery only and an absent superficial epigastric artery in 35%, and (3) separate origins of the two vessels in 17%. In 17% of the dissections the vessels arose from a regional artery other than the common femoral artery.

When both vessels arise from a common trunk, this trunk is the first branch of the common femoral artery and usually lies within 3 cm of this ligament (Fig. 11-1). The superficial circumflex iliac artery is the most commonly used vessel because the superficial epigastric system exhibits such variability. The course of the superficial circumflex iliac vascular axis is on a line just below the inguinal ligament, extends laterally toward the anterior superior iliac spine, and continues toward the angle

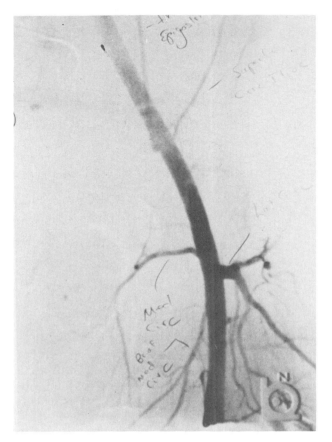

Fig. 11-1. Arteriogram showing superficial circumflex iliac and superficial epigastric arteries as the first branches of the common femoral artery.

of the scapula. It commonly remains beneath the deep fascia until the lateral border of the sartorius is reached; this is a critical anatomic point in flap dissection. Its course can be traced several centimeters from the femoral artery laterally toward the anterior superior iliac spine with the aid of a Doppler flowmeter.

The superficial epigastric artery pierces the deep fascia below the inguinal ligament and passes cranially just superficial to the deep fascia. It lies deep to and closely parallels the easily demonstrable superficial epigastric vein. There are extremely rich anastomoses between the superficial circumflex iliac and superficial epigastric systems, constituting a "cobweb" that fans from the rectus abdominis muscle to the greater trochanter.

The region of the groin flap is drained by both a superficial and deep venous system. The superficial system is composed of veins (either superficial circumflex iliac or superficial epigastric) that are part of the "spokewheel" of veins that drain into

the saphenous bulb. These are 2 mm in diameter and are suitable for microvascular repair. The deep system comprises the venae comitantes with the superficial circumflex iliac or superficial epigastric arteries, which are much smaller, although usable if necessary.

Recently Taylor et al. have recommended the use of the deep circumflex iliac vessels as the better pedicle for free groin flap transfer, especially for osteocutaneous flaps.[14,15] This vascular pedicle is larger, averaging 2 mm in diameter, and longer than the superficial systems commonly used in the past. The deep circumflex iliac artery arises from the lateral or posterolateral surface of the external iliac artery opposite the inferior epigastric artery just above the inguinal ligament and passes obliquely upward and laterally toward the anterior superior iliac spine for 5 to 7 cm. It pierces the transversalis fascia and curves along the medial lip of the iliac crest to a point 6 to 9 cm from the anterior superior iliac spine, where it pierces the transversus abdominis muscle and anastomoses with other regional vessels. Throughout its course the artery gives off nutrient branches to adjacent muscle and iliac crest bone as well as a segment of the overlying skin. A large vena comitans parallels the artery and empties into the external iliac vein.

FLAP DISSECTION

We have used the osteocutaneous groin flap as described by Taylor both in this volume (see Chapter 14) and elsewhere,[15] and will concern ourselves here with only the free groin skin flap dissection. Depending upon the recipient site, most free groin flaps are performed with two surgical teams operating simultaneously on the donor and recipient sites. The central axis of the flap is on a line drawn from approximately 2.5 cm below the inguinal ligament on the femoral artery and runs laterally toward the anterior superior iliac spine. It can be continued toward the angle of the scapula if necessary. A 10 by 20 cm flap can be designed within the axial vascular territory and will still achieve primary donor site closure (Fig. 11-2).

The dissection may be performed either lateral to medial or vice versa (Fig. 11-3). When one is coming from the lateral direction, a key point is to go beneath the fascia at the lateral margin of the sartorius muscle to keep the vessel in the flap. When the surgeon is using the medial to lateral approach, the common femoral artery must be isolated and carefully dissected below the inguinal ligament to allow identification of the first branches, which will be the vascular axis of the groin flap.

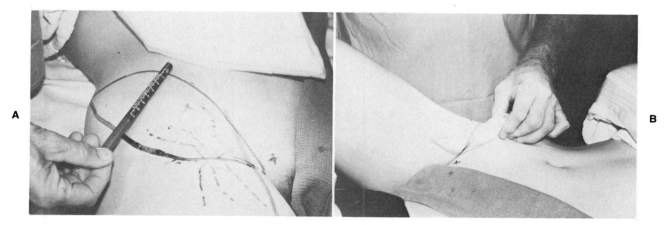

Fig. 11-2. A, Outline of groin flap; scratches are along dopplered superficial circumflex iliac artery. **B,** Ten centimeter flap may be closed with some hip flexion.

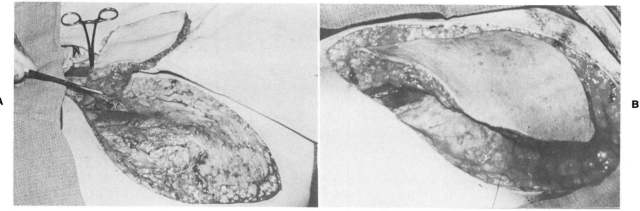

Fig. 11-3. A, The flap elevated; vascular pedicle is very short and of small caliber. Note exposed sartorius muscle; the fascia has been elevated with the flap. **B,** Flap on its donor bed.

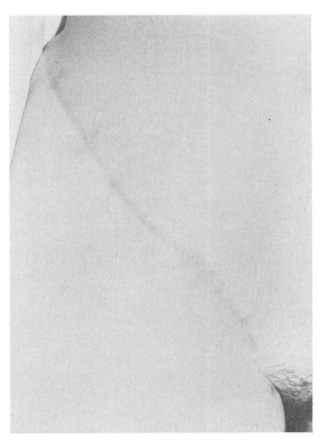

Fig. 11-4. Postoperatively the donor site scar is acceptable.

Table 11-1. Free groin flaps performed from 1974 to April 1981

Year	Skin	Osteocutaneous
1974	4	
1975	6	
1976	8	
1977	13	
1978	9	
1979	11	
1980	9	6
1981	4	1
TOTAL	64	7

Table 11-2. Free groin flap transfer sites

Leg	24
Hand	12
Foot	11
Face	11
Scalp	4
Arm	4
Breast	3
Chest	2

Table 11-3. Free groin flap failure rate

Result	Number	Percent	Number	Percent
Success	57	81	52	81
Partial loss	6	8	5	8
Total loss	8	11	7	11

When one is coming from either direction, the lateral femoral cutaneous nerve will be encountered piercing the fascia at about the anterior superior iliac spine. This can sometimes be preserved, but often it must be sacrificed to ensure continuity in the dissection. The groin flap itself does not have a sensory nerve on a predictably reliable basis to consider it an innervated flap.

After the flap is removed, the donor site is closed primarily in the majority of cases. The patient's hip may need to be flexed to accomplish closure. This position may have to be maintained for several days. Donor site morbidity is low, and this remains one of the best aesthetic donor regions (Fig. 11-4).

CLINICAL EXPERIENCE

A review of all free groin flaps performed at the Ralph K. Davies Medical Center from 1974 through April 1981 is presented in Tables 11-1 to 11-3. All flaps were done under the direction of one surgeon, Dr. Harry J. Buncke, Jr. Seven free osteocutaneous groin flaps based on both the deep and superficial circumflex iliac vascular systems are included from 1980 and 1981. A total of seventy-one flaps were performed in thirty-seven males and thirty-four females (Table 11-1). The recipient sites varied, with the lower extremities leading the list (Table 11-2). The total failure rate (including the osteocutaneous flaps) was 11% (Table 11-3). Of particular note is that five of the seven total skin flap failures occurred during a single 6-month period in 1978 and 1979. A single cause has not been determined for this, but a common factor certainly could have played a part.

Some representative cases are shown to illustrate both the versatility and aesthetic value of the groin flap. Its aesthetic advantages apply to both the donor and recipient sites. It has literally been used from head to toe to provide durable, well-contoured coverage where this has been lacking (Figs. 11-5 to 11-13). *Text continued on p. 83.*

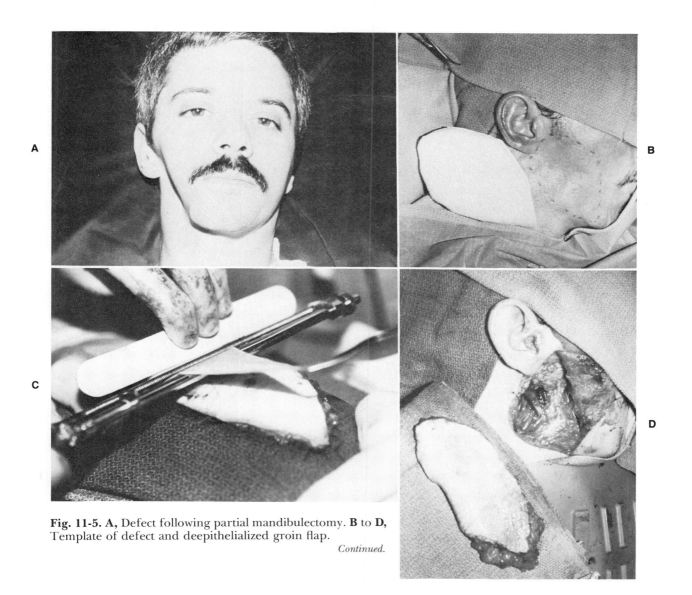

Fig. 11-5. A, Defect following partial mandibulectomy. **B** to **D,** Template of defect and deepithelialized groin flap.

Continued.

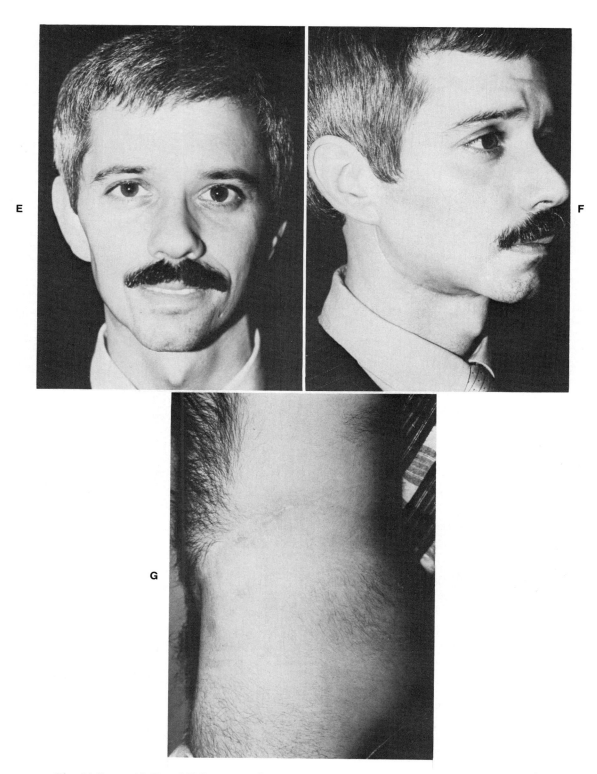

Fig. 11-5, cont'd. E and **F,** Postoperative result; defatting has been performed. **G,** Donor defect.

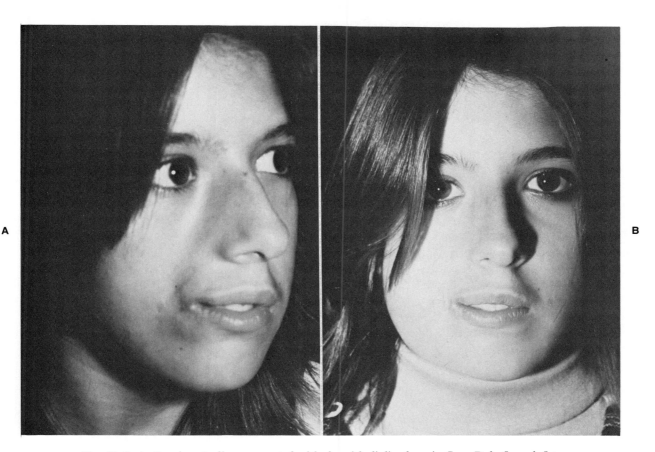

Fig. 11-6. A, Romberg's disease treated with deepithelialized groin flap; **B,** before defatting procedure.

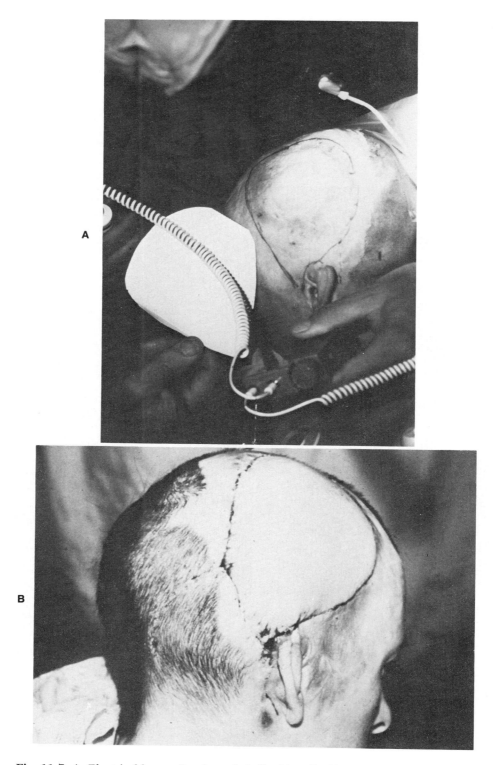

Fig. 11-7. A, Electrical burn of scalp and skull with split-thickness skin graft on dura. **B,** Coverage with free groin flap; split rib cranioplasty was subsequently performed beneath flap.

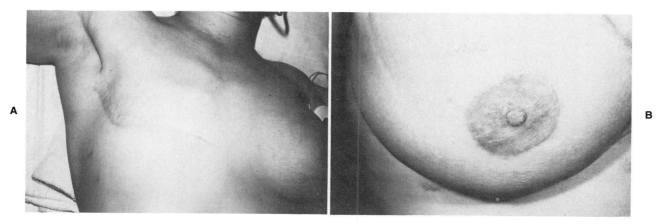

Fig. 11-8. **A** and **B,** Free groin flap for postmastectomy breast reconstruction.

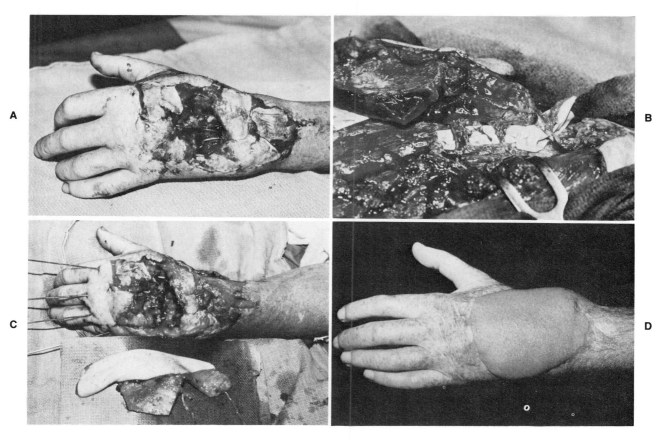

Fig. 11-9. **A,** Status 6 days after gunshot wound to hand with osteocutaneous defect. **B** to **D,** Osteocutaneous groin flap based on both deep and superficial circumflex iliac vessels to provide coverage; extensor tendon grafts were provided at a second stage.

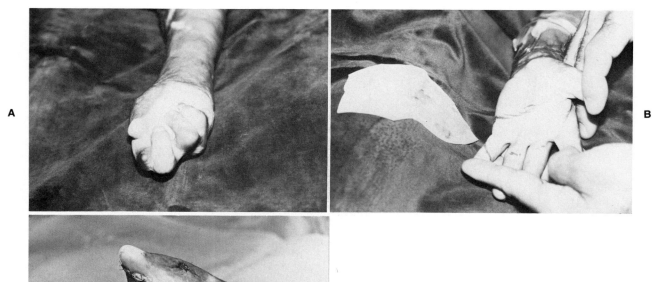

Fig. 11-10. A, Seven-year-old male with hand burn contractures. **B,** Flap template made from creases on opposite hand. **C,** Release and coverage with free groin flap.

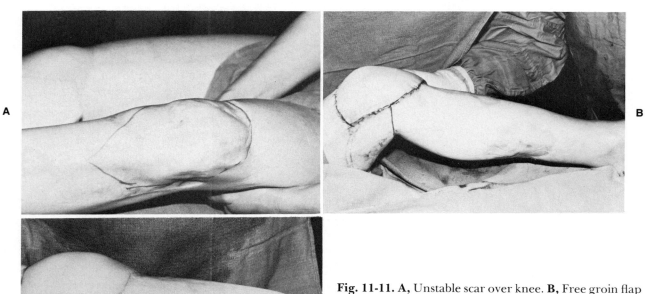

Fig. 11-11. A, Unstable scar over knee. **B,** Free groin flap gives stable coverage. **C,** Depressed lower leg defect covered with second free groin flap in same patient at a second procedure.

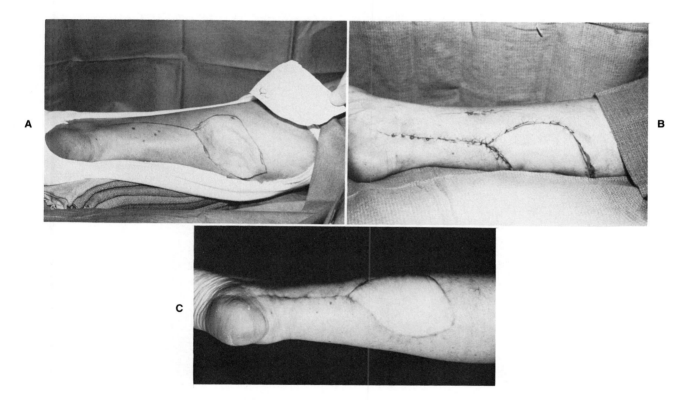

Fig. 11-12. A to **C,** Melanoma excision defect covered secondarily with free groin flap for contour improvement.

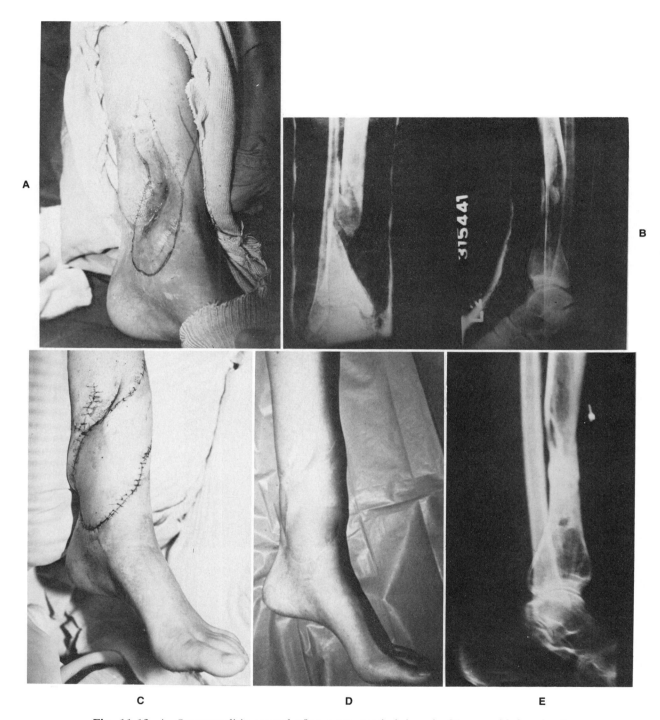

Fig. 11-13. A, Osteomyelitic wound after a traumatic injury in 21-year-old female. **B,** Radiograph shows nonunion. **C,** Free groin flap for coverage; **D,** 5-year postoperative result. **E,** Bony union after secondary grafting under free groin flap.

SUMMARY

The free groin flap was the first to be used for microvascular composite tissue transplantation. Its advantages include its highly aesthetic donor and recipient site capabilities. Disadvantages are a difficult dissection, anatomic variability, and a small, short vascular pedicle. Other flaps with larger and longer pedicles have supplanted some of its indications, but its potential as a versatile, useful flap remains. Iliac crest may be included to produce a vascularized osteocutaneous flap.

REFERENCES

1. Bakamjian, V.Y.: A two-stage method for pharyngo-esophageal reconstruction with a primary pectoral flap, Plast. Reconstr. Surg. **36**:173, 1965.
2. Baudet, J., Lemaire, J., and Guimberteau, J.: Ten free groin flaps, Plast. Reconstr. Surg. **57**:577, 1976.
3. Daniel, R.K., and Taylor, G.I.: Distal transfer of an island flap by microvascular anastomoses, Plast. Reconstr. Surg. **52**:111, 1973.
4. Harii, K., et al.: Free groin skin flaps, Br. J. Plast. Surg. **27**:225, 1975.
5. McGregor, I.A., and Jackson, I.T.: The groin flap, Br. J. Plast. Surg. **25**:3, 1972.
6. McLean, D.H., and Buncke, H.J., Jr.: Autotransplant of omentum to a large scalp defect with microsurgical revascularization, Plast. Reconstr. Surg. **49**:268, 1972.
7. O'Brien, B.M., et al.: Successful transfer of a large island flap from the groin to the foot by microvascular anastomoses, Plast. Reconstr. Surg. **52**:271, 1973.
8. Ohmori, K., and Harii, K.: Free groin flaps: their vascular basis, Br. J. Plast. Surg. **28**:238, 1975.
9. Serafin, D., Rios, A.V., and Georgiade, N.: Fourteen free groin flap transfers, Plast. Reconstr. Surg. **57**:707, 1976.
10. Shaw, D.T., and Payne, R.L.: One-stage tubed abdominal flap surgery, Gyn. Obstet. **83**:205, 1946.
11. Smith, P.J., et al.: The anatomical basis of the groin flap, Plast. Reconstr. Surg. **49**:41, 1972.
12. Taylor, G.I., and Daniel, R.K.: The anatomy of several free flap donor sites, Plast. Reconstr. Surg. **56**:243, 1975.
13. Taylor, G.I., and Watson, N.: One-stage repair of compound leg defects with free revascularized flaps of groin skin and iliac bone, Plast. Reconstr. Surg. **61**:494, 1978.
14. Taylor, G.I., Townsend, P., and Corbett, R.: Superiority of the deep circumflex iliac vessels as the supply for free groin flaps: experimental work, Plast. Reconstr. Surg. **64**:595, 1979.
15. Taylor, G.I., Townsend, P., and Corbett, R.: Superiority of the deep circumflex iliac vessels as the supply for free groin flaps: clinical work, Plast. Reconstr. Surg. **64**:745, 1979.

Chapter 12

Free omental homografts with skin autografts for repair of wounds

Hsu Hsi Cheng
Shu Lan Chia
Da Ching Yin

Since the advent of microsurgery, free flaps, free myocutaneous flaps, and free omental grafts (surfaced with a skin graft) have been added to our choices for repair of a wound.

Transplantation of the omentum with microvascular anastomoses was initially used by McLean and Buncke in 1972.[2] Its clinical application was started in our hospital in 1977.[1] A major advantage of the omentum is that it will readily fit a wound of any configuration; the major disadvantage is that it requires a laparotomy with its attendant potential for complications and morbidity. Even though the omentum had an early clinical trial, it has been applied to patients with far less frequency than other types of free flaps.

The problem of rejection of homografts has not yet been solved, although immunosuppressive drugs have been useful in kidney transplants and for split skin grafts in potentially fatal burns.

We performed experiments on free omental homografts surfaced with autologous skin grafts in April 1978, basing our work on the following hypothesis: If immunosuppressive drugs are used to delay the rejection of omental homografts, the omentum will furnish a satisfactory recipient bed for an autologous skin graft. Thus the skin graft would develop a good vascular supply before rejection of the omentum started, and vascular ingrowth from the edge of the wound would furnish sufficient blood supply for permanent survival of the autologous skin graft, even after rejection of

the omentum. The homografted omentum would thus be an effective means of furnishing a temporary blood supply to gain permanent coverage in a wound that presented difficulties.

METHOD

Rabbits weighing 2,500 to 3,000 g were used for the experiments. The apex of the animal's skull was denuded down to bare bone by excising all the soft tissues, creating a 3 by 5 cm defect. The avascular bed of this wound would not support a free skin graft.

EXPERIMENTAL GROUP
Vascularized omental allograft with free autologous skin graft in animals treated with azathioprine and prednisone

An omental flap was taken from one rabbit and was placed on the scalp defect of another rabbit by microvascular anastomoses between the left gastro-epiploic vessels and the auricular vessels. A split skin autograft was taken from the trunk of the rabbit and was sutured to the raw external surface of the omentum. The skin graft was sutured to the wound edges and was covered with a light tie-over dressing.

Azathioprine (Imuran), 10 mg, and prednisone, 3.3 mg, were administered daily for 3 weeks postoperatively. The dressing was removed on the seventh to the ninth postoperative days.

Of the thirty-two experimental rabbits, four

died 3 to 5 days postoperatively; in thirteen rabbits the autografts did not survive because of failure of revascularization of the omentum resulting from anastomotic failures. The autografts failed to survive in an additional two rabbits for unknown reasons. The skin grafts survived in thirteen rabbits; the area of survival was 100% in seven rabbits, over 90% in five, and over 80% in one. The average area of coverage with viable autograft was 86.6% in the fifteen cases (Fig. 12-1).

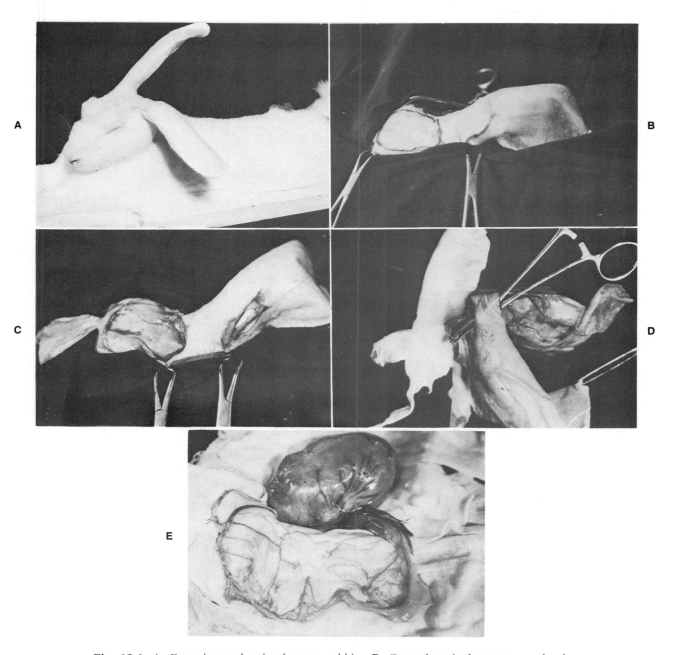

Fig. 12-1. A, Experimental animals were rabbits. **B,** Central auricular artery and vein divided in preparation for omental anastomoses. Scalp defect of 3 by 5 cm created. **C,** Vascular bundle of rabbit ear exposed. **D,** Periosteum in scalp defect removed, exposing bare skull. Recipient vascular bundle introduced into the area of the defect through a subcutaneous tunnel. **E,** Omentum taken from another rabbit.

Continued.

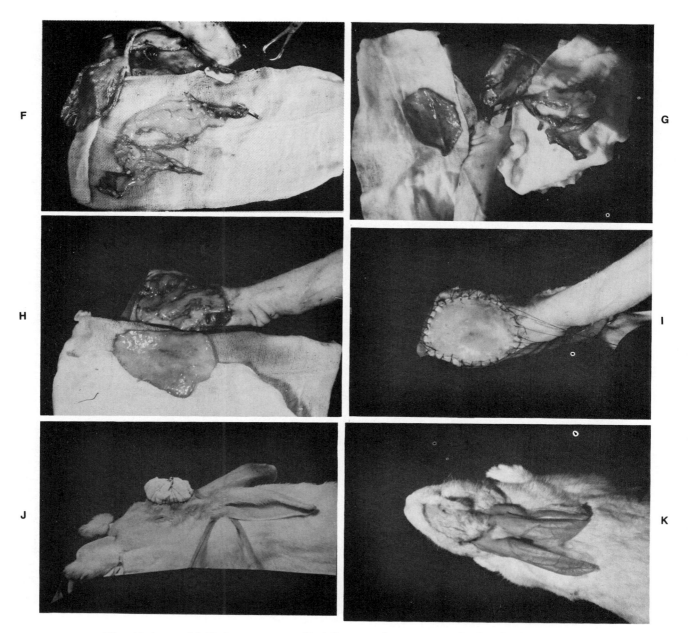

Fig. 12-1, cont'd. F, Omentum readied for vascular anastomosis. **G.** Blood supply of homograft of omentum reestablished after anastomosis of gastroepiploic vessels with central auricular vessels. **H,** Omentum placed in the scalp wound. Overlying skin graft trimmed to match defect. **I,** Skin sutured to edges of defect covering the omentum. **J,** Tie-over dressing applied over omentum. **K,** Hair growth visible on the skin graft 1 month after transplantation.

CONTROL GROUPS
Control group I: no immunosuppressive drugs

The rabbits of control group I received no immunosuppressive drugs; otherwise, they were treated identically. Of the fifteen rabbits in this group, one died 5 days postoperatively, and in three the free flap failed because of anastomotic problems. In the eleven remaining rabbits, significant areas of skin graft survived in four; the average area of surviving skin was 50% to 60% of the total area of the defect. In the remaining seven rabbits there was essentially complete loss of the skin grafts; only small areas survived at the junc-

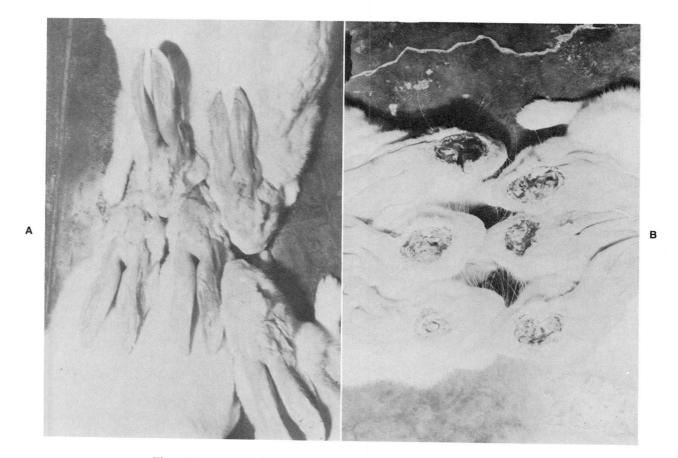

Fig. 12-2. Results of experimental group **(A)** and control group **(B).**

tion of the graft with the normal skin edge. Dead omentum and liquefied fat were seen beneath these necrotic grafts.

Control group II: omental transplant without vascular anastomoses

In the rabbits of control group II the omentum was placed in the defect without the benefit of vascular anastomoses. Skin grafts were applied to the surface. Complete necrosis of the omentum and the skin graft occurred in each rabbit.

Control group III: autologous skin graft placed on bare skull defect

In seven rabbits of control group III thick split skin grafts were applied to the exposed skull. Necrosis of the skin grafts was virtually complete. Only a few scattered, isolated spots of skin graft survived in a few cases.

CONCLUSIONS

1. Free skin grafts applied to the cortical bone in rabbits necrosed.

2. Free skin grafts placed on nonvascularized omental homografts necrosed.
3. Skin grafts applied to vascularized omental homografts without the use of immunosuppressive drugs survived in fewer than 40% of the animals and with an area of less than 80% of the recipient bed in any individual animal.
4. In animals in which the recipient bed was prepared with a vascularized omental homograft and immunosuppressive drugs were administered, over 80% of the grafts survived and the area of survival averaged 86.6% (Fig. 12-2).

ANGIOGRAPHY

Injection of auricular artery (recipient vessel) 3 weeks after transplant. Peking black ink was injected into the auricular artery in one of the experimental rabbits and the graft immediately turned black. The black color promptly faded and disappeared. With a repeat injection the same cycle was again observed. This showed that the skin graft derived its blood supply through the vascular pedicle of the omentum (Fig. 12-3).

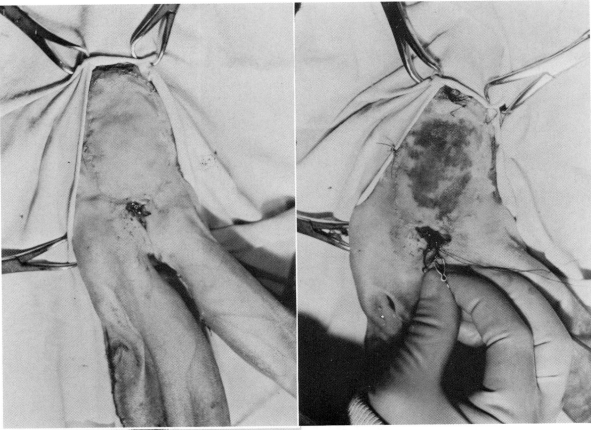

Fig. 12-3. Experimental rabbit 3 weeks postoperatively who received injection of Peking black ink into auricular artery. Ink particles in graft demonstrate establishment of vascular connections between the graft and the omentum.

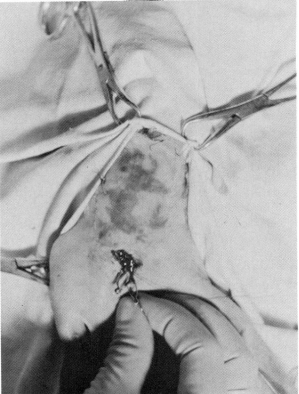

Injection of the lateral cervical artery 4 months after omental transplant in the experimental group. Peking black ink was injected into the lateral cervical artery of one of the experimental rabbits 4 months after the vascularized omental homograft had been performed. The entire scalp and skin graft turned black immediately after injection of the ink. This showed that circulation had been established between the skin graft and the surrounding skin.

HISTOLOGIC OBSERVATIONS

Studies were carried out by Dr. Liu Chia-chi and Dr. Li Sheng-mei, Department of Pathology, Chi Shui Tan Hospital, Peking. Their observations follow.

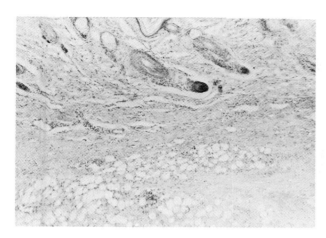

Fig. 12-4. Histologic section 3 weeks postoperatively. Fibroblasts and capillary sprouts (granulation tissue) are seen in the area of the omentum. Coagulation necrosis and associated inflammatory cellular infiltrate is seen in the rest of the omentum. Ink particles in both capillaries and small vessels.

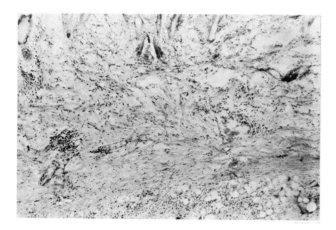

Fig. 12-5. Histologic section 1 month postoperatively. Skin graft surviving and integrated into wound with granulation tissue. Chronic inflammatory cellular infiltrates seen in dermis. Large amount of coagulation necrosis of omentum.

Three weeks after omental transplant. A rabbit was injected with Peking black ink in the auricular artery and then sacrificed. Walls of larger blood vessels showed necrosis but ink was seen in the lumen. The skin graft showed evidence of survival. Black ink was seen in subcutaneous vessels and in the capillary and small vessels of the granulation tissue and in the surrounding normal skin. Thus there was well-established circulation in the free skin graft and between the graft in its bed and surrounding normal skin (Fig. 12-4).

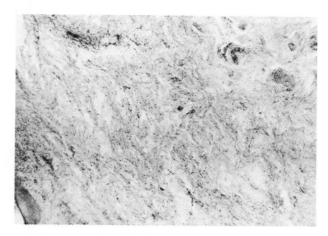

Fig. 12-6. Histologic section 3 months postoperatively. Necrotic omentum has disappeared. Granulation tissue has become scar tissue. Skin graft has acquired appearance of normal skin.

One month postoperatively. Histologic evidence of further necrosis and disintegration of the omental homograft was seen with thrombosis of larger vessels and destruction of the vessel walls. Further proliferation of granulation tissue was seen. The skin graft showed evidence of survival (Fig. 12-5).

Two to three months after grafting. The changes were basically the same as in the animals studied earlier. The entire omentum had been absorbed and was no longer visible. The granulation tissues had turned to scar tissue. The grafted skin and its bed had the appearance of normal dermis and subcutaneous tissue. The skin graft had coalesced as one piece in continuity with the surrounding skin and with the scar tissue underneath. It was identifiable only by the presence of fewer hair follicles than would be seen in normal skin (Fig. 12-6).

PRELIMINARY CONCLUSION

If a skin autograft is placed over a revascularized omental homograft in a rabbit receiving immunosuppressive drugs, the skin graft will be supported initially by blood supply from the omentum. After rejection takes place the skin graft will have gained a permanent blood supply from the surrounding skin and the wound bed. The omental homograft thus plays the role of a temporary source of blood supply for the free skin graft. This experiment provided the basis for clinical application of this principle. An obstacle in clinical application is the problem of storage of a fresh homograft of omentum.

CASE REPORT (Fig. 12-7)

A 24-year-old male electrician sustained electrical burns of both hands from a high tension current of 1,100 volts. Initial treatment was carried out elsewhere with debridement of the skin and extensor tendons of the dorsum of the right hand. There had been two attempts at coverage with free skin grafts.

At the time of admission the patient showed an unstable 6 by 6 cm scar of the dorsum of the right hand. There was no active extention of the metacarpophalangeal joint of the index, middle, ring, or small fingers.

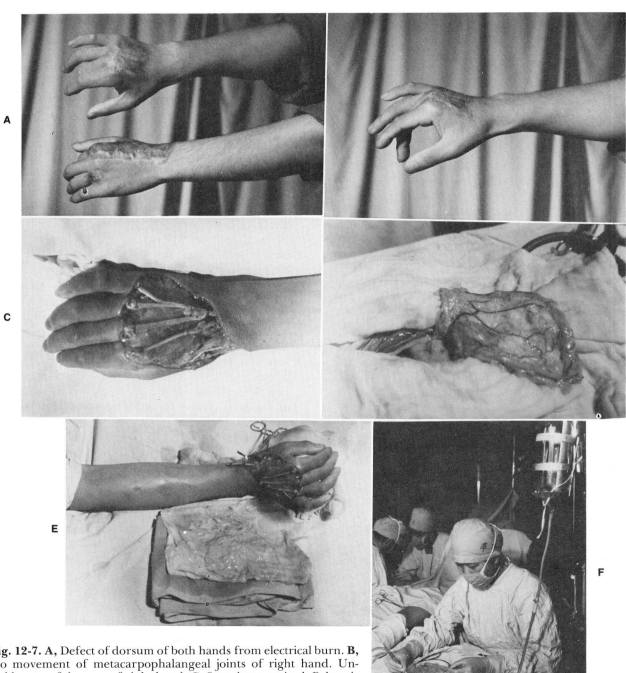

Fig. 12-7. A, Defect of dorsum of both hands from electrical burn. **B,** No movement of metacarpophalangeal joints of right hand. Unstable scar of dorsum of right hand. **C,** Scar tissue excised. Palmaris longus tendon used to bridge tendinous gaps. **D,** Fresh omental homograft is harvested. **E,** Omentum is irrigated with Ringer's solution. **F,** Omentum in hand prepared for vascularized homograft.

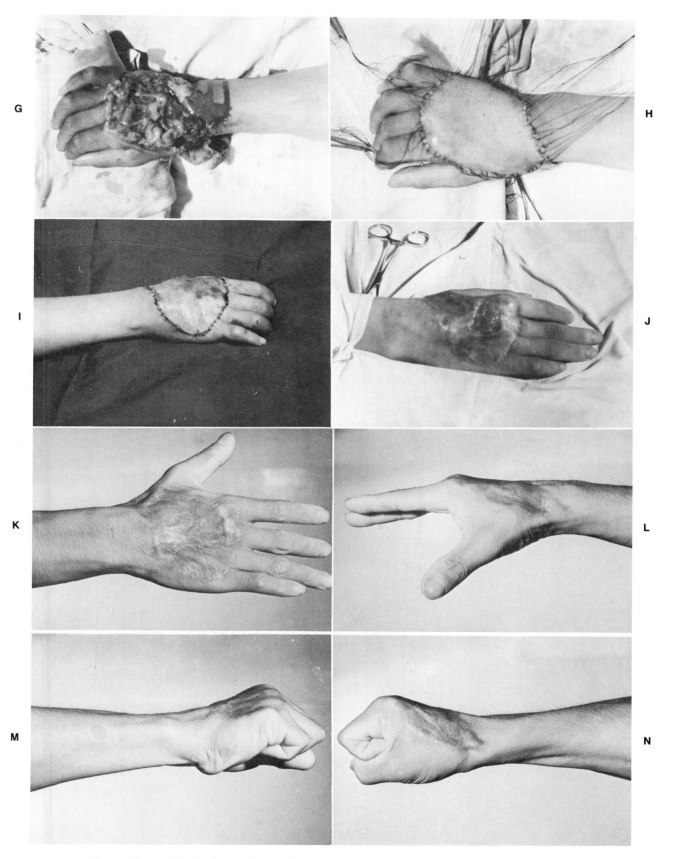

Fig. 12-7, cont'd. G, Omental vessels anastomosed to the cephalic vein and the radial artery. **H,** Split-thickness skin graft applied. **I,** Fifteen days postoperatively. The majority of the graft has taken. A 4 by 4 cm area of graft necrosis at level of second metacarpal. **J,** Residual granulating wound. **K,** Graft has survived completely. **L,** Full extension is present. **M** and **N,** Full flexion is present.

Operation. Three weeks after the patient's admission the scar on the dorsum of the hand was excised; the extensor tendons were found to have gaps extending from the distal edge of the dorsal carpal ligament to the proximal edge of the extensor hoods. The defects of the extensor tendons were bridged by autologous palmaris longus tendon grafts joined end to end.

A homograft of omentum was placed. (The graft was matched to the patient by blood type.) The right epiploic vein was anastomosed to the cephalic vein, and the left epiploic artery was joined to the radial artery. Immediate vascularization was observed when we removed the clamps. The surface of the omentum was covered with a split skin graft that had been taken from the thigh. A tie-over dressing was applied, and the hand was immobilized with a plaster slab. Ischemic time of the omentum was 2 hours and 15 minutes.

Thirteen days postoperatively the dressings were removed; most of the graft had survived. A small patch of graft distal to the second metacarpal appeared nonviable, and there were a few punctate spots of necrosis scattered over the graft. After a few dressing changes the punctate spots healed completely and the area at the second metacarpal formed a granulating wound 4 by 4 cm in size. This healed after application of split skin grafts 3 months postoperatively. Throughout the postoperative course no necrosis nor liquefaction of the omentum was seen. The skin-grafted area was 9 by 7 cm, and the area of necrosis was 4 by 4 cm. The area of graft survival was 74.6% of the total area.

Administration of immunosuppressive drugs. During the operation intravenous cyclophosphamide, 200 mg, and dexamethasone, 80 mg, were given. Postoperatively azathioprine (Imuran), 200 mg, and prednisone, 80 mg, were given daily. One week postoperatively these doses were reduced to azathioprine, 150 mg, and prednisone, 50 mg. Five weeks postoperatively the azathioprine was discontinued, and after another month the prednisone was discontinued.

Symptoms that could have been side effects of the drug therapy were nausea, loss of appetite, and some mild excitation and insomnia. These disappeared within a week of cessation of the drugs. The white blood cell count was always within normal limits, and films of the head of the femur (to detect any loss of blood supply) were normal.

Two years postoperatively the grafts were in good condition. The range of active flexion-extension at the metacarpophalangeal joint was 70 degrees at the index finger, 50 degrees at the middle finger, 50 degrees at the ring finger, and 35 degrees at the small finger.

REFERENCES

1. Cheng, Hsu Hsi, et al.: Free omentum transplant to treat skin defect of the extremities, Symposium of the Ninth National Surgical Conference (a summary), Peking, 1978, Chinese Medical Association, p. 106.
2. McLean, D.H., and Buncke, H.J.: Autotransplant of omentum to a large scalp defect with microsurgical revascularization, Plast. Reconstr. Surg. **49:**268, 1972.

Part IV

Facial reconstruction

Chapter 13

Reconstruction of the maxilla and mandible with vascularized rib-periosteal and rib-osteocutaneous transplantation: indications and alternatives

Donald Serafin
Vincent E. Voci
Ronald Riefkohl
Ivan Thomas
Nicholas G. Georgiade

Changing concepts in mandibular and maxillary reconstruction during recent years have made it necessary to define the specific indications and the relative advantages of several new procedures.

Segmental losses of the maxilla and mandible have been reconstructed with conventional nonvascularized bone grafts for many years. Frequently, however, a deficiency in the quantity of soft tissue or the relative avascularity of the recipient bed limits the success of this procedure.[11,12]

A series of patients who have undergone vascularized rib-periosteal and rib-osteocutaneous tissue transplantation to reconstruct the mandible or maxilla is presented in this chapter, and the advantages and disadvantages of these procedures are detailed. In addition, alternative sources of donor tissue are discussed and their relative role in reconstruction assessed.[22]

PRESENT SERIES

Fourteen patients underwent reconstruction of the maxilla (three) or mandible (eleven) with vascularized composite tissue (Table 13-1). The defect to be reconstructed resulted from bone and soft tissue loss either following extirpation of an intra-

oral squamous cell carcinoma (seven patients, Figs. 13-1 and 13-2) or trauma (gunshot wound in seven patients, Figs. 13-3 and 13-4). Four patients with primary intraoral malignancy also received postoperative irradiation. In addition to the bone and soft tissue loss resulting from the initial injury or disease, four of these patients had undergone unsuccessful conventional (nonvascularized) bone grafts. Six patients had also undergone reconstruction with random flaps to replace a deficient skin or mucosal envelope.

A quantitative or qualitative deficiency of healthy well-vascularized tissue, either skin or oral mucosa, necessitated vascularized bone replace-

Table 13-1. Location of recipient defect

Maxilla	3
Mandible	11
Anterior	(6)
Body	(3)
Ramus	(2)

From Serafin, D., Riefkohl, R., Thomas, I., and Georgiade, N.G.: Vascularized rib-periosteal and osteocutaneous reconstruction of the maxilla and mandible: an assessment, Plast. Reconstr. Surg. **66**(5):718, 1980.

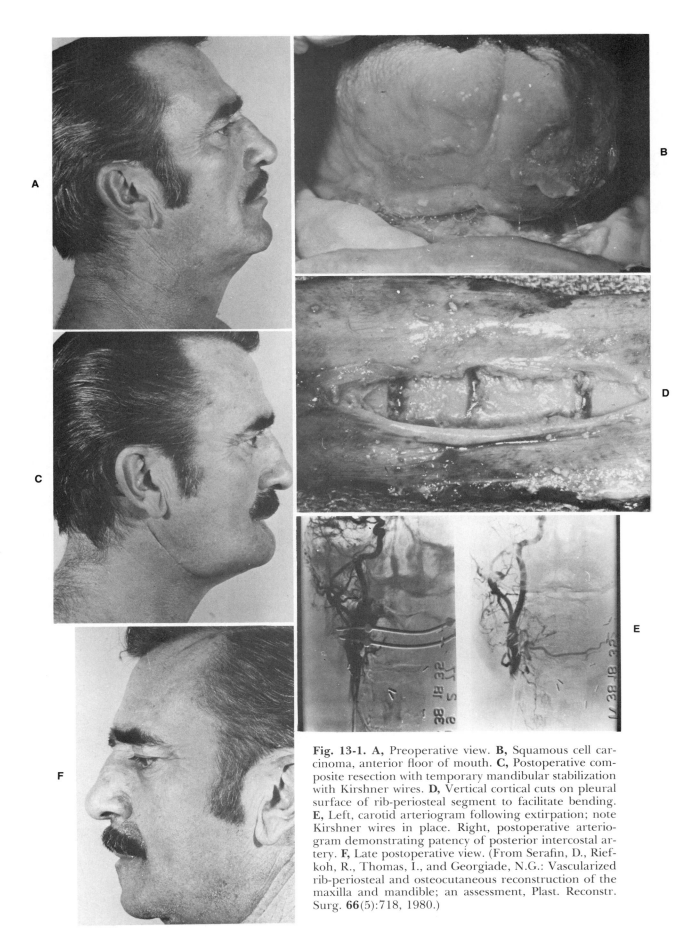

Fig. 13-1. A, Preoperative view. **B,** Squamous cell carcinoma, anterior floor of mouth. **C,** Postoperative composite resection with temporary mandibular stabilization with Kirshner wires. **D,** Vertical cortical cuts on pleural surface of rib-periosteal segment to facilitate bending. **E,** Left, carotid arteriogram following extirpation; note Kirshner wires in place. Right, postoperative arteriogram demonstrating patency of posterior intercostal artery. **F,** Late postoperative view. (From Serafin, D., Riefkoh, R., Thomas, I., and Georgiade, N.G.: Vascularized rib-periosteal and osteocutaneous reconstruction of the maxilla and mandible; an assessment, Plast. Reconstr. Surg. **66**(5):718, 1980.)

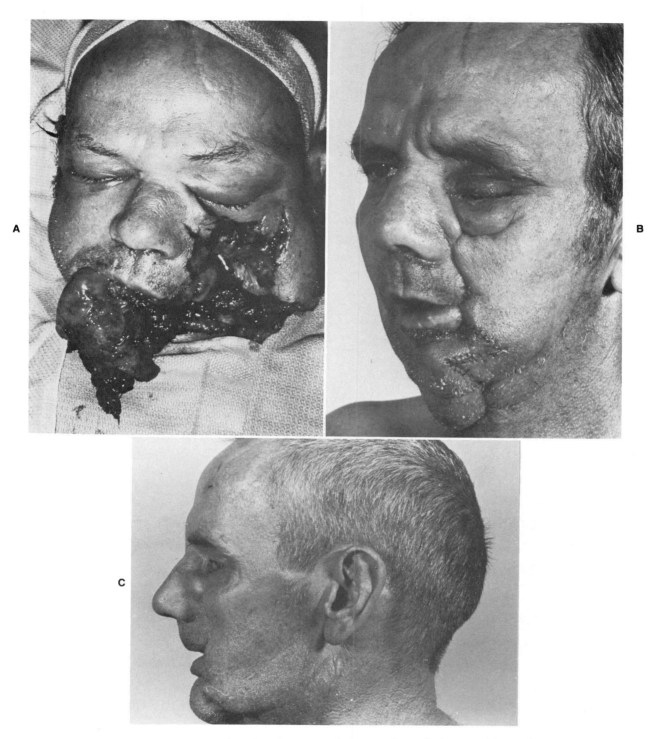

Fig. 13-2. A, Intraoperative view demonstrating extensive soft tissue and bone destruction following a gunshot wound. **B,** Postoperative view following debridement and closure; note segmental deficiency of mandible. **C,** Late postoperative view demonstrating restoration of mandibular continuity with vascularized rib-periosteal segment. (From Serafin, D., Riefkohl, R., Thomas, I., and Georgiade, N.G.: Vascularized rib-periosteal and osteocutaneous reconstruction of the maxilla and mandible: an assessment, Plast. Reconstr. Surg. **66**(5):718, 1980.)

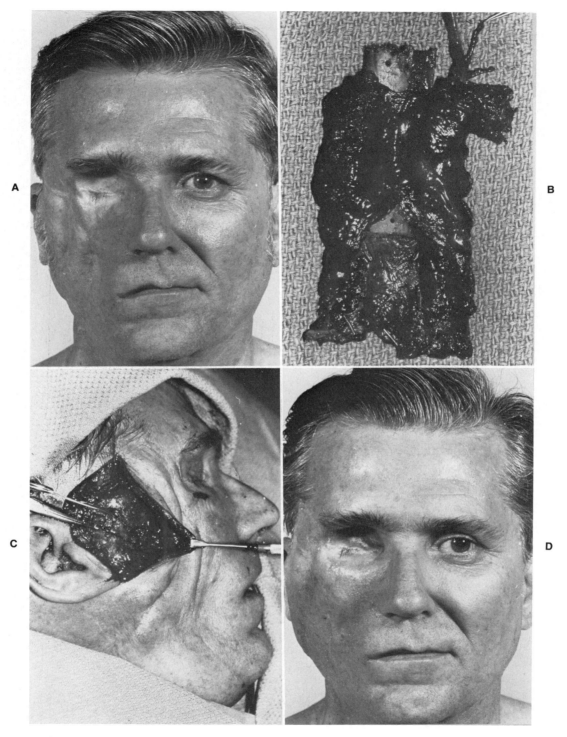

Fig. 13-3. A, Preoperative view demonstrating skeletal deficiency of orbit and maxilla following previous trauma. **B,** Intraoperative photograph demonstrating rib-periosteal segment; note clips on the periosteum. **C,** Intraoperative view demonstrating recipient vasculature superficial temporal artery and vein and creation of subcutaneous pocket for placement of rib-periosteal segment. **D,** Late postoperative view. (From Serafin, D., Riefkohl, R., Thomas, I., and Georgiade, N.G.: Vascularized rib-periosteal and osteocutaneous reconstruction of the maxilla and mandible: an assessment, Plast. Reconstr. Surg. **66**(5):718, 1980.)

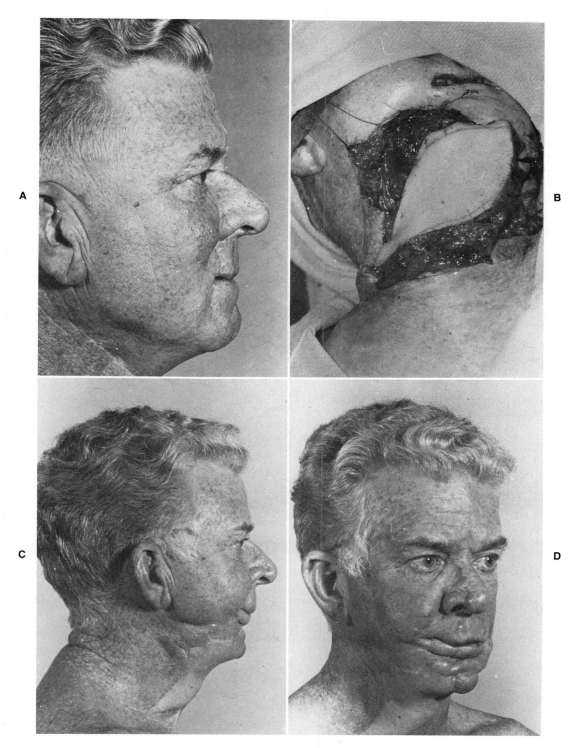

Fig. 13-4. A, Preoperative view before excision of intraoral carcinoma and radiation therapy. **B,** Intraoperative view demonstrating island latissimus dorsi cutaneous flap with attached rib-periosteal segment (revascularized) to restore mandibular continuity and replace deficient skin envelope. **C** and **D,** Late postoperative views. (From Serafin, D., Riefkohl, R., Thomas, I., and Georgiade, N.G.: Vascularized rib-periosteal and osteocutaneous reconstruction of the maxilla and mandible: an assessment, Plast. Reconstr. Surg. **66**(5):718, 1980.)

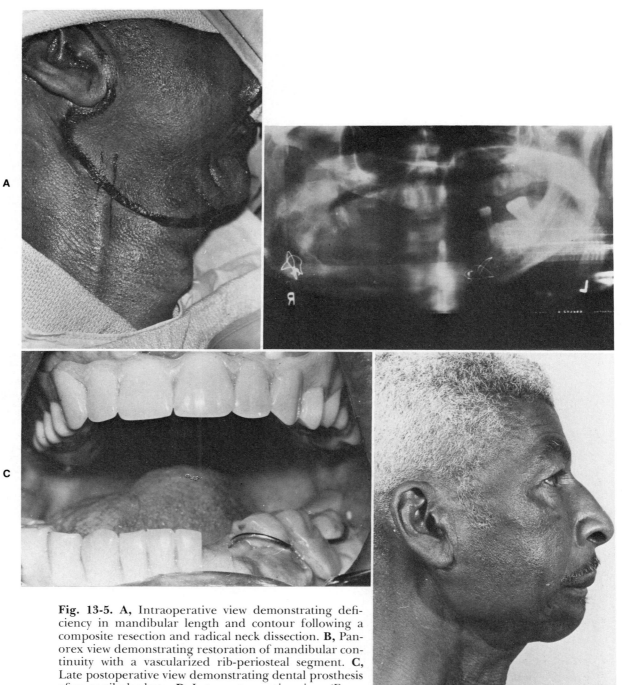

Fig. 13-5. A, Intraoperative view demonstrating deficiency in mandibular length and contour following a composite resection and radical neck dissection. **B,** Panorex view demonstrating restoration of mandibular continuity with a vascularized rib-periosteal segment. **C,** Late postoperative view demonstrating dental prosthesis after vestibuloplasty. **D,** Late postoperative view. (From Serafin, D., Riefkohl, R., Thomas, I., and Georgiade, N.G.: Vascularized rib-periosteal and osteocutaneous reconstruction of the maxilla and mandible: an assessment, Plast. Reconstr. Surg. **66**(5):718, 1980.)

ment (Table 13-2). Two patients were selected for rib-osteocutaneous flaps. Two additional patients had cutaneous cover provided by an island latissimus dorsi musculocutaneous flap to which was attached, by loose areolar connective tissue, the rib-periosteal segment (Fig. 13-5). Revascularization of the rib-periosteal segment was accomplished by anastomosis of the posterior intercostal artery and vein to suitable recipient vasculature. The remaining ten patients underwent vascularized rib-periosteal reconstruction (Table 13-3).

The anterior approach was employed in only one patient. The remaining thirteen patients underwent reconstruction with a rib-periosteal segment from the posterolateral approach. Usually the ninth or tenth rib was selected as donor tissue.

SURGICAL APPROACHES

Three surgical approaches are advocated for the microsurgical transplantation of a rib-periosteal or composite rib-osteocutaneous segment (Table 13-4).

Anterior approach

The anterior approach was first described by McKee[13,14] and then by Ariyan.[2] The advantages include large (2 to 3 mm) external diameter donor vessels and excellent pedicle length. Disadvantages include the bulk of the associated portion of pectoralis muscle that must accompany the rib-periosteal segment if skin is also required for the reconstruction. The blood supply to the skin from the anterior perforating branches of the internal mammary artery is usually good. The dissection is moderately difficult, but access to the head and neck region is facilitated by the anterior location of the donor site. Theoretically sensation, at least to the medial portion of the flap, can be restored if a recipient nerve is sutured to the posterior intercostal nerve or to its anterior perforating branch.

Posterolateral approach

The posterolateral approach was first described by Buncke et al.[4] and then by Serafin et al.[24] and Harashina et al.[9] It has the advantage of a relatively easy dissection and a long bony segment. The posterior intercostal vessels, measuring approximately 1 to 2 mm in external diameter, are isolated anterior to the paraspinal musculature and can be removed en bloc with the entire rib-periosteal segment. Additional dissection of the neurovascular pedicle from the attached rib is done with the aid

Table 13-2. Rationale for reconstruction*

Deficiency in quantity of skin or mucosa	3
Deficiency in quality of recipient bed (avascularity or fibrosis)	11
Trauma	
Multiple operative procedures	(2)
Conventional pedicle flaps	(2)
Extensive soft tissue destruction	(4)
Irradiation	
Relative avascularity	(1)
Osteoradionecrosis	(1)
Orocutaneous fistula	(1)

From Serafin, D., Riefkohl, R., Thomas, I., and Georgiade, N.G.: Vascularized rib-periosteal and osteocutaneous reconstruction of the maxilla and mandible: an assessment, Plast. Reconstr. Surg. **66**(5):718, 1980.
*Categories overlap; only the most important reason has been selected.

Table 13-3. Type of composite tissue

Osteocutaneous	2
Rib-periosteal	10
Rib-periosteal and island latissimus dorsi–musculocutaneous	(2)

From Serafin, D., Riefkohl, R., Thomas, I., and Georgiade, N.G.: Vascularized rib-periosteal and osteocutaneous reconstruction of the maxilla and mandible: an assessment, Plast. Reconstr. Surg. **66**(5):718, 1980.

Table 13-4. Comparison of surgical approaches

	Anterior	Posterolateral	Posterior
Size of donor vasculature	2-3 mm external diameter	1-2 mm external diameter	2.0-2.5 mm external diameter
Length of pedicle	11-15 cm	11-15 cm	5-10 cm
Accessibility	Excellent	Good	Fair
Ease of dissection	Moderately difficult	Relatively easy	Difficult
Major thoracotomy required	Probable	Yes	Yes
Cutaneous reliability	Good	Questionable	Questionable
Length of rib-periosteal segment	10-20 cm	10-20 cm	10-20 cm
Neurosensory flap	Yes*	Yes	Yes
Quality of medullary blood flow	Good*	Good*	Excellent*

From Serafin, D., Riefkohl, R., Thomas, I., and Georgiade, N.G.: Vascularized rib-periosteal and osteocutaneous reconstruction of the maxilla and mandible: an assessment, Plast. Reconstr. Surg. **66**(5):718, 1980.
*Theoretic advantage not demonstrated in sufficient clinical series.

of the operating microscope (Fig. 13-3). Depending on the amount of rib-periosteal segment required in reconstruction and the desired pedicle length, an appropriate segment of bone is removed subperiosteally and either discarded or used as a conventional nonvascularized bone graft. A skin paddle based on the neurovascular territory of the lateral cutaneous branches of the posterior intercostal vessels and nerves may also be added if innervated skin is desired in reconstruction. Vascular insufficiency, particularly venous, has been more of a problem than with the anterior approach because of the absence of direct anterior perforating branches to the skin. A previous "delay" procedure or additional cutaneous venous anastomoses have been suggested to improve viability of the skin.[24]

Posterior approach

The posterior approach was first described by Östrup and Fredrickson[18] and then popularized by Daniel.[5] This procedure includes the posterior nutrient artery to the rib-periosteal segment, with theoretic advantages of improved medullary blood flow and therefore better nutrition.[6] The posterior approach was not used in our present series. In all our patients, however, cortical blood supply appeared sufficient to maintain osteocyte viability, even though the nutrient artery was not included. No resorption was noted if the anastomoses remained patent. Good callus formation at the osteotomy sites was demonstrated in follow-up radiographs. Recent experimental data by Berggren et al. support these clinical observations.[3] They found no difference in bony union when comparing vascularized posterior (medullary nutrient artery included) and posterolateral (cortical-periosteal blood supply only) bone grafts in dogs.

Inclusion of the nutrient artery limits the length of the vascular pedicle and increases both the difficulty and the morbidity of the dissection. Careful, deliberate dissection to avoid injury to the artery of Adamkiewicz[5] is essential. Sensation is possible through the lateral cutaneous branch; its use in paraplegics has been demonstrated.[8] A vascularized, innervated osteocutaneous flap from the posterolateral approach has the same sensory possibilities.

RESULTS

Twelve patients (86%) in our present series underwent successful transplantation. There were two failures (14%). Preoperative planning was in-

Table 13-5. Complications

		Number*	Patients
Pulmonary		14	9
Effusion	9		
Atelectasis	3		
Pneumonia	1		
Empyema	1		
Recipient wound		4	2
Hematoma	1		
Partial dehiscence	1		
Orocutaneous fistula	2		
Upper gastrointestinal bleeding		3	3
Duodenal ulcer	2		
Curlings or anticoagulants	1		

From Serafin, D., Riefkohl, R., Thomas, I., and Georgiade, N.G.: Vascularized rib-periosteal and osteocutaneous reconstruction of the maxilla and mandible: an assessment, Plast. Reconstr. Surg. **66**(5):718, 1980.
*More than one occurred in five patients

adequate with one patient. The section of rib that was removed had been previously fractured, but this did not come to light until an explanation was sought for the abnormal and inadequate vessels. The other failure occurred during the postoperative period when the vascular anastomoses were disrupted, probably as a consequence of severe, persistent vomiting.

Although there were no deaths in the present series, the pulmonary complications were especially significant (Table 13-5). Pleural effusion and atelectasis were very common; pneumonia and empyema were also encountered. All fourteen patients responded rapidly to aggressive pulmonary care and antibiotics. Two patients who developed an orocutaneous fistula were treated successfully with local flap revision and secondary closure. Three patients developed significant gastrointestinal bleeding. Two of these patients had a bleeding duodenal ulcer, which was demonstrated angiographically. All responded to nonoperative therapy.

DISCUSSION

Segmental mandibular deficiencies are best replaced with nonvascularized bone grafts unless the recipient bed is relatively avascular, in which case vascularized bone grafts are indicated.

Because the vascularity of the recipient bed is improved, other conventional procedures may be performed later with an increased likelihood of success. In the present series a nonvascularized bone graft was employed in one patient to augment deficient rib volume anteriorly. In another a vestibuloplasty on the cutaneous surface of the rib-periosteal segment was performed to deepen the buccal alveolar sulcus, permitting the construction of dentures by a prosthodontist (Fig. 13-5, *C*).

Mandibular contour in an anteroposterior direction can be restored by making several vertical cuts in the cortex on the pleural surface of the rib, which is then forcefully bent. Consequently long segmental defects can be successfully bridged and both form and contour can be reestablished (Fig. 13-1).

Vascularized rib-periosteal donor tissue has several disadvantages, including structural weakness and volume deficiency of the transplanted bony segment (Fig. 13-5, *B*). The cutaneous portion of the composite tissue is also unreliable, particularly when the posterior or posterolateral approach is used.

An additional disadvantage of rib-periosteal donor tissue is the obligate periosteal blood supply, particularly with the anterior and posterolateral segments. Because the muscle cuff must remain attached to the underlying bone, any sculpturing is quite limited. In addition, the skin and mucosal envelope must be of sufficient dimension to accommodate the increased bulk.

The frequency of complications should be emphasized as well, and carefully considered when this method of reconstruction is being contemplated (Table 13-5). Certainly this operative procedure should not be undertaken by surgeons lacking a solid background in thoracic surgery, pulmonary physiology, and management of postoperative thoracotomy patients.

A malunion necessitating osteotomy of the vascularized rib was required in three patients as a result of inadequate intermaxillary fixation and splinting until solid bone union occurred. In this context, bone union occurs as in a mandibular fracture, requiring immobilization for 4 to 6 weeks.

ALTERNATIVE SURGICAL PROCEDURES
Iliac crest

Vascularized iliac crest osteocutaneous donor tissue, based on the deep circumflex iliac artery and vein as described by Taylor et al., is an important contribution.[26,27] Precise sculpturing is possible because a portion of the attached muscle and its periosteal communicating vessels can be discarded. Medullary circulation is provided by associated nutrient arteries. A large area of cutaneous tissue can

be included if required, and long segments of bone may be obtained. The morbidity from pulmonary complications is less than that reported using vascularized rib, and there is minimal donor site morbidity.

A segment of iliac crest nourished by the superficial circumflex iliac artery has certain limitations and is less reliable than that based on the deep circumflex iliac artery.[7,25,26,27] There is more obligate muscle mass, and a cutaneous segment must accompany the bone, even if deepithelialized; this increases the bulk and may create difficulty in placement. The limited length of the vascular pedicle also restricts placement, making an interpositional vein graft necessary at times. The vessels are smaller and flow is less reliable.[26] Bone sculpturing is possible, except at the site of cutaneous attachment.

A segment of iliac crest bone can be attached to a tensor fascia lata musculocutaneous unit supplied by the lateral femoral circumflex artery and vein.[15,16] A major disadvantage is the bulk of the obligate soft tissue. The accompanying soft tissue limits placement even more than a similar segment of iliac crest nourished by the superficial circumflex iliac artery. The long vascular pedicle, however, facilitates placement of the flap if the soft tissue can be accommodated within the defect.

The vascularized iliac crest has many advantages in reconstruction of the mandible. It is reliable, the bony segment is long and strong, its contour is similar, and sculpturing is easily done. The method employing the deep circumflex iliac vessels appears to be the most versatile and reliable.

Second metatarsal–dorsalis pedis flap

The second metatarsal–dorsalis pedis flap has been used in reconstruction of the mandible in a small number of patients.[17] There are many disadvantages—it cannot be contoured or sculptured easily, it is bulky, the osseous segment is only 5 cm long, and there is significant donor site morbidity.

Vascularized soft tissue flap and nonvascularized bone

Various vascularized soft tissue flaps have been used successfully in head and neck reconstruction.[10,21,23] A well-vascularized recipient bed is created and the restriction of a tight skin envelope is removed. Nonvascularized bone, either rib or iliac crest, can then be placed in a second stage to reconstruct the maxilla or mandible. Defects of smaller dimensions and intraoral defects can be treated successfully by microsurgical composite tissue transplantation.

Musculocutaneous flaps

The tremendous versatility, reliability, and ready availability of the pectoralis major and latissimus dorsi musculocutaneous flaps for head and neck reconstruction have made the other methods of cutaneous transfer (particularly vascularized cutaneous tissue) less applicable.[1,19] Nonvascularized bone grafts can be transplanted at the time of flap placement or at a later date. Transferring rib attached to a musculocutaneous flap has also been described.[2,20] Periosteal circulation from a latissimus dorsi flap, however, appears inadequate to support osteocyte viability in a significant segment of rib.[20] This is probably not the case when an island or pedicle pectoralis major osteomusculocutaneous flap is employed.[1] More experience with a larger series is necessary, however.

SUMMARY

Three approaches using rib-periosteal or rib-osteocutaneous composite tissue to reconstruct the mandible and maxilla are described. These methods appear to be useful in providing viable bone and improving the vascularity of the wound, but the disadvantages are significant. Bulk of the transplanted soft tissue, volume deficiency of bone, and unreliable cutaneous tissue (especially with the posterior and posterolateral approach) are serious problems. There is significant patient morbidity, and pulmonary complications are notable.

Currently vascularized rib-periosteal transplantation is most often indicated to replace large segmental defects of mandibular continuity when the recipient bed is relatively avascular, but the quantity of cutaneous cover is adequate. Reconstruction with musculocutaneous flaps and conventional nonvascularized bone grafts is indicated in patients with deficient soft tissue and only a small segmental defect.

With extensive deficiencies of both soft tissue cover and mandibular or maxillary continuity, an iliac osteocutaneous flap based on the deep circumflex iliac vessels may be the most effective, with less morbidity.

REFERENCES

1. Ariyan, S.: Further experiences with the pectoralis major myocutaneous flap for immediate repair of defects from excision of head and neck cancers, Plast. Reconstr. Surg. **64:**605, 1979.
2. Ariyan, S., and Finseth, F.J.: The anterior chest approach for obtaining free osteocutaneous rib grafts, Plast. Reconstr. Surg. **62:**676, 1978.
3. Berggren, A., Weiland, A.J., and Dorfman, H.: Free vascularized bone grafts: factors affecting their survival and ability to heal to recipient bone defects, Plast. Reconstr. Surg. **69:**19, 1982.
4. Buncke, H.J., Furnas, D.W., Gordon, L., and Achauer, B.M.: Free osteocutaneous flap from a rib to the tibia, Plast. Reconstr. Surg. **59:**799, 1977.
5. Daniel, R.K.: Free rib transfer by microvascular anastomoses (letter to the editor), Plast. Reconstr. Surg. **59:**737, 1977.
6. Daniel, R.K.: Commentary on reconstruction of mandibular defects with revascularized free rib grafts by T. Harashina, H. Nakajima, and T. Imai: The voice of polite dissent. Plast. Reconstr. Surg. **62:**775, 1978.
7. Daniel, R.K.: Mandibular reconstruction with free tissue transfers, Ann. Plast. Surg. **1:**346, 1978.
8. Daniel, R.K., Terzis, J.K., and May, J.W.: Neurovascular free flaps. In Serafin, D., and Buncke, H.J., Jr., editors: Microsurgical composite tissue transplantation, St. Louis, 1979, The C.V. Mosby Co.
9. Harashina, T., Nakajima, H., and Imai, T.: Reconstruction of mandibular defects with revascularized free rib grafts, Plast. Reconstr. Surg. **62:**514, 1978.
10. Harii, K., and Ohmori, K.: Free skin flap transfer, Clin. Plast. Surg. **3:**111, 1976.
11. Ivy, R.H.: Bone grafting for restoration of defects of mandible (collective review), Plast. Reconstr. Surg. **7:**333, 1951.
12. Ivey, R.H., and Eby, J.D.: Thirty-nine and thirty-eight year follow-up of mandibular bone grafts in 3 cases, Plast. Reconstr. Surg. **22:**548, 1958.
13. McKee, D.M.: Microvascular rib transposition for reconstruction of the mandible. Presented at the Annual Meeting of the American Society of Plastic and Reconstructive Surgeons, Montreal, Canada, 1971.
14. McKee, D.M.: Microvascular bone transplantation, Clin. Plast. Surg. **5:**283, 1978.
15. Nahai, F., Hill, H.L., and Hester, T.R.: Experiences with the tensor fascia lata flap, Plast. Reconstr. Surg. **63:**788, 1979.
16. Nahai, F., Silverton, J.S., Hill, H.L., and Vasconez, L.O.: The tensor fascia lata musculocutaneous flap, Ann. Plast. Surg. **1:**372, 1978.
17. O'Brien, B.M., Morrison, W.A., MacLeon, A.M., and Dooley, B.J.: Microvascular osteocutaneous transfer using the groin flap and iliac crest and the dorsalis pedis flap and second metatarsal, Br. J. Plast. Surg. **32:**188, 1979.
18. Östrup, L.T., and Fredrickson, J.M.: Distant transfer of a free living bone graft by microvascular anastomoses, Plast. Reconstr. Surg. **54:**274, 1974.
19. Quillen, C.G., Shearin, J.C., Jr., and Georgiade, N.G.: The latissimus dorsi myocutaneous flap in head and neck reconstruction, Plast. Reconstr. Surg. **63:**664, 1979.
20. Serafin, D.: Unpublished observations, 1978.
21. Serafin, D., Georgiade, N.G., and Peters, C.R.: Microsurgical composite tissue transplantation: a method of immediate reconstruction of the head and neck, Clin. Plast. Surg. **3:**447, 1976.
22. Serafin, D., Riefkohl, R., Thomas, I., and Georgiade, N.G.: Vascularized rib-periosteal and osteocutaneous reconstruction of the maxilla and man-

dible: an assessment, Plast. Reconstr. Surg. **66**(5): 718, 1980.

23. Serafin, D., and Villarreal-Rios, A.: Versatility of composite tissue transplantation in soft tissue reconstruction of the head and neck. In Serafin, D., and Buncke, H.J., editors: Microsurgical composite tissue transplantation. St. Louis, 1979, The C.V. Mosby Co.

24. Serafin, D., Villarreal-Rios, A., and Georgiade, N.G.: A rib-containing free flap to reconstruct mandibular defects, Br. J. Plast. Surg. **30**:263, 1977.

25. Tamai, S.: Osteocutaneous transplantation. In Serafin, D., and Buncke, H.J., Jr., editors: Microsurgical composite tissue transplantation, St. Louis, 1979, The C.V. Mosby Co.

26. Taylor, G.I., Townsend, P., and Corlett, R.: Superiority of the deep circumflex iliac vessels as the supply for free groin flaps, Plast. Reconstr. Surg. **64:** 595, 1979.

27. Taylor, G.I., and Watson, N.: One-stage repair of compound leg defects with free revascularized flaps of groin skin and iliac bone, Plast. Reconstr. Surg. **61:**494, 1978.

Chapter 14

Reconstruction of the jaw with free composite iliac bone grafts

G. Ian Taylor

Reconstruction of the jaw with free nonvascularized bone grafts is a time-proven technique, provided there is intact lining and external cover and the recipient bed is sterile and well vascularized. However, the success rate falls dramatically when there is an associated soft tissue defect that requires flap coverage. The myocutaneous flap, when combined with vascularized segments of rib, scapula, sternum, or clavicle, has solved many of these problems. Nevertheless there is a nucleus of carefully selected cases for which a free composite graft of iliac bone with appropriate soft tissue attachments, transferred in one stage by microvascular techniques, offers a viable alternative, especially where the bone defect is large or where previous procedures have failed.

When one designs the mandible on the *deep* circumflex iliac vessels, the entire iliac crest and the majority of the blade of the ilium are available.[3,4] The supplying vessels are large and the pedicle is long, thus facilitating the microvascular repairs. Because the blood supply approaches the ilium from its *medial* cortex, bone can be sculptured from the outer cortex to provide an exact replica of the jaw. Alternatively, for smaller grafts, the hip bone can be split, taking the inner cortex only as the graft and leaving the outer surface for normal hip contour. Step or wedge osteotomies of the iliac crest may be performed to reconstitute the chin prominence without compromise to the blood supply, if the integrity of the medial periosteum and the muscle attachments along the inner lip of the iliac crest are preserved.[5,6]

Our experience in eight cases in which there was an associated soft tissue defect of mucosa or skin has been most encouraging (Fig. 14-1). In five patients the ramus and body of the mandible were reconstructed. In three of these patients the graft was extended across the midline, incorporating a step or a wedge osteotomy of the bone to reconstitute the chin. In the remaining three patients the body or central segment of the mandible was reconstructed, and in one of these, the jaw was replaced from angle to angle. In every case an associated soft tissue defect was present.

In seven patients the reconstruction followed tumor resection, and in two of these cases the tissues had been heavily irradiated. In four patients the repair was performed at the time of resection, and in three it was done as a secondary procedure. In the remaining case the transfer was done to correct the soft tissue and bony deformity of hemifacial microsomia. One graft failed because of arterial thrombosis. In the remaining seven cases clinical union of the bone was seen between 4 and 6 weeks.

The bone graft size varied from 9 by 3 cm to 21 by 7 cm and the skin flap from 10 by 3 cm to 27 by 14 cm. The donor site was closed as a linear scar in every case, with minimal contour deformity of the hip. There was no instance of abdominal herniation.

DESIGNING THE GRAFT

The lower jaw can be planned as a living graft in one of two ways (Fig. 14-2). As suggested by Manchester,[1] the ramus of the mandible can be

All figures for this chapter are from Taylor, G.I.: Reconstruction of the mandible with free composite iliac bone grafts, Ann. Plast. Surg. **9**(5):361, 1982, Little, Brown & Co. Reprinted by permission.

106

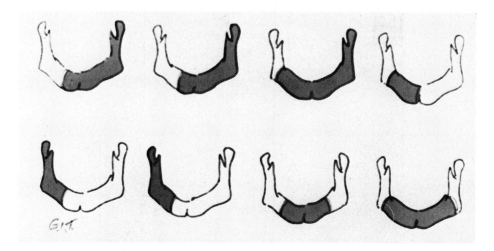

Fig. 14-1. Segments of jaw reconstructed in eight patients. Note that three grafts cross the midline.

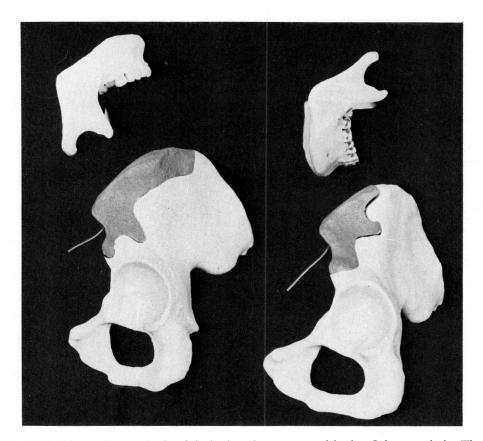

Fig. 14-2. Alternative methods of designing the ramus and body of the mandible. The second method provides short body segments only, but either hip is available, whereas the ipsilateral hip must be used in the former.

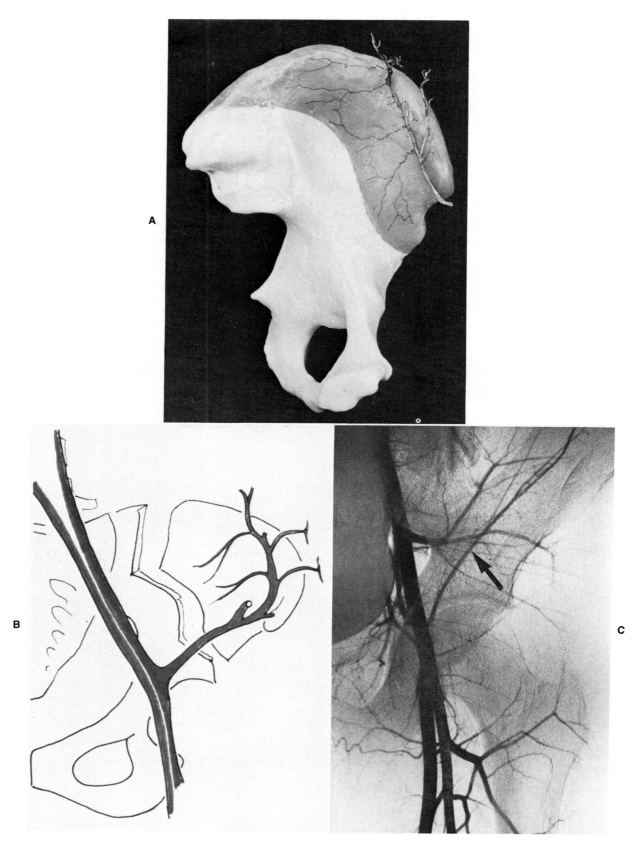

Fig. 14-3. Deep circumflex iliac artery (**C,** *arrow*) with its periosteal and musculocutaneous branches, is demonstrated on a model of the hip bone after a resin injection of the artery (**A**), diagrammatically (**B**), and on angiography (**C**).

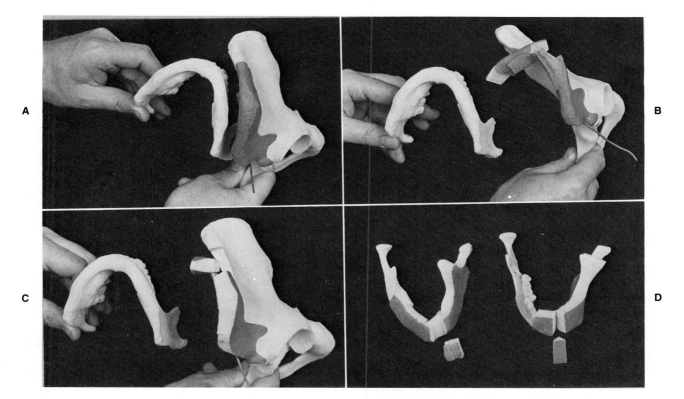

Fig. 14-4. Reconstruction of the mandible across the midline planned with bone models. **A,** Curvature of the ipsilateral hip matches the mandible to the point of the chin, but beyond this it veers away. To correct this, a step osteotomy **(B)** or a wedge osteotomy **(C)** can be made, preserving the medial periosteum and muscle attachment and then designing rectangular or wedge "keystones" **(D)** to complete the shape of the graft.

designed from the buttress of bone between the anterosuperior and the anteroinferior iliac spines, and the body of the mandible can be designed from the iliac crest. If the ipsilateral hip is used, the curvature of the jaw will be correct. Since the entire iliac crest is nourished by the deep circumflex iliac system, sufficient bone is available to reconstruct the jaw to the opposite angle (Fig. 14-3). However, if this is contemplated, it will be found that the curvature of the ilium is in the wrong direction beyond the tuberosity of the iliac crest. This is why a wedge or a step osteotomy must be made in this area to correct the curvature in two planes, thus providing the normal prominence of the chin (Fig. 14-4).

Alternatively, the pattern can be reversed, with the ramus of the jaw designed from the iliac crest (Fig. 14-2, right). However, this will provide only a short body segment. Either hip is available for this technique: if the ipsilateral hip is used, the vessels and soft tissues will be superficial; if the contralateral hip is used, they will be deep.

When planning the graft it is advisable to have a replica of the hipbone and the jaw on hand, with the position of the vessels tagged to avoid confusion. A methylmethacrylate model of the graft can be made; this can be sterilized and used in the operating room to check the size and shape of the graft at both the donor and recipient sites *before transfer*. Trial operations in cadavers are suggested until experience is obtained. All incisions should be planned before surgery.

DISSECTING THE GRAFT

Dissecting the graft has been described elsewhere,[3,4] but the important steps will be highlighted.

1. The blood supply to the skin is from a row of musculocutaneous perforators that emerge through the external oblique muscle adjacent to or just above the upper border of the anterior iliac crest. They appear at approximately 2 cm intervals, commencing near the anterior superior iliac spine (ASIS).

The largest perforator, which is usually a continuation of the main vessel, is situated 6 to 8 cm beyond the ASIS. Thus the skin flap should be centered over this point, with two thirds of its area placed above the iliac crest and its long axis along a line that joins the ASIS to the inferior angle of the scapula. Although we have raised the flap in several cases as far medial as the femoral artery, this end of the flap has often been cyanotic for a day or so. Hence we would advise designing the flap lateral to the ASIS in most cases.

2. The skin is incised over the inguinal canal and the upper border of the flap to expose the external oblique. The loose areolar layer over this muscle is dissected and preserved with the flap, since it contains a rich anastomosis between the perforators of the deep circumflex iliac artery (DCIA).

3. The external oblique is divided in the line of its fibers, two fingersbreadth above its attachment to the iliac crest, and the incision is curved medially into the inguinal canal.

4. The pedicle is then isolated by dividing the internal oblique and transversus muscles from the inguinal ligament laterally and retracting the cord or round ligament medially. The external iliac artery is palpated and the deep circumflex iliac vessels are identified in an areolar sheath parallel and deep to the inguinal ligament. The deep circumflex iliac vein always diverges upward from its artery 1 to 2 cm lateral to the external iliac artery and passes either in front of or behind that vessel. At some point, usually 1 to 2 cm medial to the ASIS, a large ascending branch is given off that pierces the transversus muscle and ascends obliquely between this muscle and the internal oblique. It is important not to mistake this for the main vessel, since it supplies skin in only 10% of cases and has little contribution to the bone. Except in rare cases, the main artery lies deep to the transversus muscle throughout its course. It runs in a groove between this muscle and the iliacus muscle until it reaches a point 6 to 8 cm beyond the ASIS, where it pierces the muscles of the abdominal wall, anastomoses with the subcostal artery, and provides the largest perforator to the skin.

5. Next the internal oblique and transversus muscles are divided beyond the ASIS, 1.5 cm above and parallel to the iliac crest. The transversalis fascia is incised, and the abdominal viscera are retracted medially to expose the iliacus muscle. Finally this muscle is incised 1.5 cm medial to the line formed by the fusion of the iliacus fascia and the transversalis fascia, and its fibers are swept medially by blunt dissection to preserve the periosteum and its supplying vessels.

6. The lower border of the flap is divided, and the superficial circumflex iliac vessels are identified medially and tagged as a precaution to provide a reserve lifeline. The thigh muscles are detached from the outer lip of the iliac crest, preserving periosteum only. If a thin graft is required, this can be achieved by splitting the hip and taking the inner cortex alone; this is possible because the inner cortex is supplied from its medial aspect. The bone graft is then sectioned with an oscillating saw.

7. Before the vascular pedicle is divided, the bone graft is contoured to match the methylmethacrylate model. To do this, one removes the outer cortex and rim of the iliac crest where necessary to provide an exact replica of the jaw. This has the advantage of shortening the surgical maneuvers—and hence the ischemic time—after detaching the graft.

8. It is important when closing the donor defect to repair the transversus muscle and its fascia to the iliacus muscle and its fascia to prevent abdominal herniation. Then the muscles are repaired to the buttock and thigh muscles. The tightest layer is the external oblique, and if necessary this can be released by an incision over the rectus sheath.

CASE REPORT

Four cases will be presented to illustrate the various refinements of this method of jaw and soft tissue reconstruction and are summarized in Fig. 14-5.

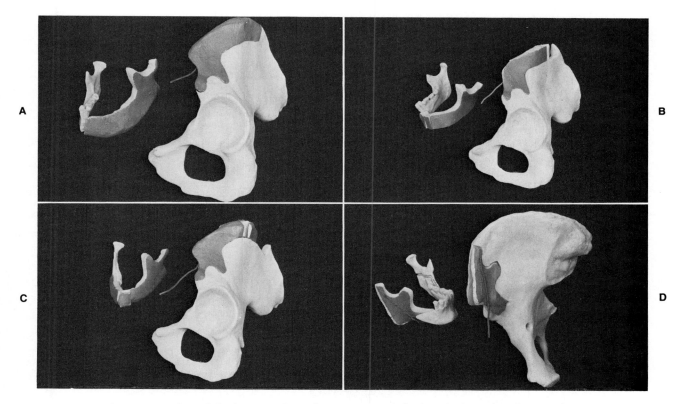

Fig. 14-5. Design of the bone graft used to reconstruct the jaws in **A,** patient I; **B,** patient II; **C,** patient III; and **D,** patient IV. NOTE: In patient II the rim of the iliac crest and a portion of the ASIS have been discarded to provide a more accurate replica of the jaw. In patient IV the hip bone and its apophysis have been split, designing the graft from the inner cortex. The position of the deep circumflex iliac artery is simulated in each case.

Patient I

In July 1978 a 19-year-old male was seen with a recurrent osteosarcoma of the left jaw (Figs. 14-6, *A,* and 14-8). Resection of this tumor required an extended left hemimandibulectomy, crossing the midline to the opposite premolar tooth, together with extirpation of soft tissues of the floor of the mouth and the attached muscles of mastication (Fig. 14-6, *B*).

An immediate one-stage reconstruction was undertaken; we designed a composite graft from the same hip on the deep circumflex iliac vessels (Fig. 14-7). In addition to bone, the following soft tissue refinements were added, made possible by the common vascular lifeline. A segment of the rectus femoris tendon was taken to repair the capsular ligaments of the temporomandibular joint; a flap of fascia lata was designed to reattach the masseter muscle; and a skin flap was taken for lining, and the strips of abdominal muscle necessary to preserve the cutaneous circulation were used to reconstruct the muscles of the floor of the mouth. In addition, a coronoid process was sculptured from the blade of the ilium to secure the temporalis tendon. Because the ipsilateral hip was chosen, the curvature of the iliac crest matched the body of the lower jaw; this was wired across the midline to the remaining mandibular segment. The deep circumflex iliac vessels were anastomosed end to end to the facial vessels.

The donor site was closed directly and the jaw was held with intermaxillary fixation. By 6 weeks there was clinical union of the graft, with a good range of movement (Figs. 14-8 to 14-10).

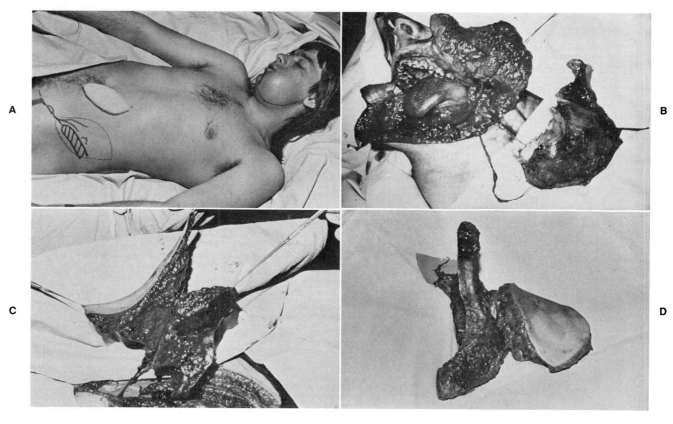

Fig. 14-6. Patient I, the operation. **A,** Incisions marked on the jaw and the hip of the same side. **B,** The tumor resected. **C,** The composite graft isolated on the deep circumflex iliac vessels. **D,** The graft shaped and ready for revascularization.

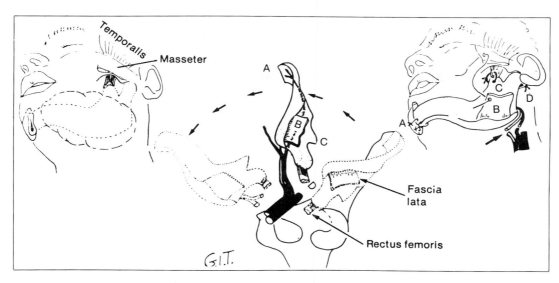

Fig. 14-7. Patient I. Diagram of the procedure showing the soft tissue and bony refinements used to reconstruct the chin *(A)*, to reattach the muscles of mastication *(B* and *C)*, and to reconstitute the capsule of the temporomandibular joint *(D)*.

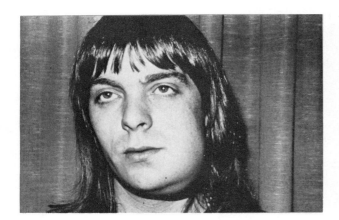

Fig. 14-8. Patient I. The problem.

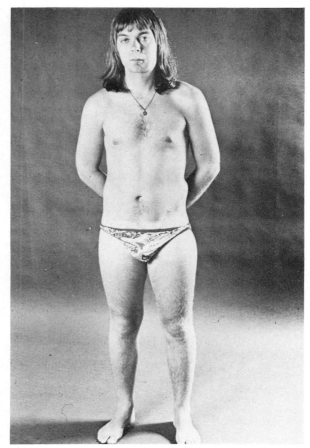

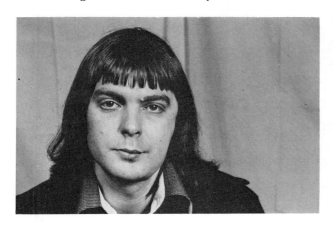

Fig. 14-9. Patient I. The final result.

Fig. 14-10. Patient I. The donor site morbidity.

Patient II

A 20-year-old male was seen by us 9 years after an extended left hemimandibulectomy with a deformity of both jaws and the associated soft tissue (Fig. 14-13). At 6 years of age the patient had had a sarcoma of the left lower lip removed and irradiated. At 11 years of age he developed an osteosarcoma of the left mandible that required resection of the jaw and associated soft tissues, crossing the midline to the opposite canine tooth. Seven years later he developed a radionecrotic ulcer over his left carotid vessels that was resected and repaired with a deltopectoral flap. There was no evidence of tumor recurrence.

During the 9-year period after his jaw resection, the right mandibular fragment had deviated to the left side, and this was associated with a similar growth deformity of his upper jaw. The plan this time was to correct the position of the lower jaw fragment, to replace the missing mandible and soft tissues with a composite graft from the same hip, and then to institute appropriate orthodontics to the maxilla to correct his dental occlusion.

The procedure was similar to that used for patient I, but with the following refinements (Fig. 14-11). The rim of the iliac crest was discarded to provide a more accurate replica of the jaw. A wedge osteotomy was made, incorporating a small keystone of bone to restore precise

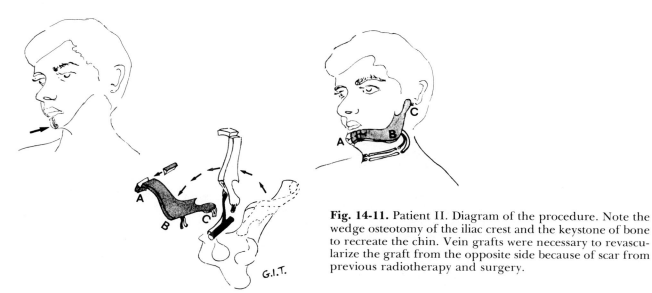

Fig. 14-11. Patient II. Diagram of the procedure. Note the wedge osteotomy of the iliac crest and the keystone of bone to recreate the chin. Vein grafts were necessary to revascularize the graft from the opposite side because of scar from previous radiotherapy and surgery.

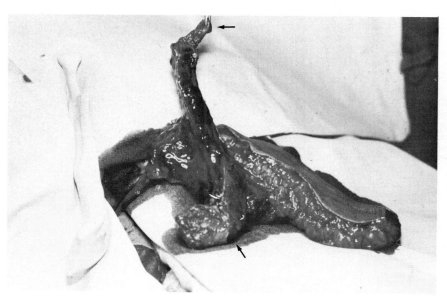

Fig. 14-12. Patient II. Graft contoured to shape while still attached in the groin by its vascular pedicle. Note the segment of rectus femoris tendon and the osteotomy of the bone *(arrows)* as well as the methylmethacrylate model used in planning.

chin contour. The coronoid process was omitted from the design because it was found to "snag" in the scarred tissues, and the skin flap was used this time for external cover to replace the relative shortage of skin over the left jaw. Finally vein grafts were planned to vascularize the graft to the facial vessels in the opposite side of the neck.

A methylmethacrylate model was used to check the shape and size of the graft. The bone was contoured with a small oscillating saw and dental burrs after reflecting periosteum from appropriate areas of the outer cortex and rim of the iliac crest. Care was taken to preserve the medial periosteum, especially at the osteotomy site. This was done by sectioning the outer cortex and making a greenstick fracture of the inner table. The small

keystone of bone was then wired in position. All of these maneuvers were accomplished while the graft was still attached by its vascular pedicle (Fig. 14-12). This confirmed the viability of its constituent parts and minimized the ischemic time after transfer.

The graft was transferred, secured in position, vascularized, and held with intermaxillary fixation. Because the corrected lower jaw was now in malocclusion with the deviated upper jaw, external support was provided by constructing a box frame between the mandible and the frontal bone. This was retained for 5 weeks. The skin flap was thinned subsequently at 3 and 4 months (Fig. 14-13), and the donor site, again, was a linear scar.

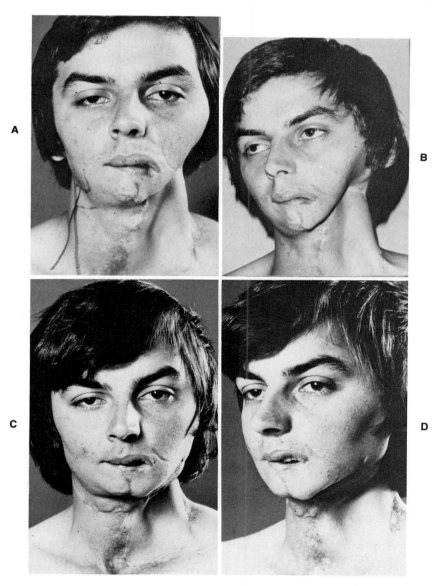

Fig. 14-13. Patient II. Preoperative problem compared in anteroposterior (**A**) and lateral (**B**) views with the postoperative result (**C** and **D**) at 6 months.

Patient III

A 54-year-old male was seen by us with recurrent squamous carcinoma of the floor of the mouth, which followed three previous attempts at excision (Figs. 14-14 and 14-15). The last procedure had included reconstruction of the mandible across the midline with a metal prosthesis, together with a block dissection of the left neck (Fig. 14-14, left).

A massive resection was required this time, including skin between the lower lip and the hyoid bone, the base and anterior segment of the tongue, the jaw prosthesis, and the entire mandible except the right ramus (Fig. 14-16).

Reconstruction was done as a primary procedure. The graft was planned from the ipsilateral hip along the lines already described (Fig. 14-14). The skin flap measured 28 by 15 cm, and the bone graft, which measured 21 by 7 cm, included the entire iliac crest. This time the chin contour was recreated with a step osteotomy in the iliac crest, which corrected its curvature in two planes. This was facilitated by a careful subperiosteal exposure of the osteotomy sites and the inclusion of a small, rectangular-shaped keystone of bone that was wired into position.

The graft was detached, transferred, and secured in place. The muscles of mastication were reattached and the capsule of the temporomandibular joint was reconstituted on the left side. The bone graft was wired to the right ramus at its angle and the graft was revascularized with vein grafts, crossing the midline to the right facial vessels. The mucosa of the floor of the mouth was closed directly (although an additional skin flap had been designed for this purpose), and the skin flap was sutured into the external defect. The graft was then immobilized with external pins, and a box frame, as before, was necessary because of the size and weight of the graft.

A bone scan and bone biopsies taken on either side of the osteotomy on the fifth postoperative day confirmed the viability of the entire graft (Fig. 14-17). At 6 weeks the external fixation was removed, at which time there was clinical union of the bone. The skin flap was thinned on two occasions at 3 and 5 months (Fig. 14-18). Sixteen months after resection of the tumor, the patient remains free of recurrence. He has very good chin contour, speech, oral continence, and jaw function.

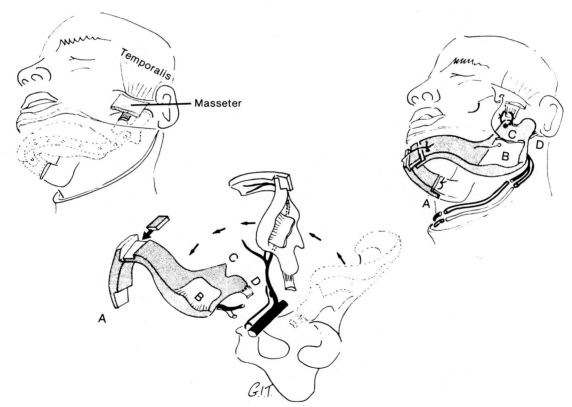

Fig. 14-14. Patient III. Diagram of the procedure. Entire mandible has been reconstructed except the right ramus using a step osteotomy and an appropriate keystone of bone to obtain the correct chin curvature. Vein grafts were necessary again to revascularize the graft from the opposite side of the neck. Note the previous jaw reconstruction with a metal prosthesis *(left)*. The soft tissue and bone refinements *(A, B, C, D)* are the same as for patient III.

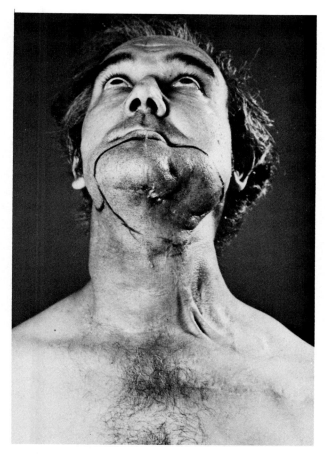

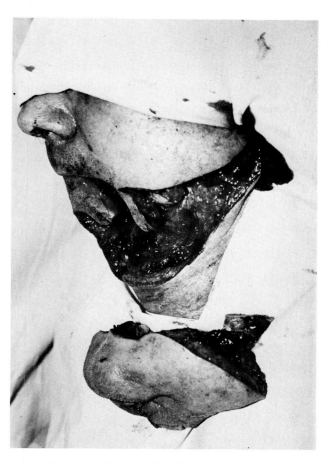

Fig. 14-15. Patient III. Preoperative problem showing recurrent squamous cell carcinoma with fistula into the floor of the mouth and the margins of skin excision.

Fig. 14-16. Patient III. The tumor resected.

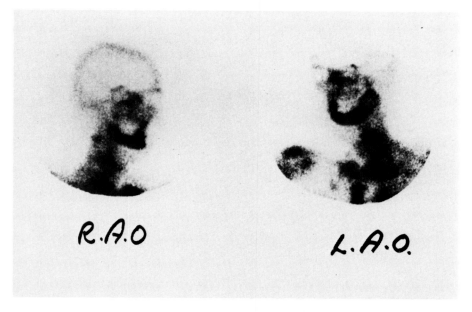

Fig. 14-17. Patient III. Bone scan on fifth postoperative day showing uptake in the graft on both sides of the osteotomy.

Fig. 14-18. A and **B,** Patient III. The result at 12 months. The flap has been thinned on two occasions.

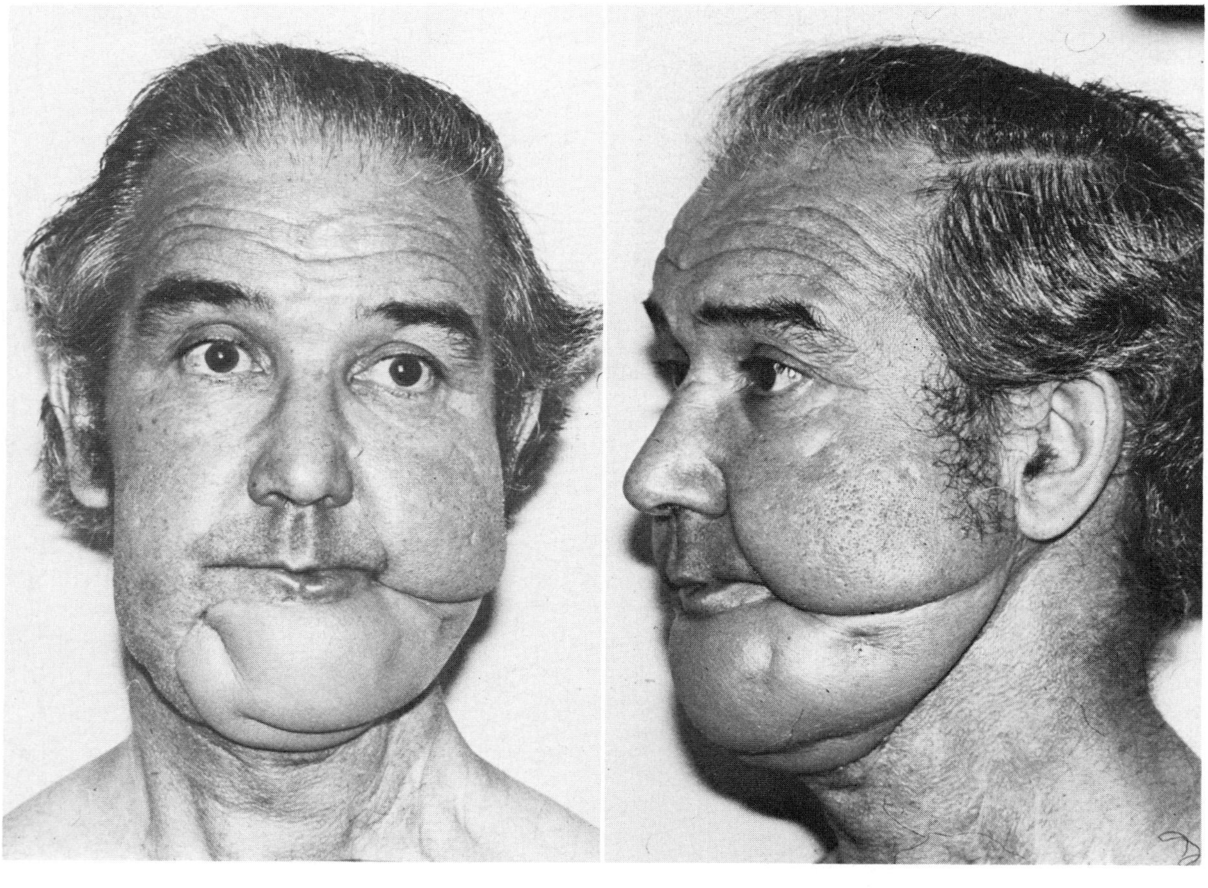

Patient IV

A 13-year-old female was seen by us with right hemi-facial microsomia, which was associated with an incomplete facial palsy on the same side (Figs. 14-19 and 14-20). The right ramus and a portion of the body of the mandible were absent; the ear and right maxilla were underdeveloped and the soft tissues of the right side of the face were deficient. Two previous attempts at reconstruction (a Silastic block spacer at 2 years of age and a conventional costochondral graft at 11 years of age) had been extruded as a result of infection.

A vascularized graft was planned to minimize the risk of infection and to reconstruct her soft tissue and bony problem in one stage. The operation was performed in August 1980.

The overgrowth of the left side of the mandible was corrected with a sagittal osteotomy to bring the chin to the midline, and a socket was contoured for the temporomandibular joint on the right side. Fortunately we knew from electrical studies that her right facial nerve was absent, and the residual function of the right facial muscles resulted from innervation from the opposite side.

A replacement for the absent segment of the mandible was then designed from the right hip. Because of her age we decided to split the apophysis along the iliac crest, together with the underlying bone, to retain normal hip development and to provide a possible growth center for the jaw. The ramus of the mandible was designed this time from the inner cortex of the iliac crest and, in addition, included a flap of apophyseal cartilage to cap the new head of the mandible. The skin flap was deepithelialized to fill out the facial contour (Fig. 14-20).

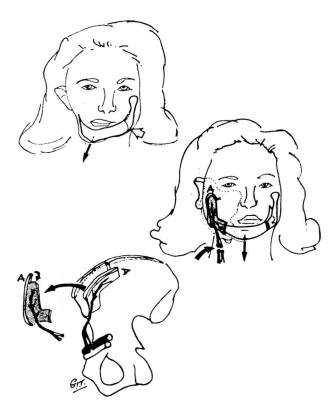

Fig. 14-19. Patient IV. The operative procedure. A sagittal osteotomy is made on the left side of the mandible to bring the chin to the midline. The right ramus and body of the jaw are designed from the inner cortex of the hip, leaving the outer surface for normal hip contour. The epiphysis has been split longitudinally and a portion of it turned as a flap to cap the new head of the mandible (A). The skin flap is deepithelialized to fill out the soft tissue contour of the face (*dotted lines*) and the graft revascularized to the facial vessels.

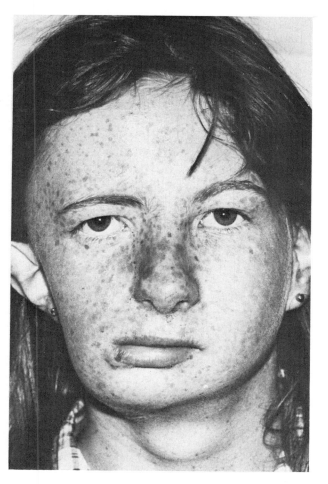

Fig. 14-20. Patient IV. Preoperative problem. Note incomplete right facial palsy.

This composite graft was isolated on the deep circumflex iliac vessels and transferred to the face. The bone graft was wired to the tapered right body of the mandible, and secured into the new temporomandibular joint with sutures to the soft tissues. The jaw was then immobilized with intermaxillary fixation, incorporating a bite plate to compensate for the underdeveloped right maxilla.

The graft was revascularized by anastomoses to the facial vessels, and the shaved skin flap was inset to fill out the facial contour, leaving a small area of its skin exposed to monitor the microvascular repairs. The donor site was closed directly. The postoperative course was uneventful, and there was clinical union of the bone graft at 5 weeks.

At 12 months there was good correction of facial symmetry, and the hip contour and function were normal (Figs. 14-21 and 14-22). No attempt has been made to correct her facial palsy.

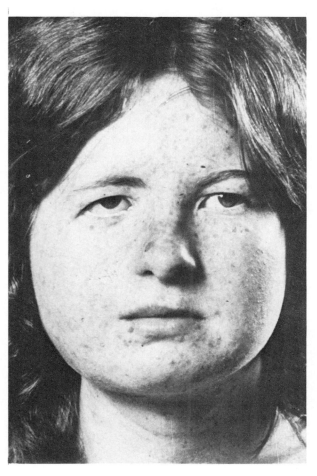

Fig. 14-21. Patient IV. Postoperative result at 12 months.

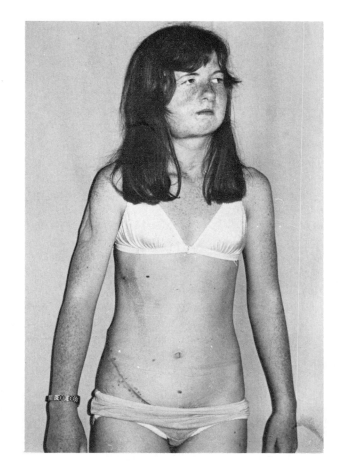

Fig. 14-22. Patient IV. Donor site scar at 4 months. Note normal hip contour.

DISCUSSION

In the last 10 years at the Royal Melbourne Hospital, 120 patients have had resection of a portion of their mandible for carcinoma or sarcoma. Of these, five have had reconstruction with conventional bone grafts and eight with free vascularized grafts. Obviously we have been highly selective in our indications for these operations, and to date we have reserved the sophisticated microvascular procedures for those patients with massive soft tissue and bony defects or for those cases in which conventional procedures had failed.

The main advantage of the free osteocutaneous graft, when it is designed on the deep circumflex iliac vessels, is the availability of a large block of composite tissue that, for jaw reconstruction, has the potential for repairing in one stage the bone, the lining, the external skin, and the other soft tissue attachments of the mandible to provide not only an aesthetic but a functional result. The other advantages are as follows:

1. The vessels are large, with diameters in excess of 2 mm, and the pedicle is long (5 to 7 cm), thus facilitating the microvascular repairs.
2. Virtually the whole iliac crest and the blade of the ilium are nourished from this stem, and, because the blood supply reaches it from its medial cortex, it is possible to remove bone from the outer surface, split the hip, or perform various osteotomies to provide an exact replica of the mandible. No other bone in the body has this potential for reconstruction of the jaw.
3. The soft tissue pedicle affords considerable flexibility to the skin flap with relation to the underlying bone. Because of this the skin flap can be rotated for lining or cover, or alternatively a strip of skin can be deepithelialized to repair both epithelial surfaces during one procedure.
4. The inclusion of other structures in the graft design that have a common blood supply—for example, fascia lata and rectus femoris tendon—allows such refinements as masticatory muscle reattachment and joint capsule repair. Hence a functional result of high standard can be achieved.
5. Despite removal of a large volume of soft tissue and bone, the donor site morbidity is remarkably small—namely a linear scar and slight contour deformity of the hip. This is of paramount importance, especially if the procedure should fail.

Nevertheless, the procedure has certain disadvantages, and these must be taken into account when assessing the individual problem:

1. The procedures are demanding of time and personnel and require a specialized center with the staff and facilities to return the patient to the operating room immediately if the anastomoses should fail. Ideally the reconstruction should be done as a primary procedure with two surgical teams—one to remove the tumor and one to repair the defect. In our small series of patients the operations have ranged from 7½ to 10 hours. However, with experience these times should diminish.
2. The color match between the groin and the face is poor, but it is preferable, in our opinion, to scarring the forehead if this is the alternative.
3. The subcutaneous layer of the abdomen, especially in obese patients, coupled with the obligatory volume of muscle necessary to preserve the cutaneous perforators, is an embarrassment that results in a bulky graft. Because of this most of our cases have required secondary procedures to thin the soft tissues. Nevertheless, the subsequent operations are relatively minor; the patients can be discharged from the hospital between operations continent of saliva, and the final results to date have been most encouraging.
4. Although the successes can be spectacular, so also may be the failures. The result, potentially, is an "all or none" phenomenon. Hence to date the majority of cases selected have been patients who were young, for whom the prognosis was very good, or for whom the alternative was depressing.

SUMMARY

In conclusion, this chapter elaborates on our new technique of one-stage reconstruction of the soft tissues and bone of the lower jaw. It uses a living composite graft of groin skin and iliac bone, designed on the deep circumflex iliac vessels and transferred by microvascular techniques. The series is small and carefully selected, but the results so far have been most encouraging. Further experience is necessary to fully assess the worth of this operation and to integrate this technique into the reconstructive surgeon's armamentarium.

REFERENCES

1. Manchester, W.M.: Some technical improvements in the reconstruction of the mandible and temporomandibular joint, Plast. Reconstr. Surg. **50:**249, 1972.
2. Taylor, G.I.: Reconstruction of the mandible with free composite iliac bone grafts, Ann. Plast. Surg. **9**(5):361, 1982.
3. Taylor, G.I., and Corlett, R.: Refinements of the free iliac osteocutaneous flap designed on the deep circumflex iliac vessels, Plast. Surg. Forum **111:**185, 1980.
4. Taylor, G.I., and Daniel, R.K.: Aesthetic aspects of microsurgery: composite tissue transfer to the face, Clin. Plast. Surg. **8:**333, 1981.
5. Taylor, G.I., Townsend, P., and Corlett, R.: Superiority of the deep circumflex iliac vessels as the supply for free groin flaps; clinical work, Plast. Reconstr. Surg. **64:**745, 1979.
6. Taylor, G.I., Townsend, P., and Corlett, R.: Superiority of the deep circumflex iliac vessels as the supply for free groin flaps; experimental work, Plast. Reconstr. Surg. **64:**595, 1979.

Chapter 15

Reconstruction of the cheek

Toyomi Fujino

Functional reconstruction of the cheek is desirable for both aesthetic and psychologic reasons after resection of a tumor of the soft tissue in the young adult or after maxillectomy and orbital exenteration for cancer of the maxillary sinus. Although many surgical procedures have been reported, a one-stage method of reconstruction is preferable to promote early rehabilitation and a short hospitalization. One-stage coverage of a total cheek defect, with the use of simultaneous temporal and deltopectoral flaps for cover and lining, has been popular.[8] Recently a trapezius musculocutaneous island flap was also reported as a useful technique.[1] However, this is often too short to reach the upper orbit and does not provide good function. We will report primary and secondary functional reconstructive methods.

PRIMARY FUNCTIONAL RECONSTRUCTION

A 20-year-old female was referred to us with a malignant lesion of short duration of her left cheek.[5] A biopsy showed a low grade fibrosarcoma of the soft tissues and skin (Fig. 15-1).

A wide en-bloc resection of the cheek lesion, together with the underlying facial muscles and branches of the facial nerve, was performed (Fig. 15-2). Frozen sections of the excised specimen showed clearance of the lesion, and the submandibular nodes were uninvolved. We therefore decided to carry out primary functional reconstruction of the cheek defect with a free, reinnervated latissimus dorsi neurovascular myocutaneous flap.

We designed and dissected the free flap, taking care to preserve the neurovascular bundle (Fig. 15-3). Microvascular anastomoses between the thoracodorsal and facial arteries and veins were done, followed by an epineural suture between the thoracodorsal nerve and buccal branch of the facial nerve.

The postoperative course was uneventful, but as a precaution we gave the patient a 12-month course of cytotoxic antitumor drugs: 1-(s-tetrahydrofuryl)-5-fluorouracil (Futraful) and a protein-bound polysaccharide preparation, PS-K, isolated from coriolus versicolor (Krestin).

One month after surgery the patient noted some movement of the upper lip; 3 months later she showed almost normal facial movement. Electromyographic studies confirmed progressive return of facial movement (Fig. 15-4), and biopsy of the transplanted muscle and adipose tissue showed an almost normal histologic picture (Fig. 15-5). It is now over 2 years since the procedure; the patient has a satisfactory functional return of facial movements and no demonstrated tumor recurrence (Fig. 15-6).

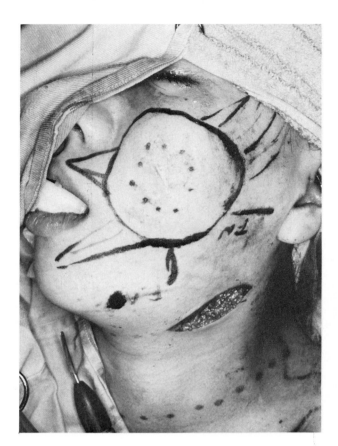

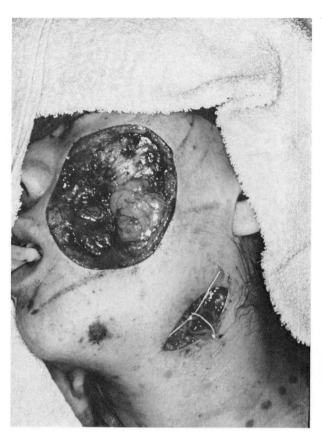

Fig. 15-1. View of the left cheek at operation. Inner dotted circle outlines the area of induration; continuous circle indicates the planned excision; triangular extensions indicate the muscle insertions in the temporal and labial regions. (From Fujino, T., Maruyama, Y., and Yoshimura, Y.: Primary functional cheek reconstruction: a case report, Br. J. Plast. Surg. **34:**136, 1981.)

Fig. 15-2. Defect in the left cheek after wide resection of the lesion. Adequacy of the excision was confirmed by frozen section of the specimen. (From Fujino, T., Maruyama, Y., and Yoshimura, Y.: Primary functional cheek reconstruction: a case report, Br. J. Plast. Surg. **34:**136, 1981.)

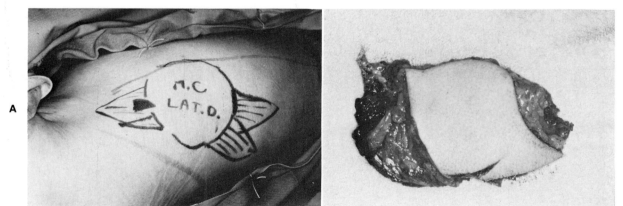

Fig. 15-3. A, Outline markings for a free latissimus dorsi myocutaneous flap, 10 by 7 cm, showing the separate muscle segments used to rejoin the divided and excised muscle segments in the cheek. **B,** The latissimus dorsi myocutaneous flap lying free before its transfer to the facial defect. (From Fujino, T., Maruyama, Y., and Yoshimura, Y.: Primary functional cheek reconstruction: a case report, Br. J. Plast. Surg. **34:**136, 1981).

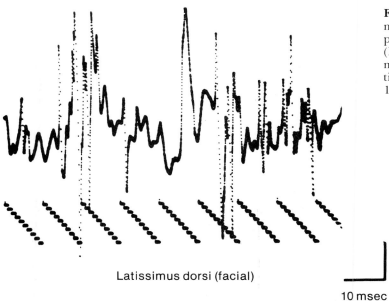

Latissimus dorsi (facial)

100 μV

10 msec

Fig. 15-4. Electromyographic tracing at maximum voluntary contraction made 4 months postoperatively shows good motor activity. (From Fujino, T., Maruyama, Y., and Yoshimura, Y.: Primary functional cheek reconstruction: a case report, Br. J. Plast. Surg. **34:**136, 1981).

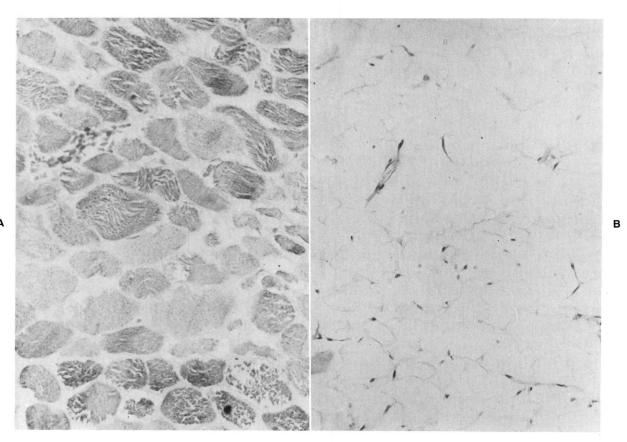

A   B

Fig. 15-5. Biopsy of the transplanted muscle **(A)** and subcutaneous adipose tissue **(B)** 4 months after the operation shows normal cellular structure. (From Fujino, T., Maruyama, Y., and Yoshimura, Y.: Primary functional cheek reconstruction: a case report, Br. J. Plast. Surg. **34:**136, 1981).

Fig. 15-6. A and **B,** Nine months after surgery. There is a good range of facial movement; at rest the mouth is symmetric. (From Fujino, T., Maruyama, Y., and Yoshimura, Y.: Primary functional cheek reconstruction: a case report, Br. J. Plast. Surg. **34:**136, 1981).

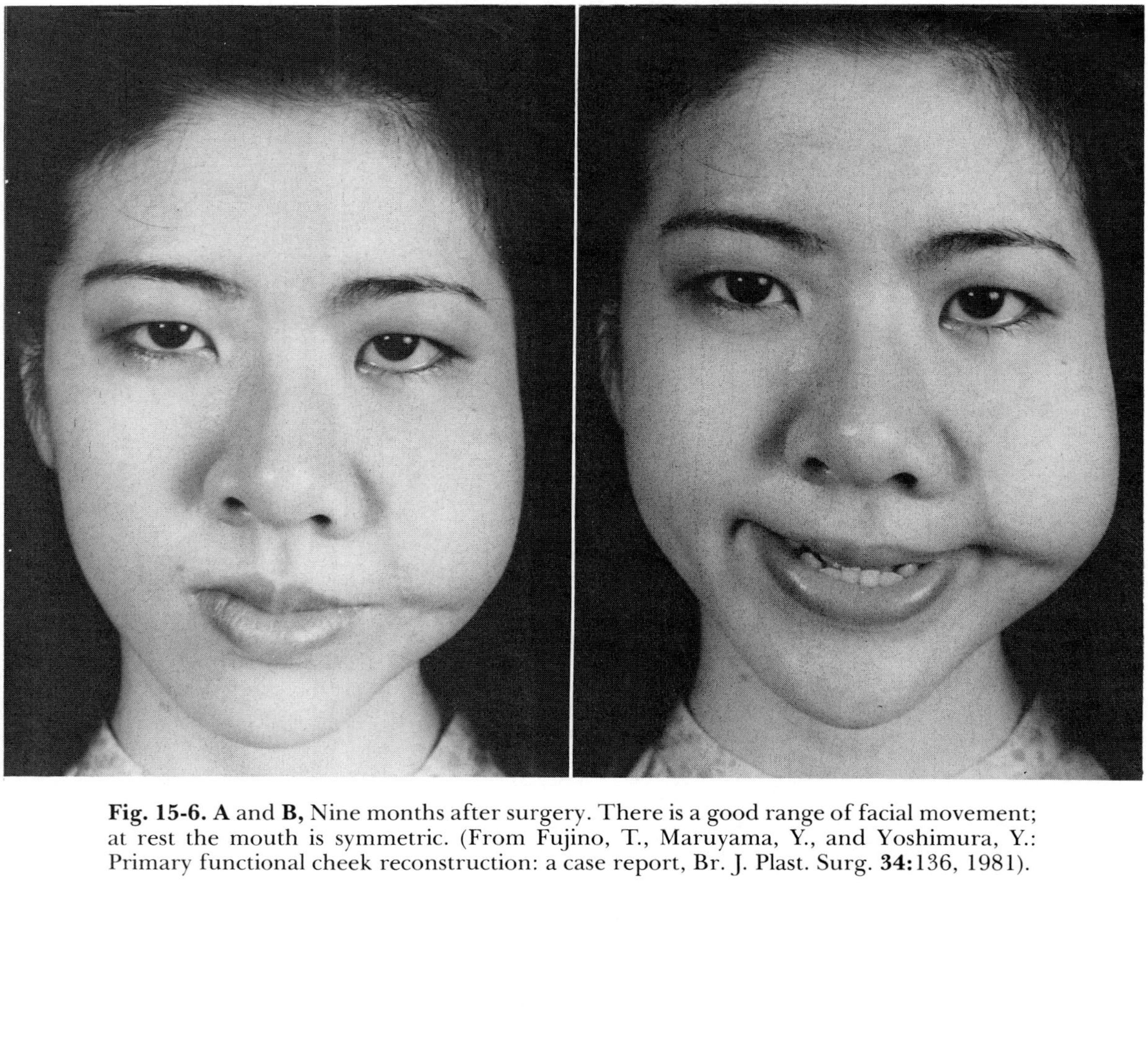

SECONDARY FUNCTIONAL RECONSTRUCTION

A 56-year-old male was initially seen with a history of epistaxis of 3 months' duration.[6] A biopsy revealed a squamous cell carcinoma of the maxillary sinus. After preoperative irradiation (with a total dose of 6,000 rads), he underwent a total maxillectomy with orbital exenteration. Six months postoperatively we carried out cheek reconstruction (Fig. 15-7). Four days before surgery an angiographic study identified the facial artery (2 mm in diameter) and the course of the thoracodorsal artery (Fig. 15-8).

A general anesthetic was administered, and reconstructive surgery was performed. The palatal defect was covered with a turnover flap from the adjacent lower cheek region. The mucosa and scar tissue covering the maxillary cavity were excised. The buccal branches of the facial nerve were identified and preserved for epineural suture. The facial artery and vein were prepared.

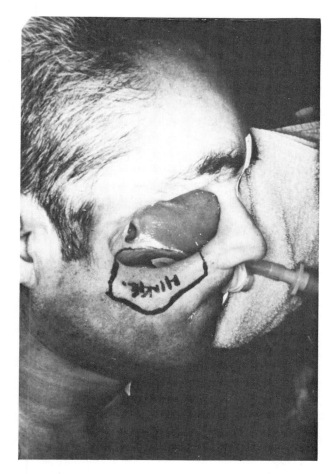

Fig. 15-7. A 56-year-old male after radical maxillectomy with orbital exenteration. Palatal defect is covered with a turnover flap (solid line). (From Fujino, T., Maruyama, Y., and Inuyama, I.: Double folded free myocutaneous flap to cover a total cheek defect, J. Maxillofac. Surg. **9:**73, 1981.)

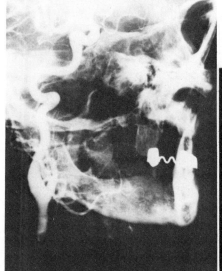

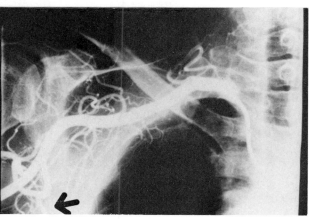

Fig. 15-8. Preoperative angiography. **A,** Good-sized recipient facial artery was identified. **B,** Thoracodorsal artery as the donor was identified *(arrow)*. (From Fujino, T., Maruyama, Y., and Inuyama, I.: Double folded free myocutaneous flap to cover a total cheek defect, J. Maxillofac. Surg. **9:**73, 1981.)

At the same time we designed a free latissimus dorsi myocutaneous flap (Fig. 15-9). The overlying skin (16 by 7 cm) was sufficient to cover the outer surface of the cheek defect and the lateral wall of the nasal cavity. We dissected the free latissimus dorsi myocutaneous flap, with its nutrient thoracodorsal vessels and nerve attached. The skin island was incised down to the level of the muscle layer to permit doubling of the flap (Fig. 15-10).

Microneurovascular anastomosis was performed. The recipient buccal branch of the facial nerve was stimulated with a nerve stimulator near the anastomosis, and, interestingly, the transplant-ed muscle contracted well (Fig. 15-11). First the lateral wall of the nasal cavity and then the cheek defect were reconstructed (Fig. 15-12). Viability of both skin surfaces was confirmed by a fluorescein technique.

Two weeks postoperatively the patient was discharged after intranasal examination revealed complete survival of the folded surface of the flap (Fig. 15-13). One month after surgery computed tomography showed a complete survival of the folded flap (Fig. 15-14). Two months after surgery both donor and recipient areas were doing well (Fig. 15-15).

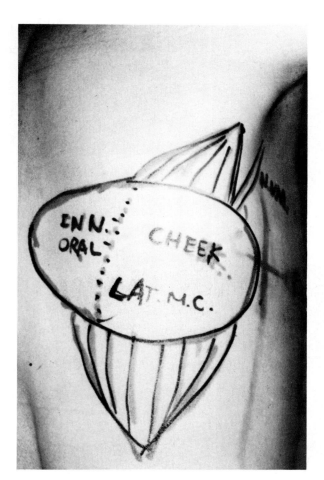

Fig. 15-9. Design of the folded free myocutaneous flap (16 by 7 cm). (From Fujino, T., Maruyama, Y., and Inuyama, I.: Double folded free myocutaneous flap to cover a total cheek defect, J. Maxillofac. Surg. **9:**73, 1981.)

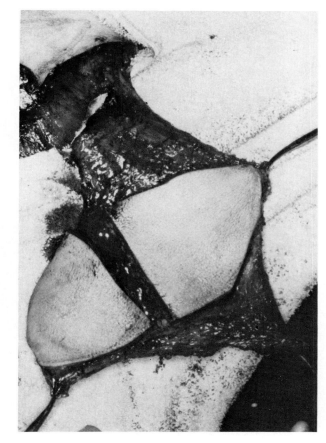

Fig. 15-10. Flap incised down to the level of the muscle layer. (From Fujino, T., Maruyama, Y., and Inuyama, I.: Double folded free myocutaneous flap to cover a total cheek defect, J. Maxillofac. Surg. **9:**73, 1981.)

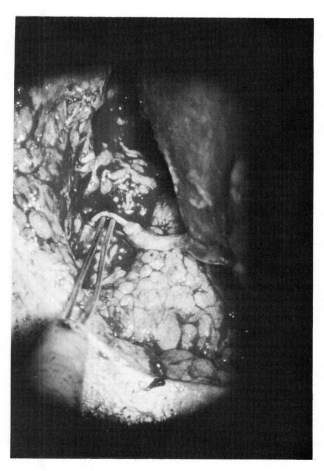

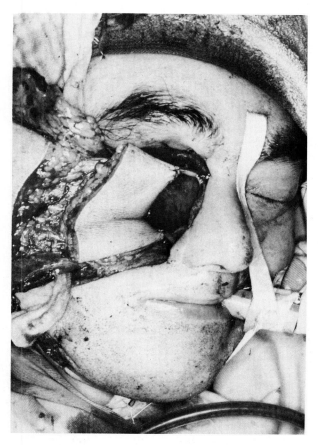

Fig. 15-11. Epineural sutures completed. Distal portion of the facial nerve near the anastomosis site was stimulated with a nerve stimulator, showing immediate contraction of the transplanted muscle. (From Fujino, T., Maruyama, Y., and Inuyama, I.: Double folded free myocutaneous flap to cover a total cheek defect, J. Maxillofac. Surg. **9:**73, 1981.)

Fig. 15-12. Folded free flap first sutured to the lateral deep wall of the nasal cavity. (From Fujino, T., Maruyama, Y., and Inuyama, I.: Double folded free myocutaneous flap to cover a total cheek defect, J. Maxillofac. Surg. **9:**73, 1981.)

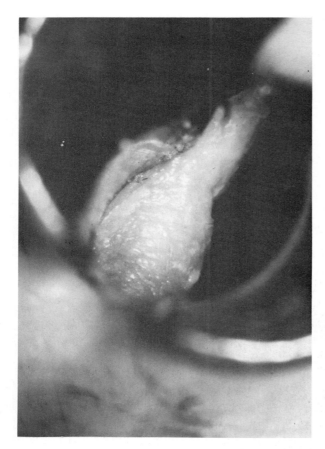

Fig. 15-13. Intranasal examination of the folded free myocutaneous flap showed pink-colored skin. (From Fujino, T., Maruyama, Y., and Inuyama, I.: Double folded free myocutaneous flap to cover a total cheek defect, J. Maxillofac. Surg. **9:**73, 1981.)

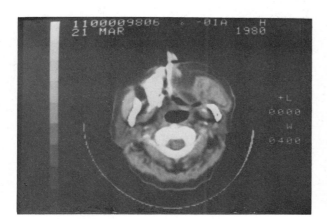

Fig. 15-14. Computed tomography at 1 month after surgery showed a complete take of the free flap. (From Fujino, T., Maruyama, Y., and Inuyama, I.: Double folded free myocutaneous flap to cover a total cheek defect, J. Maxillofac. Surg. **9:**73, 1981.)

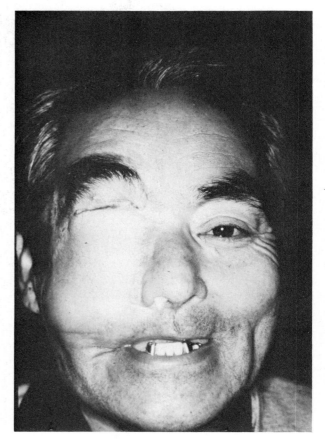

Fig. 15-15. Appearance 1 year after surgery. The free myocutaneous flap showed a complete take and the patient had a normal range of shoulder movement and regained some function. (From Fujino, T., Maruyama, Y., and Inuyama, I.: Double folded free myocutaneous flap to cover a total cheek defect, J. Maxillofac. Surg. **9:**73, 1981.)

DISCUSSION

The restoration of good facial movement is a major goal in reconstructive facial surgery. The free myocutaneous flap with neurovascular anastomoses seems to offer more natural facial expression, because the strong action of the transplanted muscle is cushioned by the overlying layer of subcutaneous adipose tissue.

The free neurovascular myocutaneous flap gained a satisfactory functional return despite a 12-month course of cancer chemotherapy. Thus chemotherapy is not a contraindication to reconstruction.

Reconstruction of a total cheek defect after radical maxillectomy with orbital exenteration in one stage is one of the most difficult procedures in head and neck reconstructive surgery. To reach the upper portion of the orbital region, a long, pedicled deltopectoral skin flap is necessary, requiring a delay procedure because the tip of the flap is a random-pattern flap. The trapezius island flap seems to work satisfactorily, but the anterior portion of the floor of the mouth and the chin are too remote to be reached by this flap. Therefore a free flap transfer with a minimal amount of donor sacrifice is the procedure of choice.

In considering a free flap transfer, we must assess the potential recipient vessels with preoperative angiography because the usual recipient vessels are often sacrificed in a radical neck dissection or injured by irradiation or infusion of chemotherapeutic drugs. We have performed preoperative angiography between 1 and 7 days before surgery with no problem. (The diameter of the anastomosed vessels has been larger than 1.5 mm in these cases.)

To provide both cover and lining, the skin of the free flap must be folded. The skin of the free myocutaneous flap can safely be incised down to the level of the muscle layer as long as the circulation of the segmental muscular vessel is unimpaired (Fig. 15-15).

Previously we transferred a free myocutaneous flap without nerve anastomosis.[2,3] Two years postoperatively a muscle biopsy showed slightly degenerated muscle striae, although morphologically the volume of the transplanted muscle had been maintained.[6] We now feel that the motor nerve should be repaired, not only to maintain bulk but also to regain function.[7]

SUMMARY

Subtotal and total defects of the cheek following the resection of a malignant tumor have been reconstructed with satisfactory functional recovery by a single- and double-folded free neurovascular latissimus dorsi myocutaneous flap.

REFERENCES

1. Bertotti, J.A.: Trapezius musculocutaneous island flap in the repair of major head and neck cancer, Plast. Reconstr. Surg. 65:16, 1980.
2. Fujino, T.: Reconstruction for aplasia of the breast and pectoral region by microvascular transfer of a free flap from the buttock, Plast. Reconstr. Surg. 56:178, 1975.
3. Fujino, T.: Primary breast reconstruction after a standard radical mastectomy by a free flap transfer, Plast. Reconstr. Surg. 58:371, 1976.
4. Fujino, T.: Double-folded free myocutaneous flap to cover a total cheek defect, J. Maxillofac. Surg. 2:73, 1981.
5. Fujino, T.: Primary functional cheek reconstruction: a case report, Br. J. Plast. Surg. 34:136, 1981.
6. Fujino, T.: Primary reconstruction of the breast by free myocutaneous gluteal flap, Int. Adv. Surg. Oncol. 4:127, 1981.
7. Maruyama, Y.: Free latissimus dorsi myocutaneous flaps in the dynamic reconstruction of cheek defects: a preliminary report, J. Microsurg. 1:231, 1979.
8. McGregor, I.A., and Reid, W.H.: Simultaneous temporal and deltopectoral flaps for full thickness defects of the cheek, Plast. Reconstr. Surg. 45:326, 1970.

Chapter 16

Reconstruction of the nose: tribulations

Douglas H. Harrison
Brian D.G. Morgan
Willi Boeckx

Squamous cell carcinomas that are treated by irradiation and then inadequately excised can leave a small nidus of tumor cells embedded in fibrous tissue that may remain clinically dormant for years. The standard 18-month delay before reconstruction may well prove inadequate. If a free flap has been used for the reconstruction and there is definitely no evidence of invasion of the free flap, then it is possible to disconnect it from the recipient area and "park it" at a distant site until a further treatment program for the tumor has been implemented. The free flap is then available for a further reconstruction once the tumor has been eradicated.

CASE REPORT

A 58-year-old male had developed a squamous cell carcinoma of the nose many years before that had been treated by irradiation and excision. On three occasions further excisions of recurrent squamous cell carcinoma were carried out, followed on each occasion, 18 months or more later, by a reconstructive rhinoplasty. On the first occasion local cheek tissue was employed, on the second occasion a forehead flap was used, and on the third occasion a Tagliacozzi reconstruction was used.

When first seen in the plastic surgery unit at Mount Vernon Hospital, the patient had developed another recurrence of the tumor that necessitated removal of the reconstructed nose; closure was achieved with skin grafts (Fig. 16-1). We hoped that the patient would be satisfied with a prosthesis, but 3 years after the excision he insisted on another reconstructive rhinoplasty. A free dorsalis pedis flap was chosen as the most suitable reconstructive maneuver under the circumstances (Fig. 16-2). The lining of the flap was to be provided by a skin graft that had been cemented to a preformed intranasal prosthesis (Fig. 16-3). Before the operation there was complete epithelialization around the margins of the nasal cavity and no clinical evidence of a recurrent carcinoma. The surgery was satisfactorily performed with the dorsalis pedis flap placed over the intranasal skin graft (Fig. 16-4).

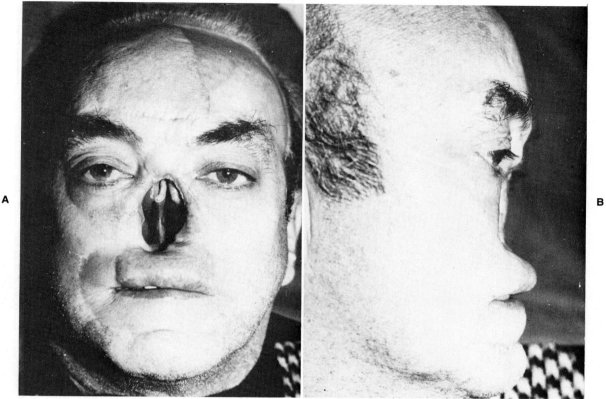

Fig. 16-1. A, Frontal view of a 58-year-old male after total excision of his nose. Scars may be seen across his forehead and face where flaps had been employed for previous nasal reconstructions. There is no evidence of ulceration around the piriform margin. **B,** Lateral view of the face showing complete loss of nasal projection.

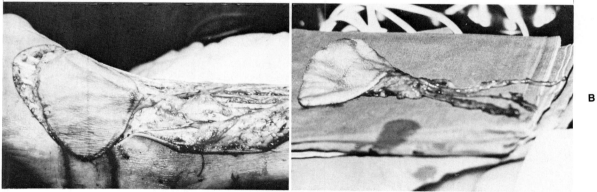

Fig. 16-2. A, Dorsalis pedis free flap being elevated from the foot, with the pedicle oriented at the future alar base. **B,** Dorsalis pedis flap disconnected from the foot, showing the length of the vascular pedicle.

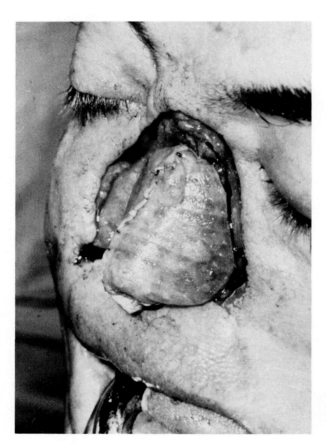

Fig. 16-3. Skin graft with its epidermal surface stuck to a preformed mould and supported on the piriform margin. The dermal surface lines the free flap transfer.

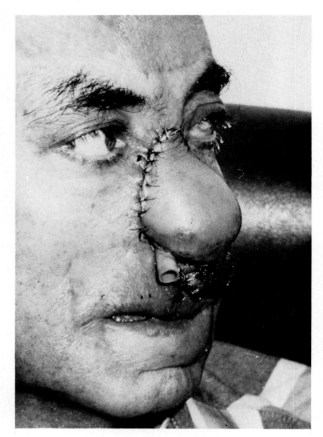

Fig. 16-4. Nasal reconstruction is complete and the dorsalis pedis flap is viable.

The early postoperative result was satisfactory and the flap remained viable. However, at the time of surgery a biopsy from the left piriform margin was sent for a histologic study. The report confirmed that squamous cell carcinoma was still present on the left side of the nose. Because it was less than a week after surgery, and clearly the flap would be unlikely to have tumor invasion, we felt it was reasonable to retain the reconstruction, but the recurrent tumor clearly needed treatment.

The dorsalis pedis flap was then disconnected from the nose, and the pedicle, which had previously been revascularized via the right facial artery, was dissected out. The flap was then transferred to the right side of the neck to await treatment of the carcinoma (Fig. 16-5). A further skin grafting procedure was required to achieve complete epithelialization. The recurrent carcinoma was treated by introducing a cannula into the left facial artery, assessing its cutaneous distribution by fluorescein staining, and then infusing a cytotoxic agent (Fig. 16-6). Tumor control was achieved by this technique, and 4 months later the dorsalis pedis flap was returned to the nose (Fig. 16-7). A satisfactory result was achieved after some final readjustments (Fig. 16-8).

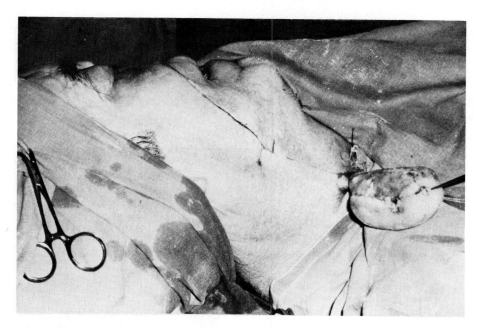

Fig. 16-5. Free flap has been removed from the recipient area on the nose and resited on the right side of the neck. Epithelialization has been achieved.

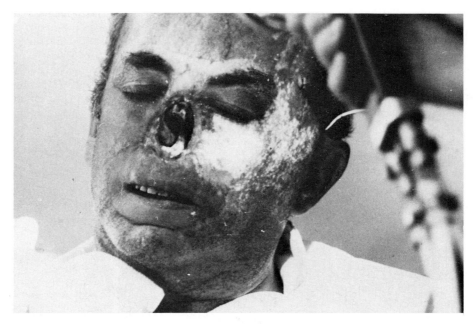

Fig. 16-6. Fluorescein staining of the left piriform margin and left cheek produced by a cannula in the left facial artery.

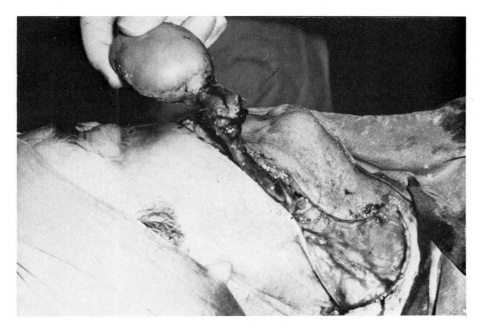

Fig. 16-7. Second reconstruction, taking the dorsalis pedis flap from the right side of the neck and replacing it on the nose.

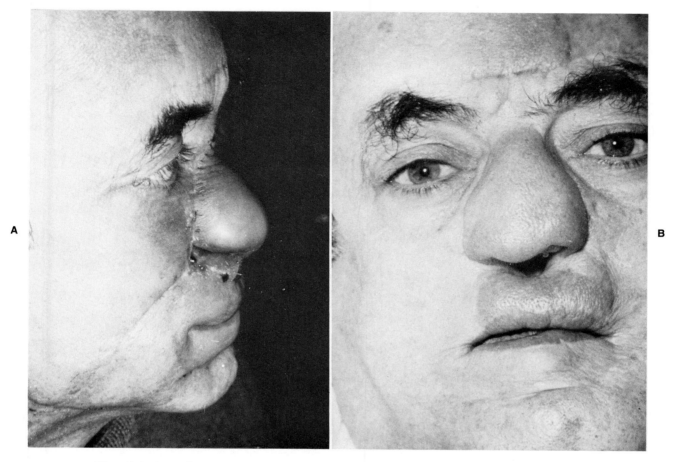

Fig. 16-8. A, Early postoperative lateral view of the nasal reconstruction. **B,** Frontal view of the nasal reconstruction 1 year after surgery.

SUMMARY

The moral of this case is clearly never to proceed to reconstruction unless you are certain that the cancer has been eradicated. However, there are occasions when, if a free flap transfer has been used, it may be stored and reused, since its vascular pedicle permits resiting at a distance from the tumor site, a maneuver not possible in cases in which a standard random pattern flap reconstruction has been employed.

Chapter 17

Microcranial surgery: microscopic control of craniofacial ostectomies and osteotomies in the treatment of congenital hypertelorism

David W. Furnas
Don R. DeFeo
John A. Kusske

We have recently used microscopic control to give precision and safety to the procedure of glabellar ostectomy and orbital craniotomies in the treatment of congenital hypertelorism in two patients.

In 1970 Edgerton et al.[3] described the glabella ostectomy as a means of correcting orbital hypertelorism without the need for a formal frontal craniotomy. We have corrected two patients with hypertelorism in whom microsurgical control was combined with the glabella ostectomy for added precision and safety. Also, we modified Edgerton's technique by moving the medial and lateral orbital walls independent of one another, a maneuver that other surgeons have used subcranially.[16]

CASE REPORT
Patient I

A hypertelorism repair with microsurgical craniotomies was carried out in a male 3 years, 9 months old with Opitz syndrome,[11] an autosomal dominant condition with hypertelorism, hypospadias, and, in 25% of cases, cleft lip–cleft palate (Fig. 17-1). The lip had been repaired at 5 months, the palate at 13 months, the short columella at 38 months, and the hypospadias at 42 months.

A preoperative cephalometric film showed a low cribriform plate and an interorbital distance of 32 mm. (The 50th percentile for his age and sex was 20 mm.[5])

Operative correction was carried out as noted under "Operating technique" (p. 142). The final interorbital distance was 16 mm. Operating time was 10 hours; 540 ml of blood was replaced (61% of the total blood volume). Drainage tubes were removed on the fifth day. The patient had a transient right abducens palsy from which he ultimately recovered. Otherwise the postoperative course was uneventful and he was discharged on the tenth postoperative day. He showed a substantial improvement from the procedure.

Fig. 17-1. A, Opitz syndrome in a 1½-year-old male: mild hypertelorism, hypospadias, and bilateral cleft lip–cleft palate. **B,** Two months after Manchester repair of cleft lip with premaxillary setback. **C,** Patient at 3½ years of age after forked flap columellar advancement and cartilage graft to nasal tip. **D,** Patient 4 months after hypertelorism repair. **E,** Posterior anterior skull radiograph 2 months before hypertelorism repair. **F,** Posterior anterior skull radiograph 2 months after hypertelorism repair.

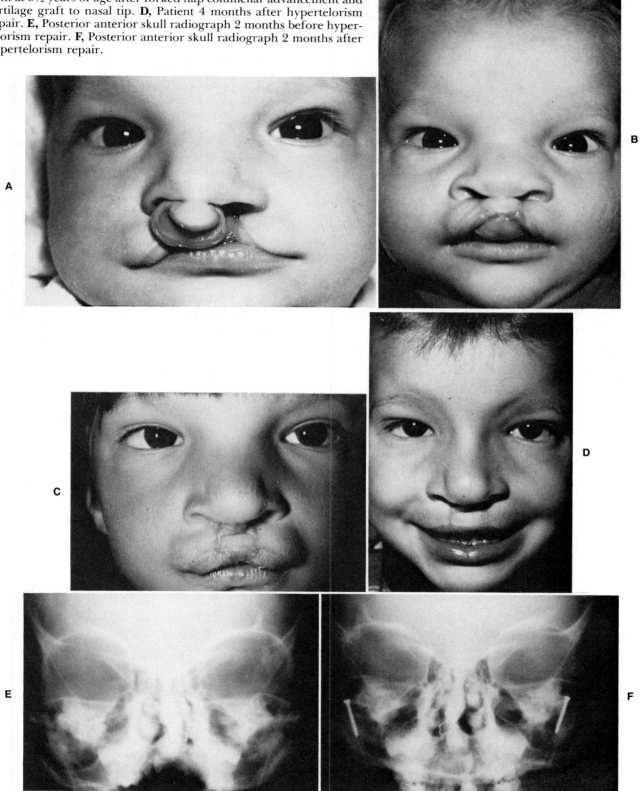

Patient II

A repair for moderately severe hypertelorism was carried out on a 12½-year-old female using a microsurgical glabellar ostectomy and orbital craniotomies (Fig. 17-2). She had been born with a severe, complete cleft of the left lip and palate. Her palate had been repaired at age 9 and the lip at age 11. She had an interorbital distance of 48 mm. (The 50th percentile for her age and sex was 24 mm.[5]) Surface anatomy showed hypertelorism that was skewed to the right. Radiographs, however, showed a wider expanse of interorbital bone on the right than on the left, as did tomography. Therefore asymmetric orbital ostectomies were planned, taking more bone on the right than on the left.

At surgery a 14 mm segment of interorbital bone was removed on the right and a 10 mm segment on the left. A 2 mm strut was left between these ostectomy sites at first, but this strut was removed early in the procedure in order to improve access for the ostectomies of the orbital roof.

Two unexpected problems added time to the operation. A large intraosseous branch of the sagittal sinus was encountered during the ostectomy. The surrounding bone was drilled away from the sinus with a diamond burr until the vessel could be controlled, a step that took several hours. Later a dural tear occurred while we were reflecting the dura from the left side of the cribriform plate. The neighboring dura was freed, and the tear was repaired with 8-0 nylon sutures, another step that required several hours.

Translocation of the medial orbital walls left gaps of 14 mm in width on the right and 10 to 11 mm on the left. The gaps were filled with split rib grafts. The final interorbital distance was 23 to 24 mm.

Nasal bone grafts were placed, the nose was narrowed, and the domes of the alar cartilages were approximated in the midline. (See "Operating technique" for details of the operation.)

On completion of the wound closures, we identified a collection of cerebrospinal fluid in the nasal wound; therefore we placed a continuous spinal drainage catheter.

Operating time was 19 hours; blood replacement was 500 ml (24% of the total blood volume).

The spinal catheter and scalp drains were removed in 1 week and no further leak was seen. The postoperative course was otherwise uneventful and the patient was discharged on the fifteenth postoperative day.

Radiographic measurements proved to be accurate for aligning the cuts with the nasal septum and the crista galli, but as the postoperative swelling subsided, undercorrection of the left orbit became obvious. Therefore 5 weeks later the patient was returned to the operating room, the left forehead flap was elevated again, the medial orbital wall was fractured inward, and the left lateral orbital wall was moved medially 4 to 5 mm further and rewired. The patient was discharged on the seventh postoperative day. No transfusions were needed.

The net effect was a major improvement in her overall appearance.

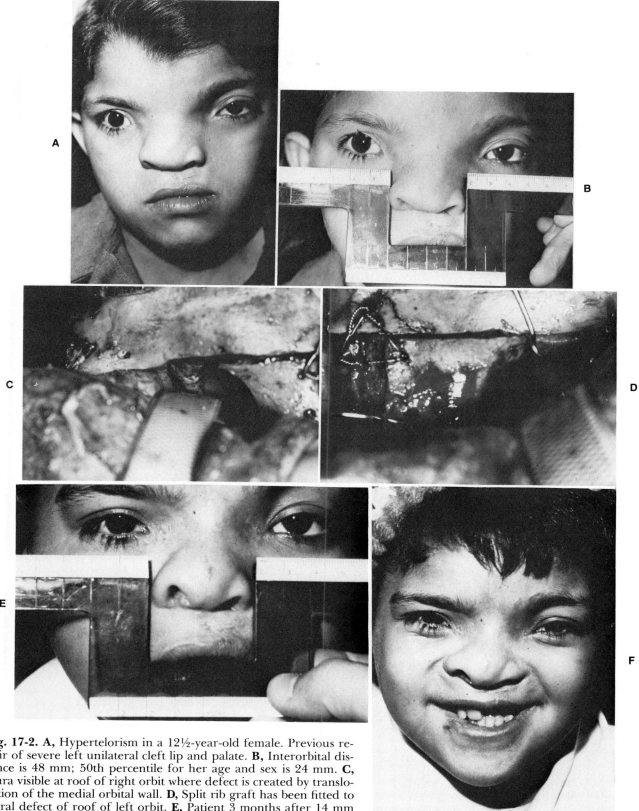

Fig. 17-2. A, Hypertelorism in a 12½-year-old female. Previous repair of severe left unilateral cleft lip and palate. **B,** Interorbital distance is 48 mm; 50th percentile for her age and sex is 24 mm. **C,** Dura visible at roof of right orbit where defect is created by translocation of the medial orbital wall. **D,** Split rib graft has been fitted to dural defect of roof of left orbit. **E,** Patient 3 months after 14 mm translocation on the right and approximately 14 mm translocation on the left. **F,** Full face 4 months postoperatively.

OPERATING TECHNIQUE (Figs. 17-3 to 17-8)

Preparation. Monitoring equipment was put in place, and the patient's head was shaved and prepared for a craniotomy.

Incision. A bicoronal incision was made from earlobe to earlobe, 1.5 cm behind the hairline. The scalp incisions were made with electrocautery to minimize blood loss. Vertical midline incisions were added for patient II for removal of excess skin.

Dissection. The forehead flap was dissected at a subgaleal level as far as the supraorbital ridge, then dissection was continued at a subperiosteal level. The temporal scalp and skin were lifted from the temporal fascia, staying beneath the upper branches of the facial nerve. Dissection was carried across the zygomatic arch and the upper part of the masseter muscle. The zygomaticofacial neurovascular bundle was divided. A 360 degree orbital dissection was carried back two thirds of the distance to the apex of the orbit. The anterior border

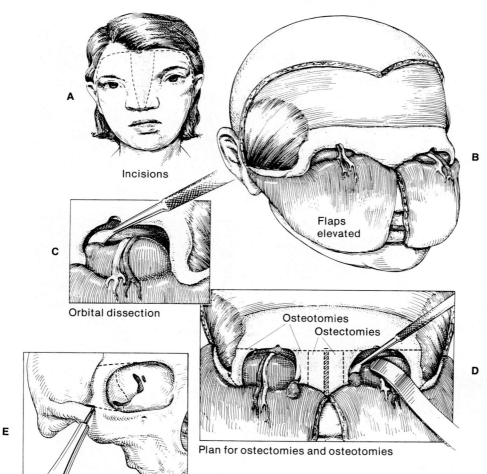

A
Incisions

B
Flaps elevated

C
Orbital dissection

D
Osteotomies
Ostectomies
Plan for ostectomies and osteotomies

E
Osteotomies of lateral orbital walls

Fig. 17-3. A, Bicoronal incision with resection of excess skin and soft tissue. **B,** Elevation of bicoronal flaps going below galea down to supraorbital ridge. Dissection of supraorbital ridge, orbits and malar arches carried out subperiosteally. **C,** Periorbita freed from wall of orbit, 360 degrees, anterior two thirds of orbits. **D,** Orbital dissection completed. Osteotomy lines placed. **E,** Cuts made in lateral orbital walls.

of the temporalis muscle was displaced posteriorly for access to the lateral orbital wall.

Osteotomies of the lateral orbital walls. Transverse cuts were made with a Midas B-3 cutter parallel and tangential to the upper and lower limits of the orbital rim. The cuts were carried posteriorly to the union of the lateral orbital wall with the cranial vault, avoiding entry into the middle fossa. The posterior part of the cut was completed with an osteotome, making a greenstick infracture.

Glabellar ostectomies. The width of the medial bone resection was determined by preoperative and intraoperative measurements. Transverse bone cuts that paralleled the upper limit of the orbital rim marked the upper limit of the ostectomies; the lower limit was the oblique free border of the pyramidal aperture. A midline segment of bone was left in front of the nasal septum and the crista galli in the first case, but none was left in the second case. The ostectomy segments were lifted out with an osteotome. The nasal mucosa was reflected downward, avoiding entry into the nasal cavity.[16]

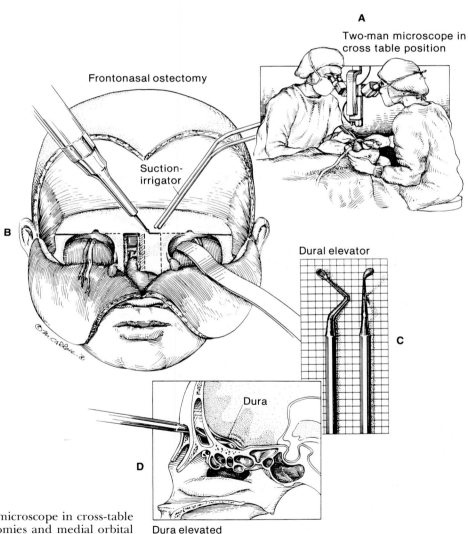

Fig. 17-4. A, Zeiss Opmi 7PH microscope in cross-table position for frontonasal ostectomies and medial orbital osteotomies. **B,** Left half of glabellar ostectomy begun. Right half completed, dura exposed. **C,** Contraangle elevator for reflecting dura. **D,** Dura is dissected posteriorly, passing elevator just lateral to the cribriform plate.

A Zeiss Opmi 7PH microscope was set up in a cross-table position. A Midas Rex air drill was used for heavier bone cuts and a Minos drill with a diamond burr was used for the ostectomies near the dura or major vessels.[13] The mucosa of the frontal sinus was identified, trimmed, and reflected downward, avoiding trapped fragments. The osteotomies were continued through the posterior wall of the frontal sinus.

Anterior fossa dissection. The dura was reflected from the floor of the anterior fossa just lateral to the cribriform plate with a small, straight elevator. The dura was reflected from the orbital plate of the frontal bone and its vertical extension with an angled elevator.

Craniectomy of excess bone bordering cribriform plate. The dura was protected with a ¼" brain retractor, and a small cutting bit was used to remove the bone just lateral to the cribriform plate. The width of the cut corresponded to the width of the segment removed from the frontonasal area.

Transverse cuts of the orbit. The dura and the orbit were protected with brain retractors, and the transverse cut was extended laterally on the frontal bone tangential to the upper border of the orbit.

Longitudinal cut of the orbital roof. Joining the transverse cut, a longitudinal cut was carried posteriorly along the roof of the orbit. It was placed at or near the highest point of the orbit to allow room for medial displacement of the globe. The cut was

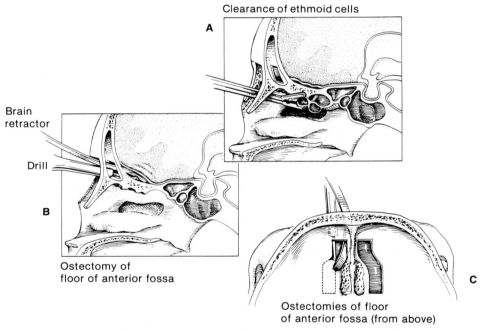

Clearance of ethmoid cells

Brain retractor

Drill

Ostectomy of floor of anterior fossa

Ostectomies of floor of anterior fossa (from above)

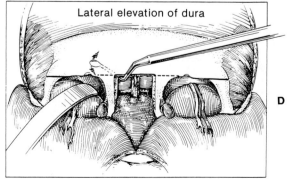

Lateral elevation of dura

Fig. 17-5. A, Clearance of ethmoid cells to make space for orbital translocation. **B,** Ostectomy of floor of anterior fossa done with drill as dura is protected with ¼" brain retractor. **C,** Ostectomy of floor of anterior cranial fossa viewed from above. **D,** Dura reflected from frontal area for transverse osteotomy.

carried two thirds of the distance to the orbital apex and was then directed medially as a posterior cut going down the medial orbital wall. The dura was protected by a brain retractor, which was inserted through the medial ostectomy site, and the globe was protected by a second brain retractor.

Posterior cut of the medial orbital wall. The cut proceeded medially along the orbital plate of the frontal bone and then along the orbital plate of the ethmoid bone. Thus the cut went from the anterior fossa to the region of the paranasal sinuses. Once this safety zone was reached, the microscope was no longer needed; 2.5× loupes and a coaxial fiberoptic headlamp were used thereafter.

Cut of the orbital floor. The cut then proceeded forward on the orbital floor, dividing the orbital rim just lateral to the lacrimal apparatus (congruent to the cut of the orbital roof).

Cut from orbital rim to pyramidal aperture. A diagonal cut was extended from the orbital rim to the lateral-most part of the pyramidal aperture.

Mobilization and approximation of medial orbital walls. These cuts were repeated on the opposite side. With digital pressure and instruments, the medial orbital walls were then mobilized inward, leaving gaps in each orbital floor, in each roof, and in each nasomaxillary area. A triangular segment was cut from the nasal bones on either side of the pyramidal aperture to retain a satisfactory nasal airway. Drill holes, number 30 interosseous wires, and 4-0 Prolene canthopexy sutures[4] were placed.

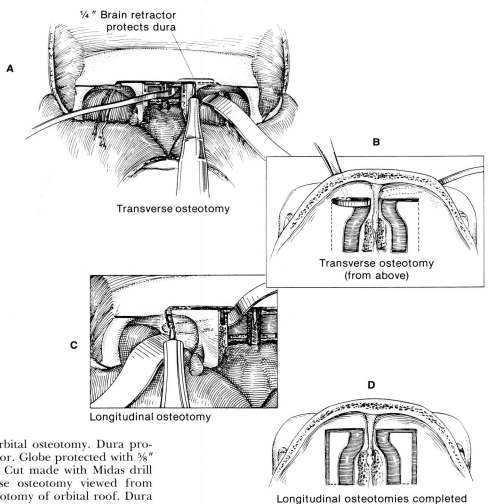

Fig. 17-6. **A,** Transverse orbital osteotomy. Dura protected with ¼″ brain retractor. Globe protected with ⅝″ silastic-clad brain retractor. Cut made with Midas drill and B-3 bit. **B,** Transverse osteotomy viewed from above. **C,** Longitudinal osteotomy of orbital roof. Dura protected with brain retractor. **D,** Osteotomy of orbital roof viewed from above. Ostectomy of anterior fossa with transverse osteotomies and longitudinal osteotomies of orbit completed. Posterior osteotomy is plotted *(dashes).*

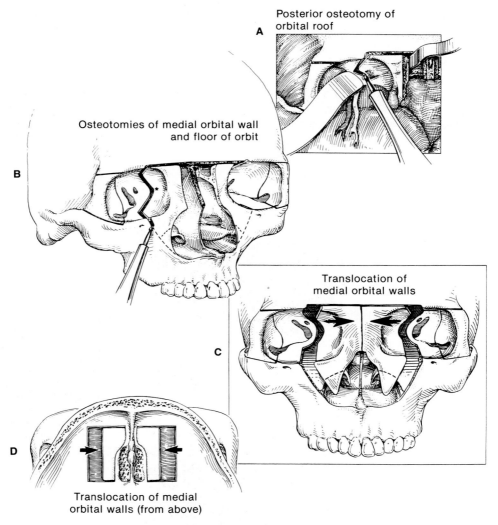

A
Posterior osteotomy of
orbital roof

B
Osteotomies of medial orbital wall
and floor of orbit

C
Translocation of
medial orbital walls

D
Translocation of medial
orbital walls (from above)

Fig. 17-7. A, Posterior cut of orbital roof and anterior floor of fossa. Dura protected with
¼″ brain retractor. **B,** Osteotomy continues down the medial wall of the orbit. As cut
passes point of asterisk it moves away from the dura and passes to the safety zone of the
ethmoid and then the maxillary sinuses. **C,** Medial orbital walls translocated. Triangle of
bone marked for removal at pyramidal aperture to maintain nasal passageway. **D,** View
from above. Medial walls of orbit are translocated medially, leaving orbitocranial defects
laterally.

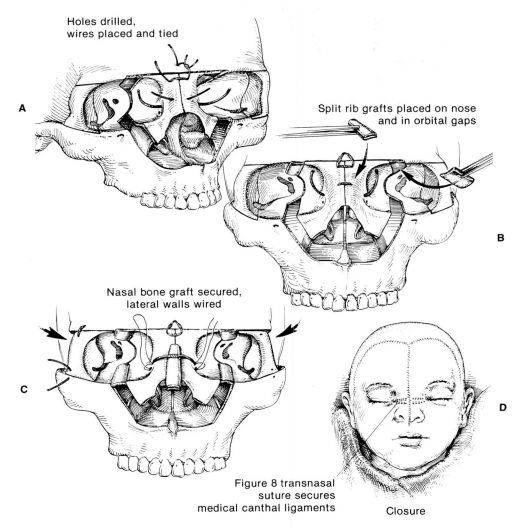

Holes drilled,
wires placed and tied

A

Split rib grafts placed on nose
and in orbital gaps

B

Nasal bone graft secured,
lateral walls wired

C

Figure 8 transnasal
suture secures
medical canthal ligaments

Closure

D

Fig. 17-8. A, Medial walls of orbit are secured with 4 No. 30 wires. An additional wire is placed for nasal bone graft. **B,** Wires tightened, split rib grafts fitted into orbital roof and orbital floor defects. **C,** Nasal bone graft secured. Gaps of roof and floor of orbit closed with bone grafts. Lateral orbital walls translocated and wired. Figure 8 canthopexy sutures ready to be tied. **D,** Final closure. Canthal ligaments are secured with figure 8 polypropylene canthopexy sutures.

The drill kerfs in the lateral orbital walls were excessively wide in our first case and the segments were not stable; therefore, Champy screws[1] were used in addition to the wire loops to buttress the medial displacement of the orbital walls.

The independent mobility of the lateral and medial walls gave added control over enophthalmos-exophthalmos—but also gave added vulnerability to error in positioning the globes. Thus position of the globes was carefully observed while the bones were fixed.

Closure. The excess soft tissues were trimmed away. The temporal scalp was then advanced as far forward as possible with figure 8 sutures that en-

gaged the temporal fascia to avoid posterior traction on the lateral canthi. Suction catheters were placed and the wounds were closed.

DISCUSSION

Microsurgical techniques for intracranial surgery were developed when House,[7,8,9] with his collaborating neurosurgeons Kurze and Doyle[10] and Hitselberger,[6] carried out over a thousand microsurgical craniotomies for acoustic neuromas and cerebellopontine angle tumors. Since then intracranial microsurgery procedures have become part of the standard neurosurgical repertoire.[12]

Conventional frontal craniotomy has been a

routine step in craniofacial surgery since its inception.[14] Advantages are wide exposure and extensive experience with the pathological anatomy.[2,17] Edgerton et al.[3] introduced the advantages of reduced blood loss and less manipulation of the frontal lobes. Tessier et al.[15] introduced the "semiopen skull" technique, which applies the same concept for osteotomies of the lateral orbit.

Our goal with the first patient was to correct a mild hypertelorism without a full-scale craniotomy. We felt that a subcranial approach would be ineffective because of a low cribriform plate, so, as a compromise, we used the glabella ostectomy with microsurgical control. After success in this case of mild hypertelorism, we employed the technique in a case of more severe hypertelorism.

Our operating time was prolonged: 10 hours in the first patient and 19 hours in the second patient. However, the patients recovered rapidly with no major complications, and the blood loss was only about 500 ml in each case. We feel that with further experience and improved instrumentation our operating time will be reduced.

The possibility that a supplementary standard frontal craniotomy might be needed for an unexpected complication is always present. Therefore the neurosurgeons on the team were prepared to proceed expeditiously with such an alternate plan at any time.

Obviously this approach is unsuitable for procedures in which full-scale craniotomies are needed anyway to correct deformities of the frontal and parietal bones, and this approach would be unnecessary in patients who have encephaloceles or bony clefts that in themselves afford access.

This work is presented as a preliminary report. We feel that it has potential advantages sufficient to recommend continued trial in selected cases.

SUMMARY

Orbital translocation was carried out in two cases of hypertelorism by a "semiopen skull" technique in which microscopic control was added to Edgerton's glabella ostectomy so that the medial orbital walls could be moved with precision without the need for a formal frontal craniotomy. The lateral walls were cut separately and moved as independent units.

ACKNOWLEDGMENT

This work was supported in part by Ninos Lisiados and in part by the U.C.I. Foundation.

REFERENCES

1. Champy, M., et al.: Mandibular osteocynthesis by miniature screwed plates via a buccal approach, J. Maxillofac. Surg. **6:**14, 1978.
2. Converse, J.M., et al.: Principles of craniofacial surgery. In Converse, J.M., editor: Reconstructive plastic surgery, Vol. 4, Philadelphia, 1977, W.B. Saunders Co., p. 2427.
3. Edgerton, M.T., Udvarhelyi, B.G., and Knox, D.L.: The surgical correction of ocular hypertelorism, Ann. Surg. **172:**473, 1970.
4. Furnas, D.W.: The pulley canthopexy for residual telecanthus after hypertelorism repair or facial trauma, Ann. Plast. Surg. **5:**85, 1980.
5. Hansman, C.F.: Growth of interorbital distance and skull thickness as observed in roentgenographic measurements, Radiology **86:**87, 1966.
6. Hitselberger, W.E., and House, W.F.: Tumors of the cerebellopontine angle, Arch. Otolaryngol. **80:**720, 1964.
7. House, W.F.: Surgical exposure of the internal auditory canal and its contents through the middle, cranial fossa, Laryngoscope **71:**1363, 1961.
8. House, W.F., editor: Transtemporal bone microsurgical removal of acoustic neuromas: Report of cases (monograph), Arch. Otolaryngol. **80:**617, 1964.
9. House, W.F.: A history of acoustic tumor surgery: 1961-1971, the dandy era. In House, W.F., and Luetje, C.M., editors: Acoustic tumors, Vol. I: Diagnosis, Baltimore, 1979, University Park Press.
10. Kurze, T., and Doyle, J.: Extradural intracranial (middle fossa) approach to the internal auditory canal, J. Neurosurg. **19:**1033, 1962.
11. Opitz, J.M., et al.: The BBB syndrome—familial telecanthus with associated congenital anomalies. In Bergsma, D., editor: Part II, Malformation syndromes. Birth Defects: Original Article Series, Vol. V, No. 2, The National Foundation—March of Dimes, New York, 1969.
12. Rand, R.W.: Microneurosurgery, ed. 2, St. Louis, 1978, The C.V. Mosby Co.
13. Shambaugh, G.E., and Glasscock, M.E.: Surgery of the ear, ed. 3, Philadelphia, 1980, W.B. Saunders Co.
14. Tessier, P., et al.: Osteotomies cranio-naso-orbito-faciales hypertelorisme, Ann. Chir. Plast. **12:**103, 1967.
15. Tessier, P.: Recent improvements in treatment of facial and cranial deformities of Crouzon's disease and Apert's syndrome. In Tessier, P., Callahan, A., Mustarde, J.C., and Salyer, K., editors: Symposium on plastic surgery in the orbital region, St. Louis, 1976, The C.V. Mosby Co.
16. Whitaker, L.A., Broennle, A.M., Kerr, L.P., and Herlich, A.: Improvements in craniofacial reconstruction: methods evolved in 236 consecutive patients, Plast. Reconstr. Surg. **65:**561, 1980.
17. Whitaker, L.A., et al.: Combined report of problems and complications in 793 craniofacial operations, Plast. Reconstr. Surg. **64:**198, 1979.

Part V

Treatment of facial palsy

Chapter 18

Overview of the treatment of facial palsy

Marcus Castro Ferreira

The surgical treatment of facial palsy remains a difficult task for the plastic surgeon, and despite the many attempts made to restore facial animation, the results are still far from ideal. We are dealing with a complex problem that results from many possible etiologic factors and that gives many possible clinical pictures, a great number features of which are poorly understood.

Microsurgery has proved to be a major advance in the treatment of facial palsy. To get an overview of the microsurgical procedures we have used since 1974, we reviewed fifty-one patients (Tables 18-1 and 18-2). Every effort was made to carry out

Table 18-1. Etiologic factors in facial palsy (fifty-one cases, 1974-1981)

Trauma	
Facial laceration	14
Temporal bone injury	4
Tumor	
Acoustic neurinoma	8
Parotid tumor	7
Facial neurinoma	1
Bell's (no recovery	15
Congenital	2

Table 18-2. Microsurgical procedures for facial palsy (1974-1982)

Reconstruction of the nerve	
Suture	2
Grafting	15
Crossface nerve grafting (two stages)	19
Crossface nerve grafting (first stage)	
Plus masseter transfer	4
or	
Plus temporalis transfer	8
or	
Plus extensor digitorum brevis transfer	1
or	
Plus gracilis transfer	2

an accurate preoperative assessment so that meaningful postoperative comparisons could be made. We divided the results into three groups—*good, fair,* and *poor:*

Good result: Symmetry of the face in repose, complete eye closure, and movement of the mouth strong enough to overcome the force of the healthy side and restore the smile

Fair result: Symmetry of the face in repose, incomplete but useful closure of the eyes, and definite improvement in motion of the mouth

Poor result: Little or no improvement

Some patients were initially seen with an incomplete palsy, usually after they had an episode of Bell's palsy. The evaluation of the result in these cases was confined to the specific area of facial nerve involvement.

The cases were divided into two groups according to whether or not reconstruction of the facial nerve itself was possible at the time of our original treatment.

RECONSTRUCTION OF THE FACIAL NERVE POSSIBLE

The first group included extratemporal injuries to the facial nerve in which either neurorrhaphy or nerve grafting was performed. The lesions were always seen and treated before 6 months had elapsed from the onset of the palsy.

The injuries were, in most instances, severe enough to produce gaps in the facial nerve trunk. Reconstruction of the nerve was accomplished by nerve grafting.[11] The facial nerve has a better prospect of recovery than most peripheral nerves, since it is a pure motor nerve; in our series, the gap in the nerve was usually not greater than 10 cm.

The problem of mass movement following nerve reconstruction can occur when the recon-

151

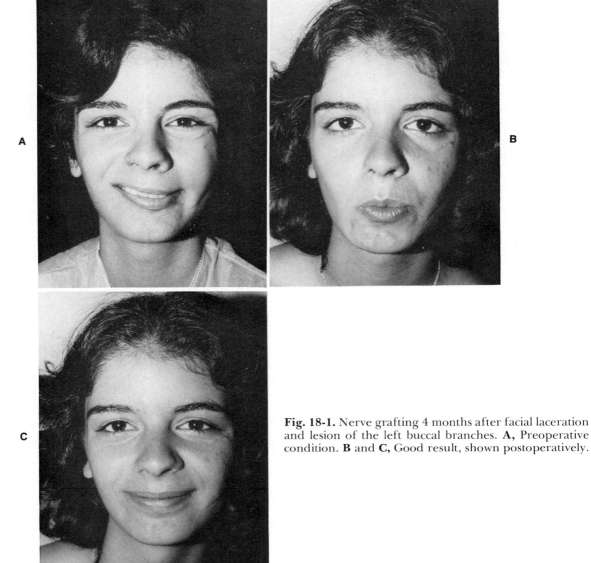

Fig. 18-1. Nerve grafting 4 months after facial laceration and lesion of the left buccal branches. **A,** Preoperative condition. **B** and **C,** Good result, shown postoperatively.

struction is done in the intratemporal part of the facial nerve or in lesions of the extratemporal trunk. In these cases the surgeon should attempt to identify the fascicles and match them to their corresponding branches.[12] Meissl's descriptions of the internal topography of the facial nerve have helped us to accomplish that task.[10]

The potential for better fascicular matching in recent lesions is an important reason for prompt repair or grafting in accidental injuries or in facial nerve excision incidental to extirpation of parotid tumors. Despite the most favorable of circum-stances, however, some degree of mass movement may occur.

In the majority of cases we have treated, the lesion was in branches of the facial nerve distal to the primary division and was seen by us after some delay (from 1 to 6 months). Fibrosis and neuromas were common, and resection of scarred nerve cre-ated gaps that required nerve grafts.

The sural nerve was used in every case, and the results were evaluated 1 year after the repair. They usually fell into the "good" category, sometime, with an almost perfect result (Fig. 18-1).

RECONSTRUCTION OF THE FACIAL NERVE IMPOSSIBLE ("DEFINITIVE" PARALYSIS)

Patients of the second group were usually referred by otolaryngologists or neurosurgeons for the palliative treatment of a facial palsy in which the patient was not a candidate for supratemporal or intratemporal procedures. We also included in this group cases of Bell's palsy with poor recovery and some cases of nerve reconstruction that had failed.

The many techniques devised to reanimate paralyzed facial muscles can be divided into two major types: (1) the use of another nerve trunk to reinnervate the facial nerve (hypoglossal, spinal accessory, phrenic, or, more recently, the contralateral facial nerve), and (2) transplants of muscle, either local or distant, with or without a nerve crossover.

In the first type of technique the hypoglossal nerve was the most widely used, and it is still strongly favored by some surgeons.[3] Most surgeons, however, feel that the procedure is unwarranted, because loss of function of the hypoglossal nerve causes a conspicuous defect in the tongue, mass movement almost always occurs after the crossover, good reeducation is often very hard to achieve, emotional control is never regained, and unpleasant synkinetic movements can result. Crossover procedures with the spinal accessory nerve may result in significant disability of shoulder movement.

The advent of microsurgery gave a better outlook to nerve grafting. The use of the contralateral facial nerve was suggested by Smith[16] and Scaramella,[15] and a clinical series was reported by Anderl.[1]

Attracted by this idea, in 1974[6] we started to use crossfacial nerve grafts in every case of facial palsy not amenable to nerve grafting or repair.[5] Among our first nineteen cases we had many disappointments. After we analyzed these cases, some interesting features came to light. Good and fair results were seen only in those cases treated within the first year of the onset of the palsy. Most cases, however, were first seen more than 1 year after the onset, and in this group the results were usually poor. It was assumed that the prolonged time of denervation of the muscle was the major factor leading to the poor result.

The number of cases with a short time interval was too small for precise evaluation, but we found fair and good results in about 50% of the cases. It is important to note that in some cases a degree of emotional control is achieved (Fig. 18-2) that is rarely seen after other crossover techniques.

We now consider the two-stage crossface nerve graft as the procedure of choice for "definitive" palsies of less than 6 months' duration. Another indication for the two-stage operation is in cases of partial palsy in which we combine a selective neurectomy[2] on the healthy side with a crossface nerve graft in an attempt to reinnervate specific territories (Fig. 18-3).

The crossface nerve graft itself survived and became reinnervated within 4 to 6 months in almost every such case. It is an excellent source of axons for the paralyzed side, and it is therefore now being used by some surgeons to innervate free muscle transplants.

In another group of patients the transfer of local muscle was used to substitute for the paralyzed mimetic muscles. The masseter, the temporalis,[14] and the platysma[4] have been used. These are satisfactory for closure of the eye but are less successful in animating the mouth; retraining the muscles is usually a problem. There is also lack of emotional control because innervation is trigeminal rather than facial.

To minimize these problems we combined the transfer of local muscles with crossface grafts, either suturing to the motor branch or with direct neurotization of the muscle.[7] We first tried using the masseter, suturing the previously placed crossface nerve graft to the masseteric nerve, but we encountered some technical problems related to the size and position of the nerve, and the functional results were not satisfactory.

Temporalis muscle transfers have frequently been used to restore eyelid closure in patients with long-standing facial palsies. More recently we added to the standard procedure a direct neurotization to the muscle coming from the crossface grafting done 6 months before. The neurovascular pedicle of the muscle remained intact. We feel that the patient regained some emotional control and that reeducation was easier to accomplish.

Reanimation of the mouth in patients with a palsy of more than 1 year's duration is still a challenging problem, and the most recent solution offered has been transplantation of a distant muscle. The free muscle graft technique was reported by Thompson,[17] and recently has been combined with a crossface nerve graft. The muscle, however, does not withstand transplantation well, and for that reason the procedure has not gained acceptance. The best technique available today is transplantation of the muscle by microvascular anastomoses.

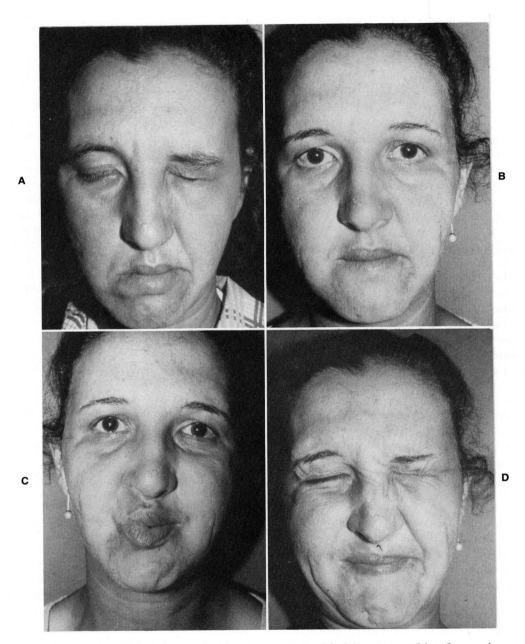

Fig. 18-2. Irreversible lesion of the right intratemporal facial nerve resulting from coles-theatoma removal. **A,** Condition before crossface nerve graft (3 months of palsy). **B-D,** Postoperative view 9 months after the two-stage crossface nerve graft. Good result.

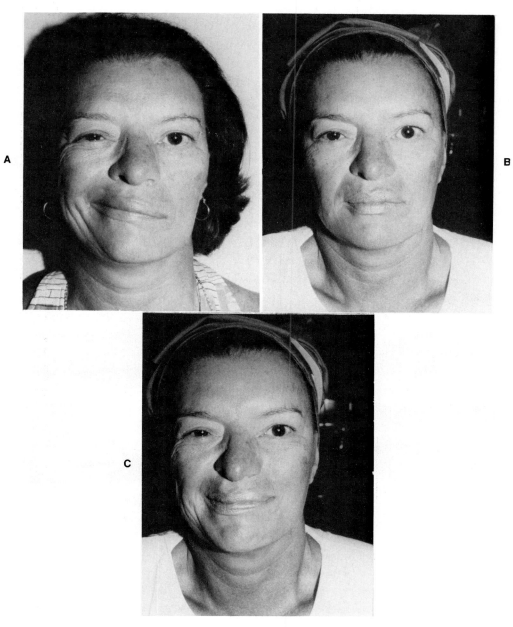

Fig. 18-3. Facial paralysis treated by spinofacial crossover. **A,** Some muscle tonus but no useful contraction of the mimic muscles around the mouth. **B** and **C,** Six months after the two-stage crossface grafting and severance of the spinofacial anastomosis. Better balance was achieved.

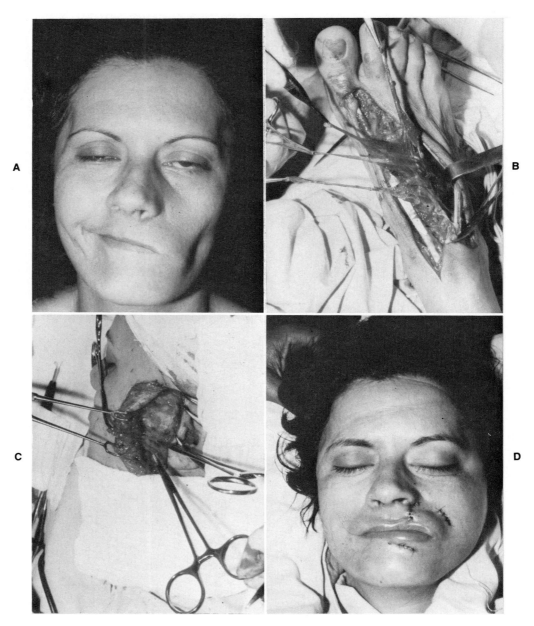

Fig. 18-4. Extensor digitorum brevis transfer to a long-standing facial palsy. **A,** Long-standing facial palsy. **B,** Dissection of the muscle of the foot. **C,** Crossface nerve grafts done 6 months before and approached by a rhytidoplasty incision. **D,** Muscle transferred by microvascular anastomoses and sutured to the mouth under some tension.

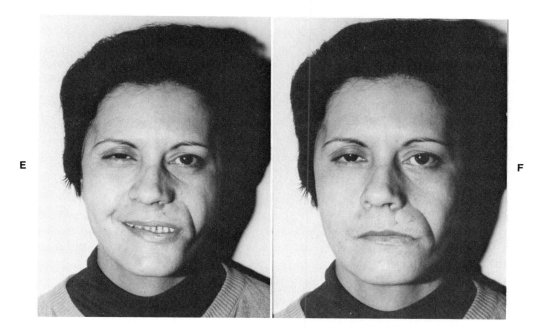

Fig. 18-4, cont'd. E and **F,** Postoperative result 1 year after the procedure—smiling.

Reinnervation can be provided by the suture of the motor nerve with a crossface nerve graft.

The gracilis transfer was first reported by Harii et al.[9] They initially used a branch of the trigeminal nerve to reinnervate the transplanted muscle. However, they now use a crossface nerve graft to regain some degree of emotional control. Results reported with this technique have been promising.[8,13] We used the gracilis in only two cases, and the follow-up is too short for an evaluation.

The extensor digitorum brevis has been used for the mouth and was reinnervated in one patient with a crossface graft done in one stage. After 1 year the patient showed good symmetry in repose and smiled with emotional control (Fig. 18-4). The muscle did not retain sufficient strength for forceful contraction of the mouth, and the donor site had conspicuous scars.

SUMMARY

In summary, we now use the following plan to achieve the best possible results in our patients:

I. Reconstruction of the facial nerve possible
  A. If there is no tension—neurorrhaphy
  B. If there is a gap or excessive tension—nerve grafting
II. Reconstruction of the facial nerve impossible
  A. If the interval between onset of the palsy and surgery is less than 6 months—two-stage crossface nerve grafting

(three grafts); (possible exception—older patients)
  B. If there is a long-standing facial palsy (more than 6 months)
    1. First stage: crossface nerve graft (two grafts through the upper lip) plus selective neurectomy on the healthy side
    2. Six months later: temporalis muscle transfer to the eyelids, direct neurotization from the crossface nerve graft, and microvascular muscle transfer to the mouth area
    3. Complementary procedures whenever necessary

REFERENCES

1. Anderl, H.: Reconstruction of the face through cross-face nerve transplantation in facial paralysis, Chir. Plast. **2:**17, 1973.
2. Clodius, L.: Selective neurectomies to achieve symmetry in partial and complete facial paralysis, Br. J. Plast. Surg. **29:**43, 1976.
3. Conley, J., and Baker, D.C.: Hypoglossal facial nerve anastomoses for rehabilitation in facial paralysis, Plast. Reconstr. Surg. **63:**66, 1979.
4. Edgerton, M.T., Tuerk, D.B., and Fischer, J.C.: Surgical treatment of moebius syndrome by platysma and temporalis muscle transfers, Plast. Reconstr. Surg. **55:**305, 1975.
5. Ferreira, M.C.: Microsurgical procedures in the treatment of facial palsy, Transactions of the Seventh International Congress of Plastic and Reconstructive Surgeons, Rio de Janeiro, 1979, p. 92.

6. Ferreira, M.C., Marchese, A.T., and Spina, V.: Injertos trans faciales de nervio en el tratamiento de la paralisis facial: observaciones iniciales, Chir. Plast. Ibero Lat. Am. **3**:301, 1977.

7. Freilinger, G.A.: A new technique to correct facial paralysis, Plast. Reconstr. Surg. **56**:44, 1975.

8. Harii, K.: Microneurovascular free muscle transplantation for reanimation of facial paralysis, Clin. Plast. Surg. **6**:361, 1979.

9. Harii, K., Ohmori, K., and Torii, S.: Free gracilis muscle transplantation with neurovascular anastomoses for the treatment of facial paralysis, Plast. Reconstr. Surg. **57**:133, 1976.

10. Meissl, G.: Die intraneurale Topographic des extrakraniellen nervus facialis, Acta Chir. Austr. Suppl. 25, 1979.

11. Millesi, H.: Zum Problem der Uberbrukung von Defekten peripherer Nerven, Wien Med. Wochenschr. **9**:182, 1968.

12. Millesi, H.: Nerve suture and grafting to restore the extratemporal facial nerve, Clin. Plast. Surg. **6**:333, 1979.

13. O'Brien, B.M.: Management of facial paralysis, presented at the annual meeting of the American Society of Plastic and Reconstructive Surgeons, New Orleans, 1980.

14. Rubin, L.: Reanimation of the paralyzed face, St. Louis, 1977, The C.V. Mosby Co.

15. Scaramella, L.: L'anastomosis tra I due nerve faciali, Arch. Otolaryngol. **82**:209, 1975.

16. Smith, J.W.: A new technique of facial animation, Transactions of the Fifth International Congress of Plastic and Reconstructive Surgeons, Australia, 1971, Butterworths.

17. Thompson, N.: Autogenous muscle grafts in the reconstruction of the paralyzed face. In Converse, J.M. editor: Reconstructive plastic surgery, Philadelphia, 1977, W.B. Saunders Co.

Chapter 19

Treatment of long-standing facial paralysis by combining vascularized muscle transplantation with crossface nerve grafting

Kiyonori Harii

Crossface nerve grafting, in which a nerve graft is routed from normal facial nerve funiculi to the affected facial nerve trunk, has proved its potential for reinnervation of paralyzed facial muscles.[1,7,8] This technique may possibly be useful for the correction of a recent facial paralysis in which the facial muscles have not completely atrophied and for which timing of surgery is optimal.

In contrast, the neurovascular free muscle transfer plays its major role in long-standing facial paralysis in which the facial muscles have completely atrophied or have been excised.[4] An important factor in obtaining a satisfactory result with this method is the availability of a suitable recipient motor nerve. If the facial nerve stump is available for neurorrhaphy, contraction of the transplanted muscle will usually be synchronous with contralateral facial movements. However, if the facial nerve is unavailable and alternatives such as the deep temporal nerve or the hypoglossal nerve are used, the resulting movement appears unnatural.[3]

Therefore, when a facial nerve stump is not available at the recipient site, we recommend a free vascularized muscle transplantation combined with a crossface nerve graft. This crossface sural nerve graft conducts impulses from the normal facial nerve to the transplanted muscle and results in natural, symmetrical contractions, controlled by the contralateral facial nerve.

We introduce herein our operative technique for combined free vascularized muscle transplan-tation and crossface nerve grafting. The primary goal of this operation is to gain a natural-appearing smile. Other methods are used for correction of the paralyzed forehead and eyelids.

OPERATING PROCEDURES

The operation is done in two stages, about 8 months apart. In the first stage a sural nerve graft is tunneled to the affected cheek from selected funiculi of the buccal and zygomatic branches of the intact facial nerve. Through a preauricular incision on the normal side, a cheek flap is elevated at the level of the superficial parotid fascia. The buccal and zygomatic branches of the facial nerve are exposed distal to their exit from the parotid gland. Both the buccal and the zygomatic branches break up into plexi, from which terminal branches pass into the mimetic muscles.

Once the facial nerve plexi have been isolated, a 15 to 18 cm sural nerve graft, harvested by a second team, is tunneled subcutaneously from the normal side of the face to the affected side with a modified tendon passer. The nerve graft is usually reversed to avoid diversion and loss of regenerating axons through side branches. The proximal end of the sural nerve is anchored near the vessels that have been chosen to receive the muscle transplant in the second stage. The site of subcutaneous tunneling of the nerve graft varies according to the location of the recipient vessels. When the superficial temporal vessels in their preauricular course are used as recipient vessels, the nerve graft is passed through the upper lip; it is passed through the submental region when the facial vessels are selected as recipients (Fig. 19-1).

The sural nerve graft is reversed, placing its distal end near the buccal and zygomatic plexi of the intact facial nerve. The stump is then prepared under magnification. Each funiculus is sutured with 10-0 monofilament nylon. An average of six to seven funiculi in the sural nerve are joined to the funiculi of the facial nerve plexi. Large funiculi are coapted individually, while small funiculi are coapted collectively. Approximately one half to three fifths of the funiculi in each plexus can be used for neurorrhaphy without causing excessive

paralysis of the normal mimetic muscles. Axon growth through the nerve graft is followed by the advance of Tinel's sign. (The facial nerve includes sensory fibers that originate from the facial nerve itself or from the trigeminal nerve.) When the terminal neuroma is tapped, the patient feels mild pain or irritation at the site where the graft joins the normal plexi.

The second stage is carried out 8 to 10 months after placement of the sural nerve graft or 2 to 3 months after Tinel's sign has reached the distal stump of the nerve graft. On the paralyzed side of the face a cheek flap is elevated through a preauricular incision, and both the vessels and the distal nerve stump are identified. The cheek is under-

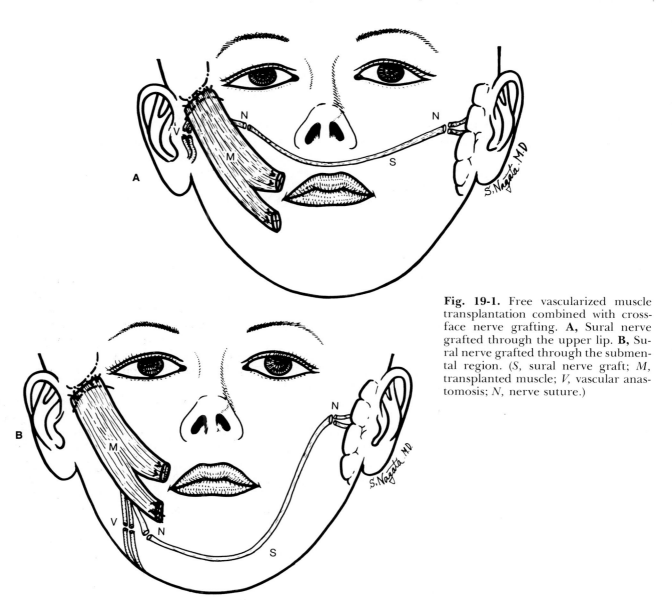

Fig. 19-1. Free vascularized muscle transplantation combined with cross-face nerve grafting. **A,** Sural nerve grafted through the upper lip. **B,** Sural nerve grafted through the submental region. (*S,* sural nerve graft; *M,* transplanted muscle; *V,* vascular anastomosis; *N,* nerve suture.)

mined sufficiently to provide space for the transferred muscle. Two to three months usually elapse after Tinel's sign has advanced to the end of the nerve graft before a sufficient number of regenerated axons is present.

Simultaneously a suitable muscle is exposed and prepared for transfer to the cheek area with neurovascular anastomoses.

Several criteria govern selection of the donor muscle:

1. The muscle should have a single neurovascular pedicle that supplies the entire muscle belly, or a definitive segment of muscle should be nourished by the neurovascular pedicle.
2. Procurement of the muscle should cause no functional loss nor significant deformity at the donor site.
3. The shape and size of the muscle should be appropriate for the functional requirements. Grafting of part of a muscle belly is usually done to restore elevation of the lips and nasolabial area.
4. The transplanted muscle must have sufficient excursion to elevate the paralyzed cheek and lips effectively. A relatively large volume of muscle will be needed, because the original volume and power of the muscle is considerably reduced after transplantation.[9]

Currently we usually choose the gracilis or latissimus dorsi muscles. Small muscles such as the extensor digitorum brevis are inadequate.[5]

Isolation of the donor muscle

Gracilis. The patient is placed on the operating table in the supine position with the knee flexed and the hip externally rotated and abducted. A 10 cm longitudinal incision is made along the upper posterior border of the adductor longus and over the dominant nutrient vessels that, after emerging from the profunda femoris vessels, enter the gracilis at its upper medial aspect (an average of 8 cm distal to the pubic tubercle).

First the fascia over the adductor longus and gracilis muscles is separated, then the vascular pedicle of the gracilis is identified and dissected toward its origin; a pedicle that is as long as possible is obtained. The motor nerve accompanying the vessels is preserved. After the neurovascular pedicle has been exposed, the muscle belly is isolated from the surrounding tissues by blunt dissection (Fig. 19-2).

Latissimus dorsi. The patient is placed on the operating table in a semilateral position. The arm on the donor side is elevated and slightly abducted. The elbow is flexed to about 90 degrees, and the forearm is fixed to a bar above the patient's head.

A skin incision is made along the anterior border of the latissimus dorsi muscle, extending to the axilla. The thoracodorsal vessels and nerve are identified in front of the anterior border of the

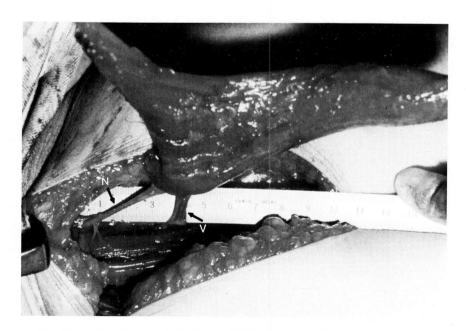

Fig. 19-2. Gracilis muscle isolated. (*V,* Nutrient vessels; *N,* motor nerve.)

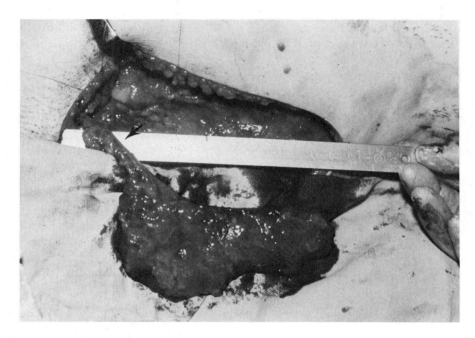

Fig. 19-3. Latissimus dorsi muscle isolated with long neurovascular pedicle *(arrow).*

muscle. The thoracodorsal vessels are then dissected distally toward their point of entry into the muscle. At this point of entry the thoracodorsal vessels give off one or two (rarely three) constant branches to the serratus anterior muscle; these branches are ligated. A neurovascular bundle of sufficient length is exposed, and then a portion of the latissimus dorsi is selected and isolated for transplantation (Fig. 19-3).

Once the muscle segment has been isolated, the muscle–neurovascular pedicle unit is immediately transferred to the face and positioned temporarily for the neurovascular anastomoses; the muscle is kept moist during the microsurgical phase of the operation. The end of the sural nerve graft is trimmed to obtain funiculi suitable for neurorrhaphy. The nerve is sutured close to its entry point into the muscle so that the regenerating axons will reach the motor end-plates promptly. The nutrient artery and vein of the muscle are simultaneously anastomosed to the recipient vessels.

After neurorrhaphy and vascular anastomoses, the muscle belly is fixed under proper tension in the cheek. The upper portion of the muscle is anchored to the zygomatic arch. The lower portion is split, and with the aid of a nasolabial incision, the muscle segments are fixed to the subcutaneous tissues of the paralyzed upper and lower lips. To accommodate the bulk of the muscle, subcutaneous fat is trimmed from the skin over the zygomatic area.

Postoperatively the patient wears an elastic bandage for about 10 days and is allowed to move the mouth freely 2 weeks after surgery. No special rehabilitative measures such as electric stimulation are used.

CASE REPORT
Patient I

A 47-year-old female suffered complete right facial paralysis following surgery for an acoustic tumor 2 years previously (Fig. 19-4). She could not elevate her eyebrow or close her eye. Her nasolabial fold was effaced and her smile was noticeably asymmetric.

As a first stage a long sural nerve graft (approximately 18 cm) was joined to healthy buccal branches and was then tunneled across the upper lip. It was anchored beneath the skin in the preauricular region close to the superficial temporal vessels. Simultaneously part of the temporal muscle and fascia was transferred to the eyelid by use of a modified Gillies' method for ectropion repair. In addition, a narrow strip of skin above the eyebrow was excised to lift the drooping eyebrow.

In the second stage 8 months later, the sural nerve stump and the superficial temporal vessels were exposed through a preauricular incision on the paralyzed side of the face. The cheek was widely undermined from the zygomatic area to the nasolabial area, making room for the gracilis muscle (which was procured from the right inner thigh by a second team). After temporarily secur-

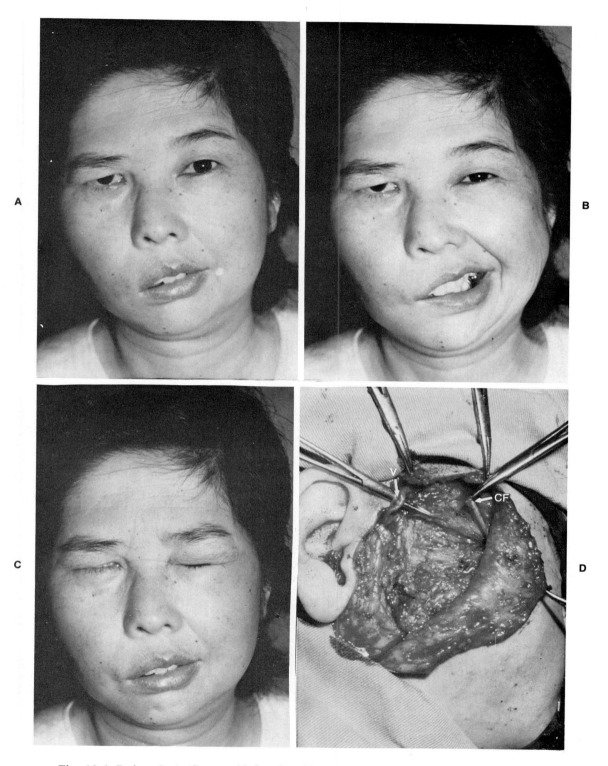

Fig. 19-4. Patient I. A 47-year-old female with complete right facial paralysis. **A** to **C,** Preoperative views. **D,** Elevation of cheek flap with identification of recipient vessels *(V)* and grafted nerve stump *(CF)*.

Continued.

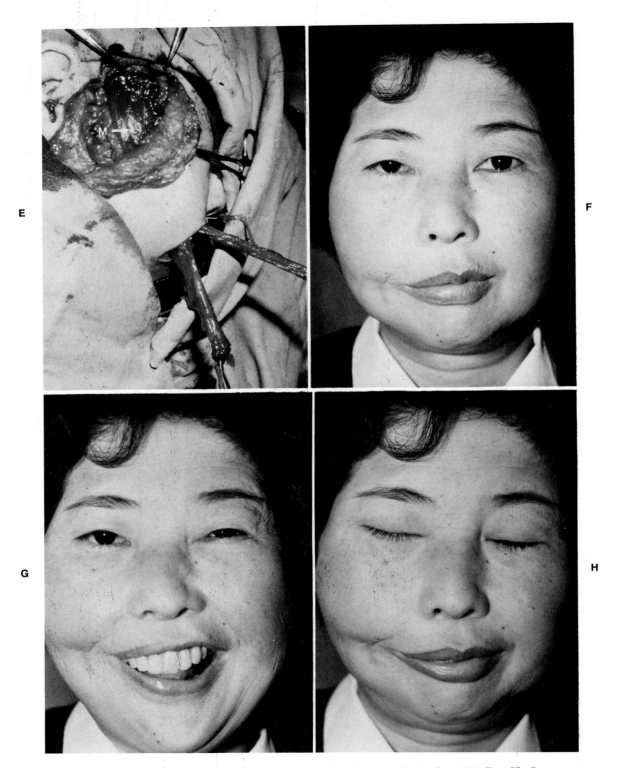

Fig. 19-4, cont'd. E, Transplanted gracilis muscle after vascularization *(M)*. **F** to **H,** One and a half years postoperatively, good facial animation was seen.

ing the muscle to the zygomatic arch, we performed neurovascular anastomoses with the use of the microscope. Ischemic time was less than 90 minutes, and revascularization of the muscle was uneventful.

Then the muscle was sutured under proper tension to the zygomatic arch proximally and to the upper and lower lips distally. Subcutaneous tissue over the zygomatic arch was trimmed to accommodate the bulk of the transplanted muscle. Approximately 7 months after transplantation the muscle showed signs of active contraction, but the range of muscle excursion was inadequate, thereby failing to satisfactorily elevate the nasolabial fold and the lips. In a secondary operation the muscle belly was shortened sufficiently to gain effective muscle contraction and satisfactory facial animation.

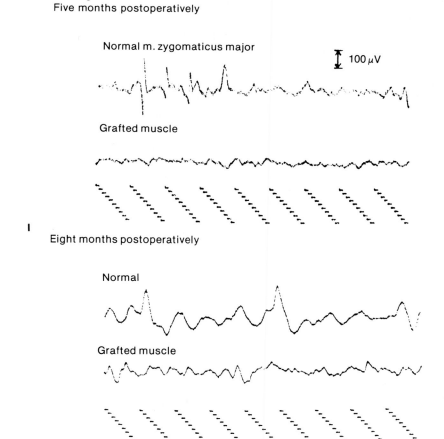

Fig. 19-4, cont'd. I, Electromyograms taken 5 and 8 months postoperatively show a rapid increase of amplitude of volitional spikes led from the transplanted muscle.

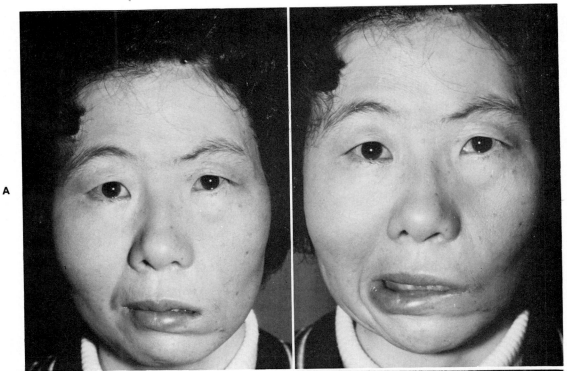

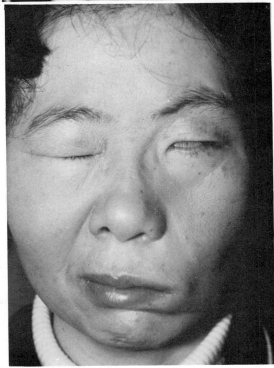

Fig. 19-5. Patient II. A 41-year-old female with complete left facial paralysis. **A** to **C,** Preoperative views.

Patient II

A 41-year-old female had complete paralysis of the left side of her face after resection of an acoustic tumor 3 years previously (Fig. 19-5). A crossface nerve graft was placed in the first stage. A free gracilis transfer and a temporal muscle transposition were performed approximately 7 months later.

Seven months after the second operation the gracilis muscle began to show signs of active contraction and the electromyogram showed positive low amplitude spikes. The patient ultimately obtained satisfactory movement of the cheek without additional surgery.

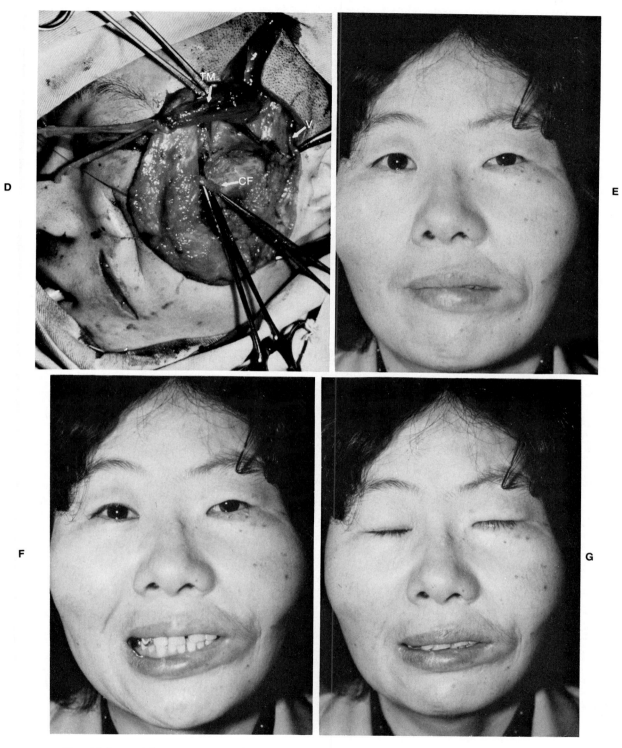

Fig. 19-5, cont'd. D, Exposure of the superficial temporal vessels *(V)* and the end of the grafted nerve *(CF)* in the recipient cheek. *TM* shows transposed temporal muscle and fascia for reconstruction of eyelids. **E** to **G,** Eleven months after the second operation.

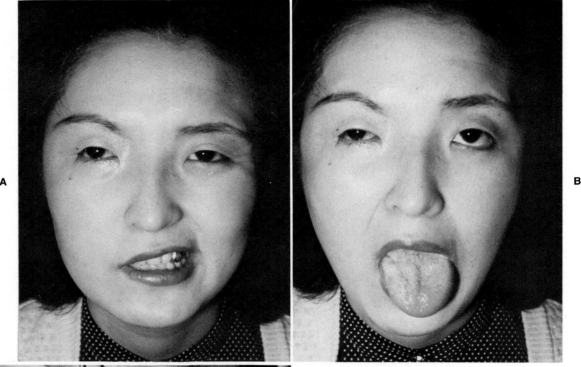

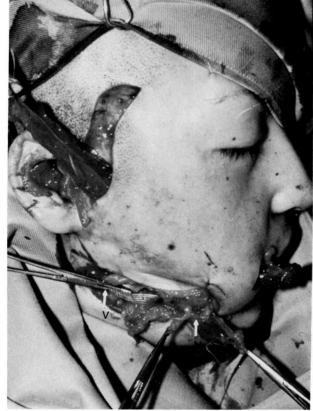

Fig. 19-6. Patient III. A 27-year-old female with right facial paralysis. **A** to **B,** Preoperative views. Movements of the tongue caused unbalanced contraction of facial muscles. **C,** Transplantation of the gracilis in the second stage operation. (*V,* site of fascular anastomoses; *N,* site of nerve suture.)

Patient III

A 27-year-old female had right facial paralysis after resection of an acoustic tumor 6 years previously (Fig. 19-6). She had been treated with a hypoglossal–facial nerve anastomosis and had gained satisfactory static balance of her face. However, the active facial movement that was present was unnatural in appearance because it was synchronous with tongue movements rather than expressive movements of the opposite side of the face.

A sural nerve graft was tunneled across the face through the submental region and was anchored close to the facial vessels at the mandibular angle. (The superficial temporal artery was not palpable in this case.) In the second stage a 9 cm portion of the right gracilis muscle was transplanted so that the zygomatic arch furnished the new origin and the distal end was inserted into the nasolabial region.

Eight months after transplantation the muscle showed active contraction; a positive evoked muscle potential was observed on electric stimulation of either the contralateral facial nerve trunk or the crossface nerve graft itself. Although the proximal part of the muscle showed some bulkiness, the patient was satisfied with the result.

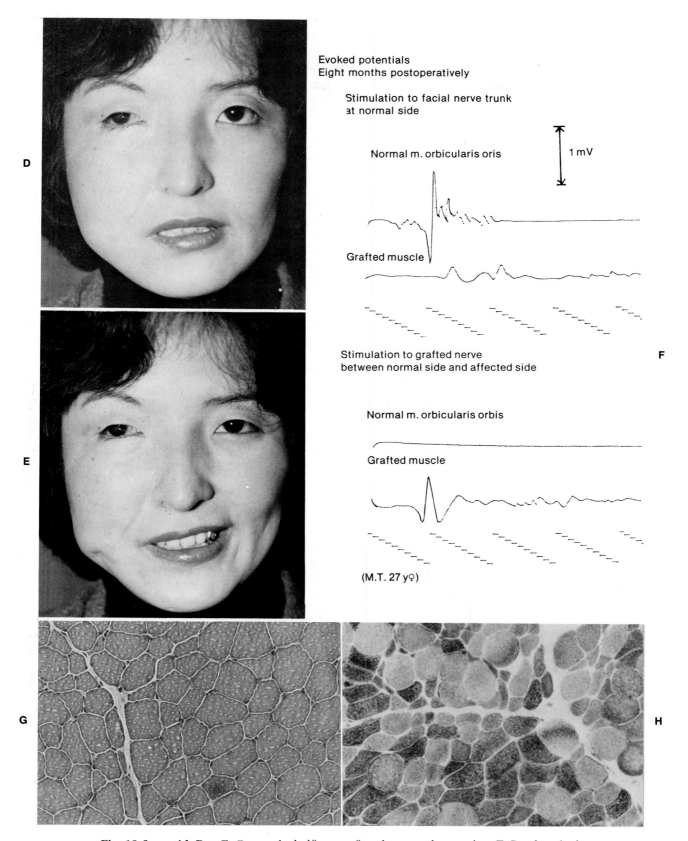

Evoked potentials
Eight months postoperatively

Stimulation to facial nerve trunk
at normal side

Normal m. orbicularis oris

1 mV

Grafted muscle

Stimulation to grafted nerve
between normal side and affected side

Normal m. orbicularis orbis

Grafted muscle

(M.T. 27 y♀)

D

E

F

G

H

Fig. 19-6, cont'd. D to **E,** One and a half years after the second operation. **F,** Good evoked potentials obtained from the muscle 8 months after transplantation. **G** to **H,** Histologic sections of the biopsied muscle 10 months after transplantation show almost normal muscle fibers (hematoxylin-eosin and NADH-tetrazolium reductase stains; ×100).

DISCUSSION

The crossface nerve graft proposed by Scaramella[7] and Smith[8] and later developed by Anderl[1] was an ingenious procedure for the correction of a fresh facial paralysis. However, the results have generally not lived up to the promise of early reports.[2,6]

We carried out crossface nerve grafting in twenty-five patients between May 1975 and March 1980. Six patients underwent surgery within 3 months after the removal of an acoustic tumor. Eight patients with facial paralysis from various causes were treated within 3 to 12 months after onset. The remaining eleven patients had had incomplete paralysis for more than 1 year. There were no significant differences in the results between those patients operated on within 3 months and those operated on 3 to 12 months after onset of paralysis. Six of the fourteen patients regained satisfactory facial contractions. The results in the patients treated more than 1 year after onset of paraysis were generally unsatisfactory (except in those few patients whose static facial balance was improved by the effect of neurectomy of the contralateral intact nerve). Detailed evaluation of the six patients with optimal results showed that spontaneous recovery of the damaged ipsilateral facial nerve fibers was the main reason for facial contraction. In most of these patients evoked potentials were obtained from the reinnervated muscles when the affected facial nerve trunk was stimulated. However, in only one patient were evoked potentials obtained by stimulating the crossface nerve graft or the contralateral facial trunk. Each of the six patients could move their left and right cheeks independently. Synkinesis was often observed.

Therefore, from a clinical standpoint, I would suggest that a crossface nerve graft alone cannot effectively activate the atrophied facial muscles. In a crossface nerve graft the axons must penetrate two scar barriers, travel the distance from one cheek to another, and perhaps pass through additional scar formation in the sural nerve graft itself. Biopsy specimens taken from the distal end of the crossface nerve grafts in five patients about 8 months after grafting showed a 40% decrease in axon diameter and a 30% decrease in counts of myelinated axon fibers. Electron microscopy examination showed that large myelinated fibers were absent, small myelinated fibers were present, and nonmyelinated fibers were present in abundance (Fig. 19-7).

Of course, some axons (perhaps 20% to 30%) may penetrate the second scar barrier to reach the denervated muscle and form new myoneural junctions. These are, however, generally insufficient to

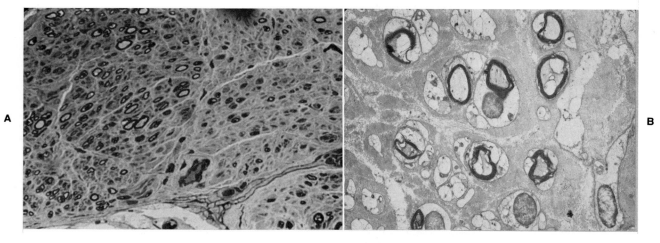

Fig. 19-7. Cross section of the end of the grafted sural nerve 1 year after neurorrhaphy in the intact side. **A,** Specimen embedded in epoxy resin and stained by toluidine blue shows scattered regeneration of myelinated axons, which are small in diameter (×350). **B,** Regenerating axons are seen on electron microscopy. They are small in diameter and are both myelinated and nonmyelinated. Collagen is appreciably increased (×2500).

form enough myoneural junctions to stimulate functional regeneration of the atrophic muscle cells. The presence of degenerative muscle atrophy gives an unfavorable prognosis for conventional crossface nerve grafting. The use of a new, healthy muscle with good vascularization materially improves the prognosis for active facial movement.

In our series the transplanted muscle was innervated chiefly by nerve fibers from the contralateral facial nerve branches. Contractions of the transplanted muscle corresponded well with contractions of the normal facial muscles of the opposite side. Evoked potentials were observed in the transplanted muscle when the contralateral facial nerve trunk was stimulated. Atrophy of the muscle in these transplants was greater than that seen in muscle transplants innervated directly by a facial nerve neurorrhaphy (without an intervening graft). Initially the muscle appeared excessively bulky, but the volume gradually reduced over a period of 8 to 10 months. Gravitational pull on the cheek often caused elongation of the muscle, necessitating a secondary procedure to shorten the muscle for effective animation.

In all of our cases the transplanted muscle was placed subcutaneously in the cheek and was anchored so that its force would elevate the paralyzed cheek and the corner of the mouth. A temporalis muscle transfer using a modified Gillies' method was performed to reconstruct the eyelids when needed.

SUMMARY

With this technique of free vascularized muscle transplantation combined with crossface nerve grafting, patients can obtain a high degree of satisfactory facial animation.

REFERENCES

1. Anderl, H.: Reconstruction of the face through crossface nerve transplantation in facial paralysis, Chir. Plast. **2:**17, 1973.
2. Clodius, L.: Personal communication, 1981.
3. Harii, K.: Microneurovascular free muscle transplantation for reanimation of facial paralysis, Clin. Plast. Surg. **6:**361, 1979.
4. Harii, K., Ohmori, K., and Torii, S.: Free gracilis muscle transplantation with microneurovascular anastomoses for the treatment of facial paralysis, Plast. Reconstr. Surg. **57:**133, 1976.
5. O'Brien, B.M., Franklin, J.D., and Morrison, W.A.: A cross-facial nerve graft and microvascular free muscle transfer for long established facial palsy, Br. J. Plast. Surg. **33:**202, 1980.
6. Rubin, L.R.: Discussion in Tolhurst, D.E., and Bos, K.E.: Free revascularized muscle grafts in facial palsy, Plast. Reconstr. Surg. **69:**760, 1982.
7. Scaramella, L.: L'anastomosi tra i due nerve faciali, Arch. Otologia **82:**209, 1971.
8. Smith, J.W.: A new technique of facial animation. In Hueston, J.H., editor: Transactions of the Fifth International Congress of Plastic and Reconstructive Surgery, Australia, 1971, Butterworth, p. 83.
9. Terzis, J., Sweet, R.C., Dykes, R.W., and Williams, H.B.: Recovery of function in free muscle transplants using microneurovascular anastomoses, J. Hand Surg. **3:**37, 1978.

Chapter 20

Facial palsy

Wayne A. Morrison

In cases of facial palsy in which spontaneous recovery cannot be expected and neither primary or secondary nerve repair nor nerve grafting can be performed, the results of surgical correction have been generally poor. The aims of treatment are to achieve not only static balance but also symmetry during both voluntary and involuntary emotion. By far the most logical and innovative approach to this problem has been the crossfacial nerve graft. Anderl[1] and Smith[4] reported that satisfactory results can be hoped for only when the procedure is performed within 18 months of the original nerve injury. Unfortunately many patients are initially seen with congenital palsy or a palsy that persists after the failure of previous surgical procedures. The outlook for correction of these cases—particularly where the palsy is complete or nearly complete—has been depressing.

At St. Vincent's Hospital since 1975 the management of long-established facial palsy has been by a two-stage procedure.[3] First, a crossfacial sural nerve graft is performed; subsequently a free vascularized muscle transplant is inserted into the paralyzed side of the face, and the previous nerve graft is connected to it. Harii[2] reported a one-stage vascularized gracilis transplant to the paralyzed side of the face, innervated by the nerve to the temporalis. Subsequently he has also used crossfacial nerve grafting for muscle innervation.

OPERATING TECHNIQUE
First stage

Via a modified face lift incision on the nonparalyzed side, the major branches of the facial nerve are identified as they emerge from the anterior border of the parotid gland. At least half of all the branches identified may be safely transected and used for innervation of the nerve grafts. Both sural nerves are removed from the legs by a second surgeon. The nerve grafts are reversed in the face so that valuable axons will not be lost by growth out through the branches. One graft is tunneled above the eyebrows, and the other is tunneled below the point of the chin to the other side of the face, where both grafts are brought out just anterior to the tragus. On the nonparalyzed side the proximal stumps of the previously divided facial nerves destined for the eye and forehead are joined to the upper sural nerve graft after its end has been split into its corresponding fascicles. Similarly the proximal stumps of half the facial nerve destined for the lower face are joined to the lower facial nerve graft. Although the course of the sural nerve grafts is considerably longer than in the conventional technique in which the grafts are tunneled across the upper lip, subsequent tunneling of the muscle graft through the upper lip risks damage to nerves in this region.

For incomplete palsies when only the lower face is being corrected, a single sural nerve graft is used and tunneled below the chin.

The progress of nerve regeneration can be monitored by tapping along the course of the nerve grafts, eliciting a tingling sensation at the site of repair on the nonparalyzed side of the face. Ultimately, when the axons have grown through the full course of the nerve graft, tapping at the opposite tragus will cause tingling on the nonparalyzed side. This usually occurs in 6 to 9 months, and it would seem logical to wait even 12 months to enable the maximum number of axons to reach the end of the nerve graft before the second-stage muscle transplant is performed so that there will be minimal delay in muscle reinnervation.

Interestingly, the degree of myelinization of the regenerated nerve fibers at the distal stump of the sural nerve grafts just before second-stage muscle transplant does not correlate with the return of motor function in this series. In the majority of cases no myelinization was present, but despite this good motor function has been achieved.

Second stage

Approximately 9 to 12 months after the first-stage crossfacial nerve graft, a vascularized muscle is transplanted to the paralyzed face. Initially we used the extensor digitorum brevis muscle, but only one out of eight cases regained significant movement. The standard muscle now transferred is the gracilis. The ipsilateral muscle is used so that the neurovascular pedicle will lie superficially on the muscle surface when inserted into the face, allowing easy vessel and nerve repair and postoperative Doppler monitoring. One team dissects out the gracilis muscle, while a second team simultaneously explores the paralyzed side of the face. A modified face lift incision is performed while the sural nerve grafts are identified. In most cases the recipient vessels are the superficial temporal artery and vein, but when only the lower face is to be corrected, the facial vessels are occasionally used. For complete facial palsy, subcutaneous tunnels are created in the eyebrow, upper and lower eyelids, alar base region, and across the upper and lower lips.

The gracilis muscle is exposed via a longitudinal incision just posterior to the adductor longus muscle; the knee is flexed and abducted. In the upper quarter of the leg, the incision is angled proximally and laterally from the line of the adductor muscle to the inguinal ligament at the point where the femoral artery can be palpated. The junction of the upper quarter and lower three quarters of the adductor muscle marks the site of the neurovascular hilum of the gracilis muscle. The anterior border of the gracilis muscle is identified and the muscle reflected medially. This rapidly exposes the neurovascular hilum. The vascular pedicle is traced deep to the adductor longus muscle where multiple branches ascending from the vessel into the muscle require division. There are no branches from the deep surface of the pedicle. The vascular pedicle is then identified on the lateral side of the adductor longus muscle, and its origin from the profunda vessels is cleared. The venous drainage of the muscle is from a vena comitans system that is bifurcate to just before its termination in the profunda vein. The nerve, although it enters in common with the vascular pedicle, arises from the obturator nerve and descends

through the obturator foramen in an axis superomedial to the vascular pedicle; 6 to 7 cm of both vessel and nerve are usually available. Conveniently, the nerve to the gracilis almost always divides just before entry into the muscle, so an interfascicular dissection can separate the nerve into two bundles. The superior division of the nerve supplies the upper one third of the muscle and the larger inferior portion supplies the posterior two thirds. This allows the muscle to be separated into an upper portion that can be further subdivided into segments that pass to the eyebrow and upper and lower lids. The lower, more substantial portion of the muscle is subdivided into slips for the alar base and upper and lower lips. A nerve stimulator is helpful during this separation.

The muscle is then transferred to the face, where its proximal tendinous end is sutured to the temporalis and preparotid fascia. The distal separated portions of the muscle are then tunneled into their appropriate positions in the eyelids and mouth and sutured under maximum tension. The redundant portions of muscle are excised. The muscle is then revascularized and the upper crossfacial nerve graft joined to the upper division of the muscle destined for the eyelids; the lower crossfacial nerve graft is joined to the lower segment. Rarely is excessive bulk a problem because the muscle is widely fanned out.

Postoperatively the viability of the muscle can be monitored through the skin with a Doppler probe.

RESULTS

Since 1973 at St. Vincent's Hospital, thirty-three cases of facial palsy have been treated by two-stage crossfacial nerve grafting and a vascularized muscle transplant. In the first eight cases the extensor digitorum brevis muscle was used, and in only one case was convincing movement achieved. From 1974 onward, only the gracilis muscle has been used, and through December 1980 twenty-five cases have been performed. In fourteen of these there was a complete paralysis of both upper and lower portions of the face, and in eleven the muscle was used to innervate only the lower face. Of the twenty-five cases performed, only twenty-one were considered to be of sufficient postoperative duration to evaluate. Of these twenty-one cases, eighteen had regained obvious strong movement. Of the three failures, one resulted from failure to vascularize the muscle, so no movement was expected in this case. Eight of the eighteen that developed movement subsequently developed in-

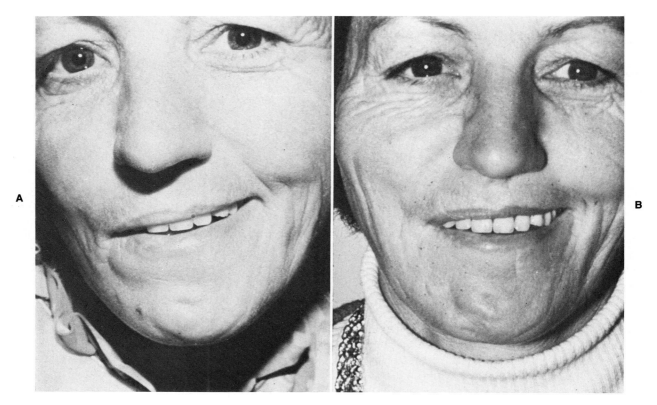

Fig. 20-1. A, Forty-two-year-old patient with a 4-year paralysis of the right side of the face following removal of an acoustic neuroma. Preoperative view. **B,** Five and a half years after crossfacial nerve graft, followed by gracilis muscle transplant to the lower face, patient shows good contraction and symmetric smile.

dependent movement of the paralyzed side, both in the upper and lower face. Also patients learned independent movement of the upper and lower face corresponding to each crossfacial nerve graft.

The average duration of the palsy before surgery ranged from 1 month to 40 years, with a mean of 8.4 years. The causes of the palsy were postsurgical Bell's palsy, congenital, and traumatic.

Some representative preoperative and postoperative cases are shown in Figs. 20-1 to 20-4.

DISCUSSION

Eighteen of twenty-one cases obtained good symmetry at rest and strong active lifting of the angle of the mouth and cheek. In the fourteen cases in which the eyelid was included in the reconstruction, satisfactory lid closure was achieved. Only three cases—and this included one where the muscle necrosed—failed to achieve movement. This result is vastly superior to any reported series using standard crossfacial nerve graft techniques alone. Furthermore, eight cases to date have obtained independent movements of the face, de-

spite the fact that it is motorized from the opposite side. There appears to be no satisfactory explanation for this at present. As the upper portion of the muscle graft is innervated by an independent nerve from the lower portion, there has also been independent movement of the eye from the cheek. Although convincing movement has been obtained in these transfers, the degree and sophistication need qualification.

Whereas the extensor brevis muscle from the foot generally proved too weak, the gracilis on occasion has continued to increase in function. In two cases the muscle became too powerful, resulting in an exaggerated grimace and giving the appearance of macrostomia. Adherence of the transplanted muscle to the overlying skin has caused some distortion on occasion, particularly of the philtrum, requiring release in two cases. The portion of the gracilis muscle tunneled into the eyelids was initially anchored at the medial canthal region, but this frequently produced webbing; the muscle is now sutured loosely into the upper and lower lids without medial attachment.

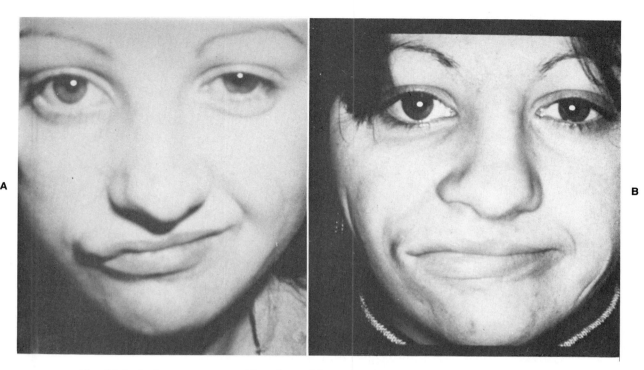

Fig. 20-2. **A,** Seventeen-year-old patient with 5-year right paralysis following skull fracture. Preoperative view. **B,** Four and a half years after two-stage gracilis transfer to lower face.

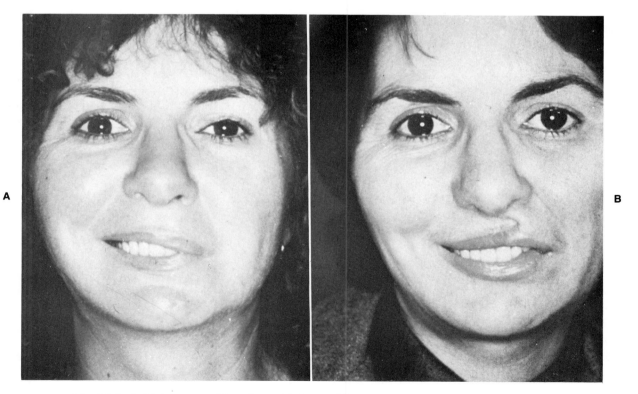

Fig. 20-3. **A,** Thirty-year-old patient with 2-year history of left paralysis following parotidectomy. Preoperative view. **B,** Three years after gracilis transfer to lower face. Some skin tethering of the upper lip required subsequent release.

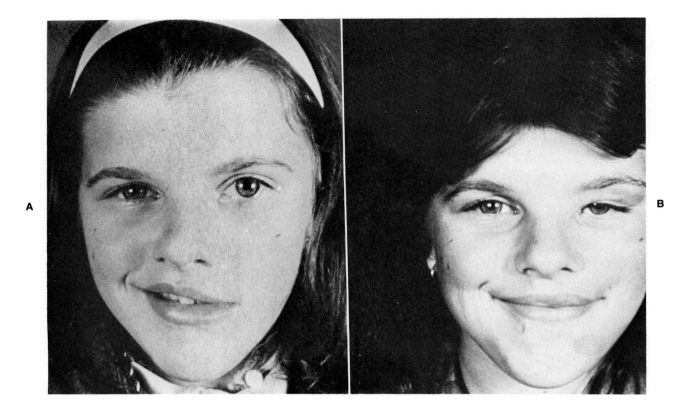

Fig. 20-4. A, Twelve-year-old female with left-sided congenital palsy. **B,** Eighteen months after gracilis transfer to upper and lower face.

Excessive bulk of the muscle graft has not been a problem, particularly when the muscle is fanned out to reconstruct the full face. A mandibular branch palsy deformity is not corrected by the procedure, since the muscle is pulling in the opposite direction, in some cases remaining the only key to the original palsy. Some dyskinetic movements are not infrequent, particularly when the patient is not concentrating, and the degree of voluntary contraction also tends to slacken if the patient is distracted. In general, movements are first detected 4 to 6 months following insertion of the muscle graft, and they continue to increase in strength with time.

SUMMARY

A two-stage method of total facial reanimation, combining a crossfacial nerve graft with a vascularized muscle transfer, generally achieves good function. The likelihood of return of movement is much greater than with standard crossfacial nerve grafting techniques, and movement is much more powerful. Complications of exaggerated movement, dyskinesia, and skin tethering are frequent and may necessitate some revisional surgery.

REFERENCES

1. Anderl, H.: Nerve repair and crossover grafting in facial nerve palsy. In Fredricks, S., and Brody, G., editors: Symposium on the neurologic aspects of plastic surgery, St. Louis, 1978, The C.V. Mosby Co.
2. Harii, K., Ohmori, K., and Torii, S.: Free gracilis muscle transplantation, with microneurovascular anastomoses for the treatment of facial paralysis: a preliminary report, Plast. Reconstr. Surg. **57:**133, 1976.
3. O'Brien, B.M., Franklin, J.D., and Morrison, W.A.: Cross-facial nerve grafts and microneurovascular free muscle transfer for long established facial palsy, Br. J. Plast. Surg. **33:**202, 1980.
4. Smith, J.W.: A new technique of facial animation. In Transactions of the Fifth International Congress of Plastic Surgery, London, 1971, Butterworth & Co. p. 83.

Chapter 21

Extensor digitorum brevis and pectoralis minor muscles in the treatment of unilateral facial palsy

Douglas H. Harrison
Bryan J. Mayou

The use of the extensor digitorum brevis muscle on a neurovascular pedicle has become less popular as unsuccessful results of this procedure have been reported.[5] We will present a series of ten cases in which we used this pedicle, describing our technique and results. We will also describe our use of the pectoralis minor muscle graft, which is presently being employed in the plastic surgery unit at Mount Vernon Hospital.

The use of crossfacial nerve grafts for restoring animation in a unilateral facial palsy appears to be a satisfactory procedure up to 1 year after nerve damage.[1] However, after this time interval the results are more variable, almost certainly because of irreversible changes in muscle infrastructure. In such cases it is necessary to introduce both the nerve and a muscle into the denervated side of the face. Thompson[8] suggested the use of the extensor digitorum brevis muscle of the foot as a suitable graft. Its size was appropriate to the distance between the modiolus of the mouth and the zygomatic arch, it was not too bulky, and the donor site defect was minimal. The muscle was denervated 2 weeks before a transplantation to effect changes in the histochemistry of the muscle rendering it capable of withstanding a prolonged period of anoxia before revascularization from the surrounding tissues.

For partial paralysis, the grafts were laid directly on the weakened facial muscle, with the nerve supply introduced into the grafted muscle by a process of muscular neurotization. In a complete unilateral palsy the anterior tibial nerve was taken with the muscle graft so that the muscle graft would be laid on the denervated side of the face and the nerve graft would be taken across the upper lip and sutured to the facial nerve on the innervated side.[9] This series is a further modification of this procedure in which the anterior tibial vessels were sutured to a recipient artery and vein to vascularize the muscle (Fig. 21-1). We hoped by this procedure to maintain the muscle bulk before reinnervation.

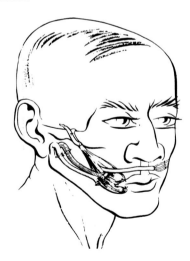

Fig. 21-1. The principles of the extensor digitorum brevis muscle graft with neurovascular anastomosis. (From Mayou, B.J., Watson, J.S., Harrison, D.H., and Parry, C.S.: Free microvascular and microneural transfer of the extensor digitorum brevis muscle for the treatment of unilateral facial palsy, Br. J. Plast. Surg. **34:**362, 1981.)

OPERATING TECHNIQUE

The surgery is carried out in two stages. At the first operation the extensor digitorum brevis muscle that has been chosen for transfer is denervated by approaching the anterior tibial nerve 10 cm above the ankle joint. The reason for this is two-fold—first, to denervate the muscle to prepare it for a period of anoxia in case of a thrombosis at the site of anastomosis, thus enabling it to survive as a free graft, and second, the anterior tibial nerve is a mixed nerve supplying motor fibers to the extensor digitorum brevis and sensory fibers to the adjacent sides of the first cleft. We had tried on many occasions to separate the sensory nerve fibers from the motor fibers in a 10 cm section of this nerve by dissection under a microscope. However, it proved extremely difficult because of frequent crossovers of axons among the three major fascicles. Therefore when there was a limited number of innervated seventh nerve fibers available, it was important to attach them to the fascicle carrying most of the motor fibers. At the time of denervation the anterior tibial nerve was dissected out into three fascicles and each of the fascicles was labeled with a code of 7V S&T sutures (Fig. 21-2). A section of each of these fascicles was then stained for acetylcholinesterase to ascertain which one of the fascicles contained most of the motor axons.[2,4] Axon counts and differential staining were carried out, and in general it was fairly easy to differentiate the axons into motor, sensory, and mixed. At the time of muscle transfer, therefore, the fascicles containing most of the motor axons could be dissected out and a contralateral innervated seventh nerve sutured to the most profitable fascicle.

Two weeks after denervation the extensor digitorum brevis muscle is dissected from the foot, dividing its origin from the tarsus and its insertion from the extensor hood of the toes (Fig. 21-3). The anterior tibial vessels and nerves are dissected on the bony plane for 10 cm above the ankle joint. The anterior tibial nerve must be dissected away from the vessels so that it may be passed into the contralateral cheek (Fig. 21-4). The nerve and muscle graft are removed from the foot, transferred to the paralyzed side of the face, and placed into a preformed tunnel between incisions in the nasolabial fold and another in the preauricular area (Fig. 21-5).

The vascular pedicle can be brought alongside the muscle graft into relation with the superficial temporal artery, which is prepared for anastomosis. The proximal bellies of the extensor digitorum brevis are attached to the angle of the mouth with

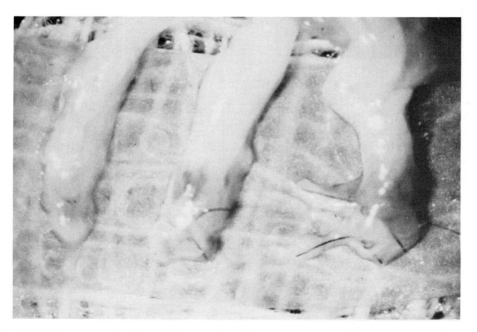

Fig. 21-2. The three fascicles of the anterior tibial nerve that had been labeled with S&T 7V sutures 2 weeks before. Note that the fascicle on the right has two sutures, the central fascicle one suture, and the fascicle on the left no sutures.

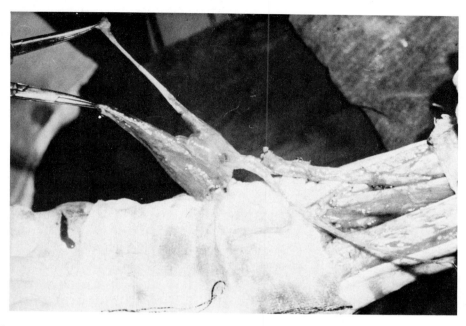

Fig. 21-3. Extensor digitorum brevis muscle delivered from the foot; note its neurovascular pedicle.

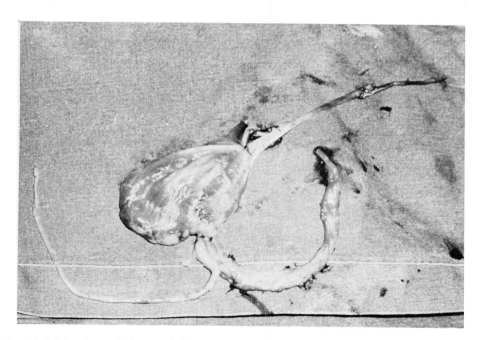

Fig. 21-4. Muscle graft removed from the foot; note its separated neurovascular pedicle.

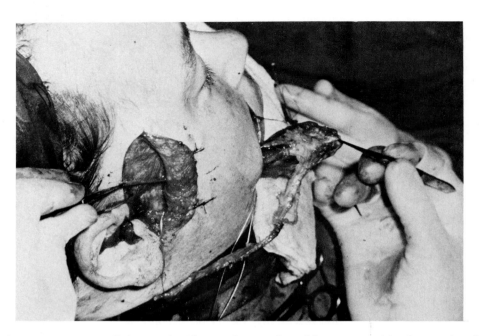

Fig. 21-5. Extensor digitorum brevis muscle transferred into a tunnel in the paralyzed cheek.

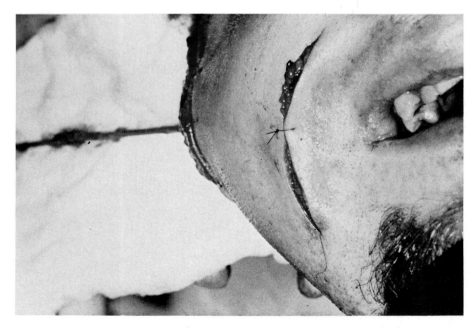

Fig. 21-6. Origin of the extensor digitorum brevis muscle has been sutured around the angle of the mouth in such a way that when tension is applied to the muscle tendon, it produces movement in the upper and lower lips and a balanced smile.

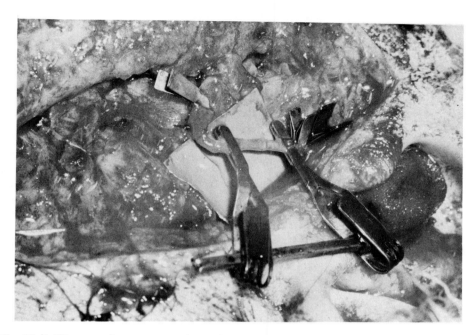

Fig. 21-7. The vascular anastomosis carried out between the superficial temporal artery and the anterior tibial artery on the paralyzed side of the face.

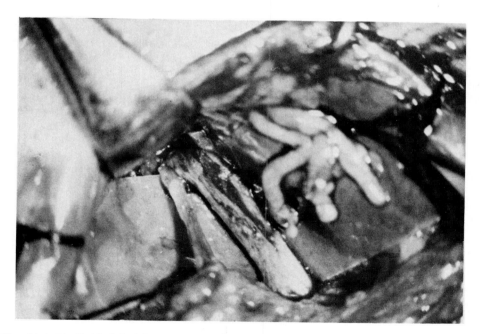

Fig. 21-8. Undivided facial nerve on the animated side of the face in the nasolabial fold. Beside these fibers note the three fascicles of the anterior tibial nerve that have been brought through a tunnel in the upper lip. The neurorrhaphy will be carried out under magnification.

nonabsorbable sutures in such a way that the inferior belly is sutured to the lower lip, the central belly into the modiolus of the mouth, and the superior belly into the upper lip. Thus when the extensor digitorum brevis tendon is placed under tension, a satisfactory elevation of the corner of the mouth is achieved (Fig. 21-6). Under positive tension the extensor digitorum brevis tendon is passed around the zygomatic arch and secured. The superficial temporal artery is then anastomosed to the anterior tibial artery, there commonly being a 1:3 disparity in vessel diameter (Fig. 21-7). In a series of ten cases, the superficial temporal artery was used in nine and a facial artery in one. The latter requires a more extensive dissection, although the caliber of the two vessels is comparable.

The anterior tibial nerve is then taken across the upper lip, through a preformed tunnel to a nasolabial incision on the contralateral animated side. The normal contralateral seventh nerve is then prepared at this level. Confirmation that the fibers found are indeed the facial nerve fibers supplying the levators of the angle of the mouth is achieved by nerve stimulation. The neurorrhaphy is carried out between the fibers of the normal seventh nerve and the fascicles in the anterior tibial nerve graft, which have been previously confirmed as carrying most of the motor axons to the extensor digitorum brevis muscle graft (Fig. 21-8). The nerve repair is carried out under the microscope, with a perineural type of suture.

RESULTS

In this series of ten cases treated by this technique, it has been apparent that positive results are often not witnessed until 2 to 3 years after surgery. Of the patients studied, four had a congenital facial palsy, four had a division of the facial nerve, and two had a Bell's palsy. The average duration of the palsy was 4½ years. Still photography is an unsatisfactory method of assessing the results of a dynamic muscle graft procedure; the series was therefore reviewed clinically by cinephotography and electromyography. Two cases had excellent excursion of the grafted muscle and approached symmetry (Fig. 21-9).

Two further cases had unquestioned muscular

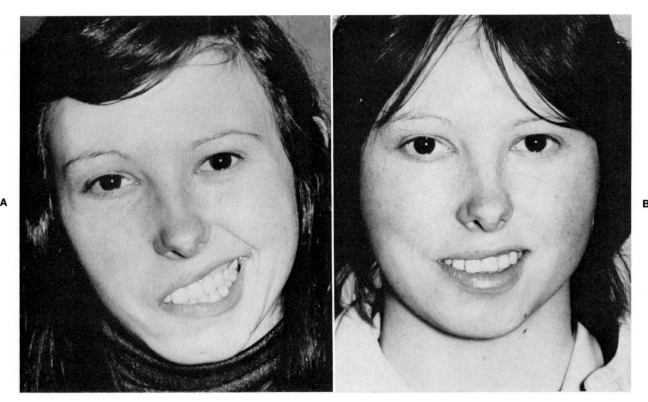

Fig. 21-9. A, Nineteen-year-old female with a right-sided facial palsy. **B,** Three years later she has developed a virtually symmetrical smile, and muscle activity can be clearly observed.

activity but were insufficient to equalize the power of the contralateral cheek. The remaining six were graded as static support only, although two had equivocal active movements. Electromyography was carried out in all the cases, with a needle placed into the muscle graft to record activity on voluntary movement. Action potentials of between 250 and 500 microvolts were recorded. This compares with an amplitude of 300 microvolts in normal facial muscles and 7 millivolts in a normal extensor digitorum brevis. With the needle electrode still in the muscle graft, the contralateral facial nerve was stimulated at the stylomastoid foramen and at the nasolabial fold at the point of nerve repair. This produced action potentials of a similar amplitude to those on voluntary movement. This procedure confirmed that muscle graft activity was mediated from the innervated side of the face rather than from any other source. The conduction velocity across the nerve graft was between 11 and 31 meters per second, compared with a normal conduction velocity of over 50 meters per second, which is consistent with regeneration. The electromyogram studies suggested that there was muscle activity in six out of ten grafts rather than four that showed clinical evidence of activity.

DISCUSSION

A success rate of two cases out of ten is hardly a commendation for a procedure that takes some 4 to 6 hours to carry out. However, the fact that it was possible to achieve some movement in four out of ten cases is encouraging, and methods of improving these results need exploring. It was of interest that the two good results occurred in the younger age groups—one patient was 19 years old and the other 22. Youth probably played a beneficial role in axon growth.

The extensor digitorum brevis is a relatively small muscle, and its tendon excursion is probably little more than 1.5 cm. Terzis et al.[7] have shown that under optimal experimental conditions the muscle will attain only 25% of its previous working capacity after transplantation. Even if the 25% quoted by Terzis is a rather pessimistic figure, the excursion of the transplanted extensor digitorum brevis under favorable conditions is unlikely to be greater than 7 mm. It would therefore be desirable to have a muscle with increased bulk that is sufficient—even if considerable reduction in power does occur after reinnervation—to elevate the modiolus of the mouth and equalize the pull on the innervated side of the face. The muscle should have enough excursion of its tendon to elevate the modiolus of the mouth by some 1.5 cm. Suitable

muscles for transfer would be the latissimus dorsi or gracilis[3,6]; however, both of these muscles are too long, although they can be sectioned if the neuromuscular hilum is not damaged. The pectoralis minor muscle presented herein has the advantages of being a suitable length and width and leaving minimal donor site deformity.

The problems of innervating the graft also require refinement. The long anterior tibial nerve passed across the cheek requires only one nerve repair, but the axons will certainly take some months to reach the nerve graft before reinnervation occurs. The long delay period increases the number of muscle fibers that will not regenerate. The solution is to carry out a preliminary facial nerve graft 6 months before transfer, which has the advantage of shorter axon growth before reinnervation. It is unfortunate that two nerve repairs are necessary, with the inevitable fibrosis and axon loss across them. The facial nerve at the level of the nasolabial fold tends to be relatively small, and therefore the nerve repair is less satisfactory. The facial nerve at the level of the parotid duct is a much larger and more well-defined structure and is very suitable for nerve repair. Virtually all the facial nerve may be divided at this level with little fear of a paralysis developing and indeed is beneficial as a selective neurectomy.

PECTORALIS MINOR TRANSFER

To improve the results of the treatment of unilateral facial palsy, we examined a number of possible muscles for transfer. The length of the muscle fibers was felt to be important so that the muscle could be placed into its new recipient site under normal tension. The muscle clearly needed to be supplied in its entirety by the hilar vessel and nerves. The length of the neurovascular pedicle should preferably be as long as possible and of sufficient caliber to facilitate easy and safe vascular repair and restore nerve continuity.

The pectoralis minor muscle has advantages of size, shape, and a suitable neurovascular pedicle, and it can be harvested without a donor site deformity. The muscle originates from the third, fourth, and fifth ribs and from the fascia over the external intercostals. The fibers pass upward into a flat tendon and insert into the coracoid process of the scapula. Its vascular supply comes largely from the lateral thoracic artery, with its vein draining directly into the axillary vein. The nerve supply is provided by the medial and lateral pectoral nerves issuing from the medial and lateral chords of the brachial plexus.

At the first stage a sural nerve graft is taken

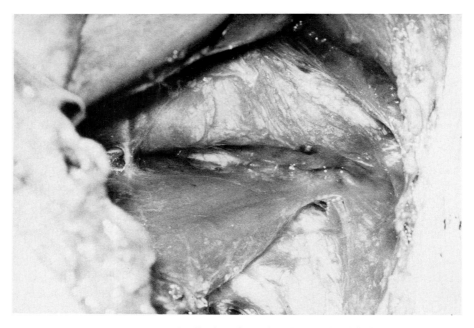

Fig. 21-10. Pectoralis minor muscle displayed on the chest wall with the pectoralis major muscle retracted from its anterior surface. The insertion to the coracoid process is on the right.

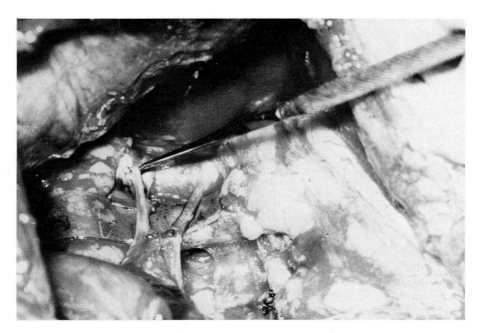

Fig. 21-11. The insertion of the pectoralis minor has been divided, exposing the hilar structures. The hook is elevating the lateral pectoral nerve, which can be seen straddling the axillary artery and joining with the medial pectoral nerve to enter the muscle. Just lateral to the nerve is the lateral thoracic artery issuing from the axillary artery. It passes over the branch from the axillary vein, which drains the muscle and may be seen at the 3 o'clock position.

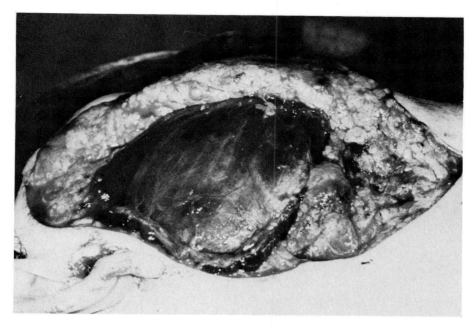

Fig. 21-12. The pectoralis minor muscle inserted into the paralyzed right cheek and revascularized by anastomosis of the hilar vessels to the facial artery and vein and reinnervated by a neurorrhaphy to a crossfacial nerve graft.

from the leg and sutured to the facial nerve at the level of the parotid duct on the innervated side via a face lift incision. The nerve is then taken across the upper lip with the use of an incision in the vermillion edge to guide the nerve. The distal end of the nerve graft is then sutured to the preauricular area on the denervated side of the face; the growth of the axons is awaited for 6 months, and the rate of growth is assessed by an advancing Tinel's sign.

Six months after the nerve graft, the pectoralis minor muscle is harvested via an incision along the anterior axillary fold, which can be taken upward into the deltopectoral groove if necessary. This incision exposes the pectoralis major muscle, which may be retracted superomedially to expose the pectoralis minor muscle (Fig. 21-10). To expose the hilar vessels of the pectoralis minor muscle, the surgeon divides the insertion into the coracoid process. When the insertion of the muscle is retracted in a downward direction, the pedicle is clearly defined. The axillary artery gives off the lateral thoracic artery, which supplies the muscle; the medial and lateral pectoral nerves issue from both sides of the axillary artery and may join together before entering the muscle (Fig. 21-11).

The neurovascular hilum is relatively short but of good caliber.

After dissecting and isolating the neurovascular hilum, one can divide the origin of the muscle from the third, fourth, and fifth ribs. Confirmation of muscle viability can be confirmed by the presence of bleeding from the origin. After dividing of the vessels, the surgeon may transfer the muscle to the face (Fig. 21-12). The preauricular incision is extended into the submandibular region, exposing the facial vessels. Via this incision the nerve graft and modiolus of the mouth may be defined. The hilar structures of the pectoralis minor are relatively short, and therefore anastomosis of the vessels and the nerve repair may need to be carried out on the deep surface of the muscle. This is done before suturing the pectoralis minor muscle into its new bed. The preauricular tissues provide the origin for the pectoralis minor transplant.

Our series at present is small, and evaluation must await the passage of time, but early results are encouraging (Fig. 21-13). The pectoralis minor muscle does seem to have many positive benefits, not the least of which is a virtually invisible donor site scar.

Fig. 21-13. A, Twenty-five-year-old male with a total right-sided facial palsy before operation. **B,** Nine months after surgery there is distinct movement in the pectoralis minor muscle graft, and tone in the right side of the face is much improved.

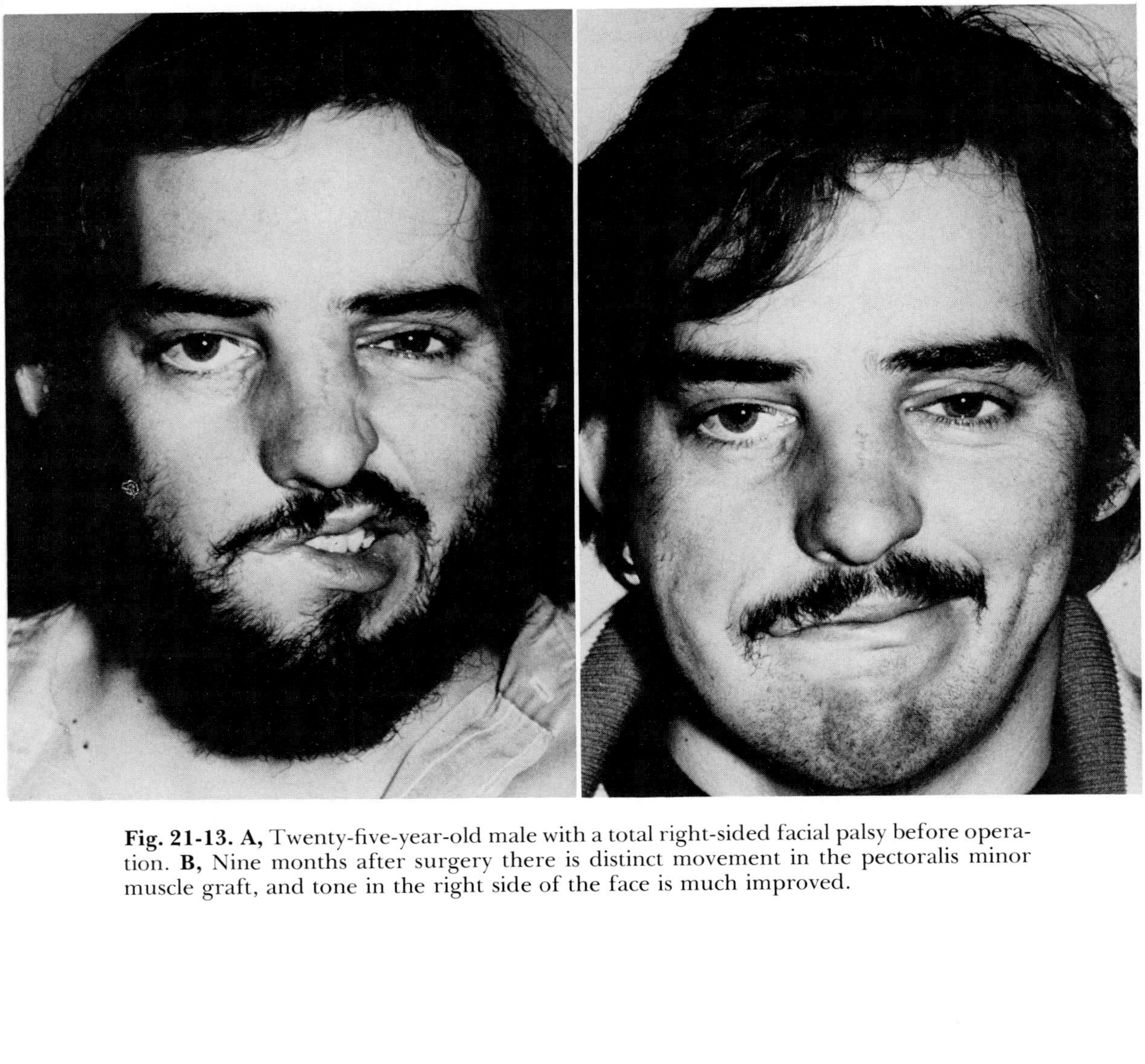

SUMMARY

The value of free muscle grafts with neurovascular anastomosis to animate the paralyzed face has been questioned. Certainly early results were not promising in view of the investment in operating time. It is clear, however, that the final result may not be fully apparent for 2 to 3 years. Techniques have become refined and more reliable results may be expected in the future. Our early experience has suggested that results will improve with the use of larger muscles with greater tendon excursion.

ACKNOWLEDGMENTS

The work on the vascularized extensor digitorum transfer was carried out in collaboration with Mr. Stewart Watson, F.R.C.S., M.R.C.P., and Dr. Wyn Parry, M.B.E., M.A., D.M., F.R.C.S., F.R.C.P., and owes much to the encouragement of Mr. Noel Thompson, M.S., F.R.C.S.

REFERENCES

1. Anderl, H.: Reconstruction of the face through cross facial nerve transplantation in facial paralysis, Chir. Plast. **2:**17, 1973.
2. Gruber, H., and Zenker, W.: Acetylcholinesterase: histochemical differentiation between motor and sensory fibres, Brain Res. **51:**207, 1973.
3. Harii, K., Ohmori, K., and Torii, S.: Free gracilis muscle transplantation with microneurovascular anastomosis for the treatment of facial palsy, Plast. Reconstr. Surg. **57:**133, 1976.
4. Karnovsky, J.J., and Roots, L.: A "direct colouring" thiocoline method for cholinesterases, J. Hist. Chem. Cytochem. **12:**219, 1964.
5. Nicolai, J.P.A.: Free muscle grafting in facial paralysis, Br. J. Plast. Surg. **34:**91, 1981.
6. O'Brien, B.M., Franklin, J.D., and Morrison, W.A.: Cross-facial nerve grafts and microneurovascular free muscle transfer for long-established facial palsy, Br. J. Plast. Surg. **57:**133, 1980.
7. Terzis, J.K., Sweet, R.C., Dykes, R.W., and Williams, H.B.: Recovery of function in free muscle transplants using microneurovascular anastomoses, J. Hand Surg. **3:**37, 1978.
8. Thompson, N.: Treatment of facial paralysis by free skeletal muscle grafts, Proceedings of the Congress of Plastic and Reconstructive Surgeons, London, 1971, Butterworth & Co.
9. Thompson, N., and Gustavson, E.H.: The use of a neuromuscular free autograft with microneural anastomosis to restore elevation to the paralysed angle of the mouth in cases of unilateral facial paralysis, Chir. Plast. **3:**165, 1976.

Part VI

Breast reconstruction

Chapter 22

Microsurgical composite tissue transplantation in postmastectomy breast reconstruction

Donald Serafin
Vincent E. Voci
Nicholas G. Georgiade

Reconstruction after mastectomy has been facilitated by techniques that employ an island latissimus dorsi musculocutaneous flap. However, in a small percentage of patients with extensive qualitative and quantitative defects, this method has excessively high flap morbidity. It is in this small subgroup of patients that reconstruction with vascularized composite tissue transplantation is indicated.

Since 1974 approximately 300 of our patients have undergone postmastectomy breast reconstruction.[4] Twenty-six of these patients (9%) were felt to be candidates for microsurgical composite tissue transplantation (Table 22-1). Fourteen patients underwent reconstruction with a vascular-

ized latissimus dorsi musculocutaneous flap. A vascularized groin flap was employed as donor tissue in twelve patients. Only one failure occurred in this series (4%); thus 96% of the cases with extensive defects were reconstructed successfully.[14]

INDICATIONS FOR MICROSURGICAL RECONSTRUCTION
Conditions precluding use of ipsilateral island latissimus dorsi musculocutaneous flap

The most common indication for microsurgical reconstruction is the presence of factors precluding the use of an ipsilateral island latissimus dorsi musculocutaneous flap. Significant injury or atrophy of the latissimus dorsi muscle alone may not obviate its use, but the addition of other local recipient wound factors may dictate the selection of alternative methods of reconstruction.

Radical mastectomy and postoperative irradiation can contribute to increased donor flap or recipient site morbidity. Although the modified radical mastectomy is the most common surgical procedure performed for extirpation of a breast malignancy, some surgeons still perform a radical mastectomy. Along with the breast, the pectoralis major muscle and axillary contents are removed through a vertical incision, frequently extending from the clavicle to the rectus abdominis fascia (Fig. 22-1, *A* to *D*). A split-thickness skin graft is sometimes required for wound closure. Edema of

Table 22-1. Indications for microsurgical composite tissue transplantation in breast reconstruction following mastectomy

Indication	Number of patients	Percentage
Conditions precluding ipsilateral latissimus dorsi musculocutaneous flap	17	65
Previous failure of an ipsilateral latissimus dorsi musculocutaneous flap	1	4
Restoration of form and contour with minimal donor deformity	8	31

From Serafin, D., Voci, V.E., and Georgiade, N.G.: Microsurgical composite tissue transplantation: indications and technical considerations in breast reconstruction following mastectomy, Plast. Reconstr. Surg. **70:**24, 1982.

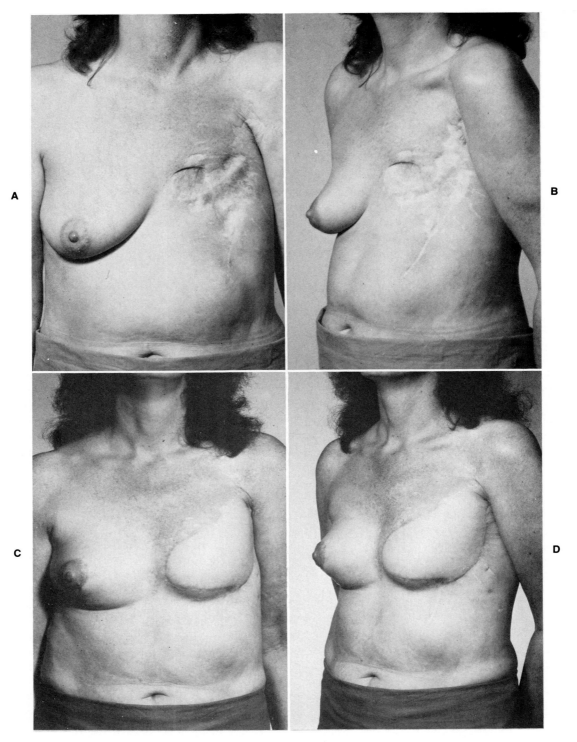

Fig. 22-1. A and **B,** Postoperative views demonstrating extensive qualitative and quantitative deficiency of skin following a classic radical mastectomy. The thoracodorsal neurovascular pedicle was sacrificed during the initial extirpative procedure. **C** and **D,** Postoperative result following contralateral vascularized latissimus dorsi musculocutaneous transplantation and reconstruction. Subtotal resection with submuscular augmentation during the second stage of breast reconstruction. (From Serafin, D., Voci, V.E., and Georgiade, N.G.: Microsurgical composite tissue transplantation: indications and technical considerations in breast reconstruction following mastectomy, Plast. Reconstr. Surg. **70:**24, 1982.)

the ipsilateral upper extremity and a decreased range of shoulder motion are known complications of the radical mastectomy. As a result of this extensive dissection, a severe qualitative and quantitative loss of skin and subcutaneous tissue anteriorly and laterally may result; in addition, the neurovascular pedicle to the latissimus dorsi muscle may be interrupted.

Fisher and Bostwick[2] have demonstrated that ligation of the muscle's dominant thoracodorsal artery will result in a reversal of blood flow from the serratus anterior muscle branch into the remaining distal thoracodorsal artery. The lateral thoracic artery then becomes the dominant blood supply to the latissimus dorsi muscle. An island musculocutaneous flap based on this blood supply can be transferred safely, but the muscle will be atrophied if it was denervated at the time of mastectomy.

Atrophy of the latissimus dorsi always follows division of its motor nerve; consequently muscle volume and bulk is reduced. This limits reconstruction of an infraclavicular depression and creation of an anterior axillary fold and may obviate immediate submuscular augmentation. A noncontracting (denervated) latissimus dorsi muscle can be easily identified preoperatively (Fig. 22-2). In patients with extensive defects to be reconstructed and who have had the thoracodorsal neurovascular bundle ligated, island transfer of an ipsilateral latissimus dorsi musculocutaneous composite tissue segment is often inadequate.

Likewise, when a major portion of the latissimus dorsi muscle has been transected (e.g., by previous thoracotomy), innervation of the isolated segment is interrupted. This portion will remain viable, but atrophy will eventually occur. Unless there is sufficient volume of the innervated portion, transfer of such a muscle to reconstruct large complicated defects is ill advised.

Axillary lymph nodes with positive pathologic findings, a medially positioned tumor, or a local incisional recurrence are often considered indications for postoperative radiation therapy. An overlap of treatment fields and/or treatment with an orthovoltage machine may contribute to tissue morbidity at the mastectomy site and in adjacent areas.[15] A qualitative deficiency of skin and subjacent tissues is added to the quantitative loss from the mastectomy. Avascularity, dense fibrosis, and induration characterize these recipient sites. In addition, osteoradionecrosis of the underlying ribs and clavicle does occur with predicted frequency.[7,9,10] Brachial plexus neuropathy, edema of the upper extremity, and a decreased range of shoulder motion also contribute to tissue morbidity at the mastectomy site.[2] Transfer of an island latissimus flap whose primary neurovascular pedicle has been previously ligated would be ill advised.

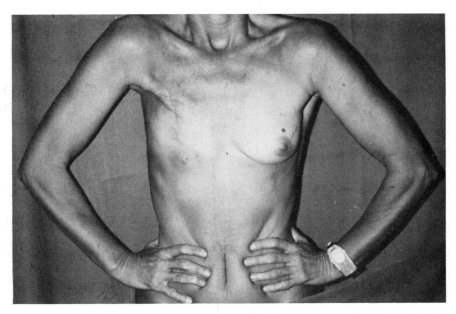

Fig. 22-2. Preoperative view demonstrating lack of visible contraction of the ipsilateral latissimus dorsi muscle following modified radical mastectomy. (From Serafin, D., Voci, V.E., and Georgiade, N.G.: Microsurgical composite tissue transplantation: Indications and technical considerations in breast reconstruction following mastectomy. Plast. Reconstr. Surg. **70:**24, 1982.)

Fig. 22-3. A, Preoperative view of a patient with a left radical mastectomy and right modified radical mastectomy. **B,** Postoperative view following failure of conventional island latissimus dorsi musculocutaneous flap. **C,** Postoperative view following contralateral vascularized latissimus dorsi musculocutaneous flap to reconstruct left breast and submuscular insertion of silicone prosthesis for right breast reconstruction. (From Serafin, D., Voci, V.E., and Georgiade, N.G.: Microsurgical composite tissue transplantation: indications and technical considerations in breast reconstruction following mastectomy, Plast. Reconstr. Surg. **70:**24, 1982.)

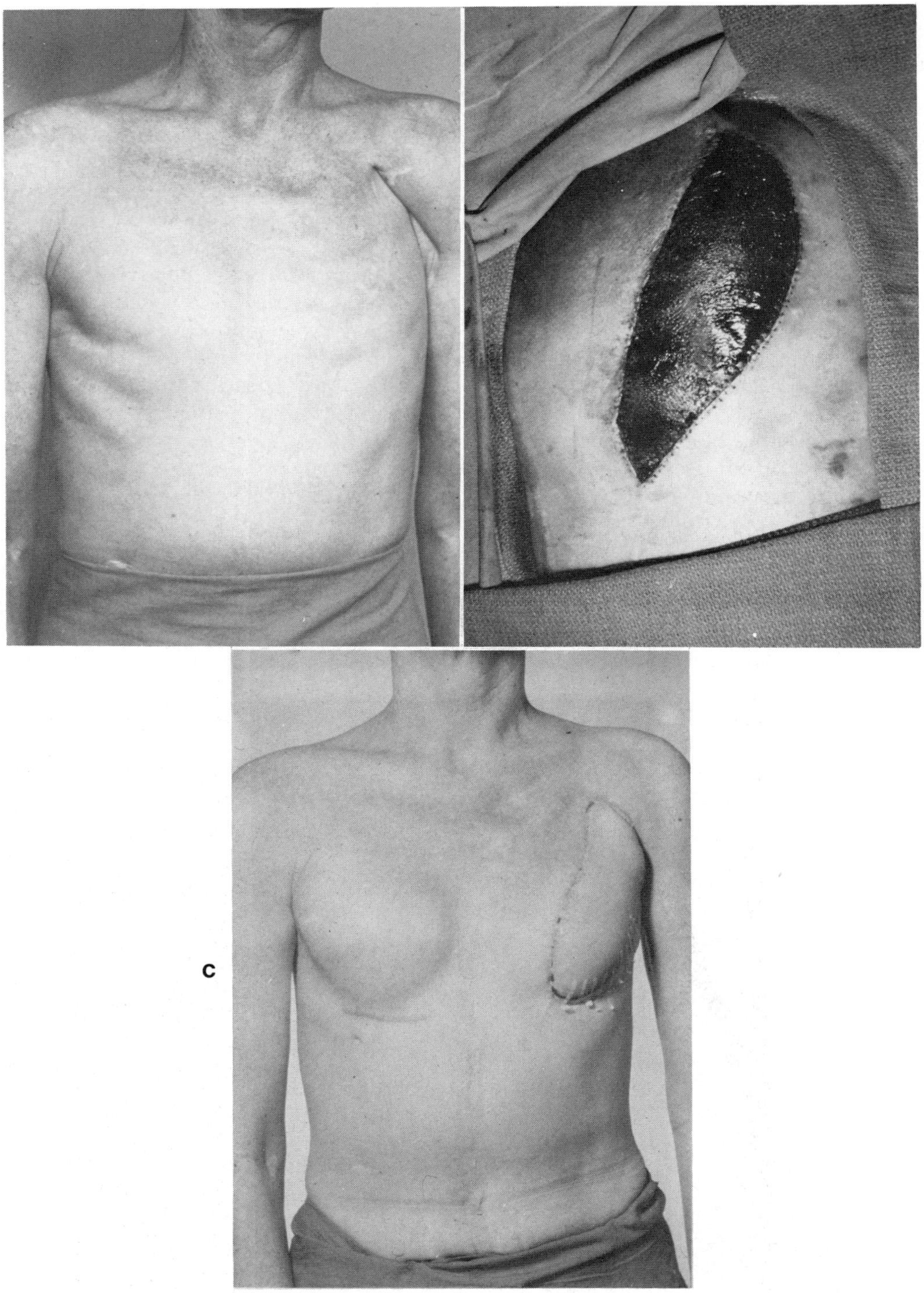

In the present series there were seventeen patients in whom the ipsilateral latissimus dorsi musculocutaneous flap could not be employed in reconstruction. Thirteen of these patients had previously undergone a standard radical mastectomy with postoperative radiation therapy. Contraction of the ipsilateral latissimus dorsi muscle could not be demonstrated clinically. Three additional patients had also undergone an extensive radical mastectomy but did not receive postoperative irradiation. A contracting latissimus dorsi muscle could not be demonstrated in this group either. Another patient had an atrophic latissimus dorsi muscle as a result of a previous thoracotomy.

Thirteen patients underwent reconstruction with a contralateral vascularized latissimus dorsi musculocutaneous flap and four with a vascularized groin flap.

Previous flap failure

Previous failure of a conventional island latissimus dorsi musculocutaneous flap is another indication for microsurgical composite tissue transplantation to reconstruct the breast after mastectomy (Fig. 22-3, *A* to *C*). Although reconstruction with a conventional island latissimus dorsi flap is a reliable method, flap morbidity does exist. Several large patient series exclusively employing a microsurgical method in reconstruction have documented patient and flap morbidity statistics.[6,13] In addition, flap morbidity data for a specific donor tissue in a variety of recipient sites have also been published.[5,6,13] Such data are also published for direct distant and indirect distant flaps.[1,8,12,17,18] However, morbidity statistics in an adequate number of patients, comparing musculocutaneous flaps at different reconstructive sites, are long overdue.

Only one patient (4%) in the present series underwent reconstruction following failure of an ipsilateral latissimus dorsi flap. One additional patient awaits reconstruction. Incorrect identification of the serratal branch and transection of the insertion of the latissimus dorsi muscle at the time of reconstruction resulted in flap necrosis. Both the thoracodorsal neurovascular pedicle and the serratal branch had been ligated during mastectomy. A vascularized latissimus dorsi musculocutaneous flap from the contralateral side was successfully transplanted 1 week later.

Minimal donor deformity

The restoration of form and contour with a minimal secondary donor deformity is yet another indication for microsurgical reconstruction. A very small number of patients seeking breast reconstruction finds any thoracic donor scar unacceptable. Most posterolateral thoracic donor site scars, even if located in a brassiere line, are wide and conspicuous. The use of the vascularized groin flap eliminates the need for additional thoracic scars. Its selection may have greater appeal in the younger age group undergoing reconstruction. The donor incision in the groin is closed primarily and can be concealed even by brief clothing.

Eight patients in this series underwent reconstruction with a vascularized groin flap to minimize the secondary deformity of the donor site.

DISCUSSION

A combination of factors can exist at the postmastectomy site that may seriously limit the effectiveness of reconstruction with an island latissimus dorsi musculocutaneous flap. Reconstruction of extensive qualitative and quantitative defects with an atrophied muscle may be ill advised. This complicated situation was encountered in approximately 6% of all patients requesting postmastectomy breast reconstruction. In addition, a smaller group of patients (3%) refused latissimus reconstruction because a thoracic donor site scar was undesirable.

Patients with complicated recipient sites present difficult problems in microsurgical transplantation as well. Most of the branches of the axillary artery and vein have often been ligated at the time of mastectomy. This complicates recipient vascular selection. In addition, the various donor tissues present technical difficulties in transplantation unique to that specific tissue. Certain technical modifications, taking into account the limitations of the specific donor tissue and existing recipient site requirements, have contributed to the success in this series. To date we have successfully used two specific types of microsurgical donor tissue in breast reconstruction. Others have been reported and will be reviewed here as well.[3,16]

Vascularized groin flap

The vascularized groin flap has a few advantages in breast reconstruction. Its primary advantage is the location of the donor deformity.[11] In addition, a large segment of composite tissue (11 by 27 cm) can usually be obtained and the donor site closed primarily. Disadvantages include a short vascular pedicle, necessitating an interpositional vein or arterial graft (Table 22-2 and Fig. 22-4, *A* to *E*). An end-to-side anastomosis between the donor artery and the recipient axillary artery is done

Table 22-2. Technical considerations: types of anastomoses

End-to-end arterial anastomosis	11
End-to-end venous anastomosis	23
End-to-side arterial anastomosis	15
End-to-side venous anastomosis	3
Interpositional vein graft	8
Neural coaptation	3

From Serafin, D., Voci, V.E., and Georgiade, N.G.: Microsurgical composite tissue transplantation: indications and technical considerations in breast reconstruction following mastectomy, Plast. Reconstr. Surg. **70:**24, 1982.

if necessary, though an end-to-end venous anastomosis can usually be done (Table 22-2). Postoperative irradiation further complicates recipient vascular selection. The only flap failure in the present series was caused by the ill-advised selection of an incompletely obstructed recipient vein in a severely irradiated axilla. Other disadvantages include difficult flap dissection and the probability of significant and sometimes confusing variations in the vascular anatomy of the donor site. A vascularized groin flap was used in twelve patients. The

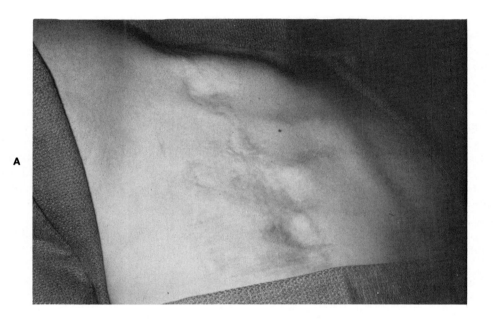

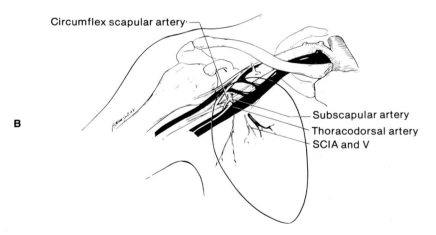

Fig. 22-4. A, Preoperative view following right radical mastectomy. Note extensive qualitative and quantitative deficiency of skin. **B,** Intraoperative findings during the first stage of breast reconstruction with a vascularized groin flap. Note ligation of thoracodorsal artery. (From Serafin, D., Voci, V.E., and Georgiade, N.G.: Microsurgical composite tissue transplantation: indications and technical considerations in breast reconstruction following mastectomy, Plast. Reconstr. Surg. **70:**24, 1982.)

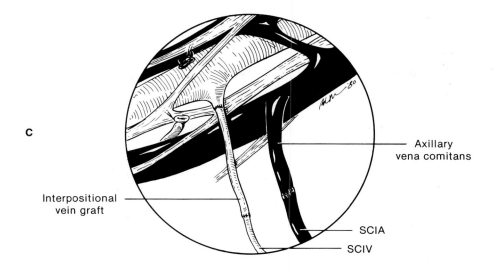

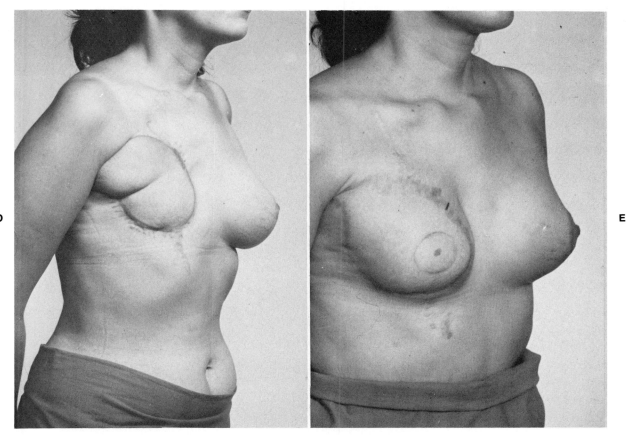

Fig. 22-4, cont'd. C, Reversed intrapositional vein graft with end-to-end anastomosis to patient subscapular artery and superficial circumflex iliac artery of the donor groin flap. An end-to-end anastomosis is performed between axillary vena comitans and the drainable vein of the groin flap. **D,** Postoperative result following the first stage of breast reconstruction with a vascularized groin flap. Note silicone prosthesis placed during the second stage of breast reconstruction. **E,** Late postoperative result following completion of breast reconstruction.

flap was positioned during the initial operative procedure. A second procedure was required to augment the flap with a silicone prosthesis and to perform a subtotal resection on the contralateral breast to provide mound symmetry. The delayed placement of the prosthesis was done to minimize the potential of postoperative extrusion and infection. Neither occurred in this series. The incidence of significant capsular contraction was noticeably higher in this series of groin flaps than in the vascularized latissimus dorsi flaps. This supports current conjecture that a lower incidence of capsular contraction occurs with submuscular techniques of augmentation.

Vascularized latissimus dorsi musculocutaneous flap

A contralateral vascularized latissimus dorsi musculocutaneous flap was employed in fourteen patients, without flap morbidity. The entire muscle is used with a smaller elliptical cutaneous paddle, making available an extensive amount of donor tissue (Fig. 22-5, *A* to *F*). With this, the infraclavicular depression is corrected and the anterior axillary fold is recreated. The prosthesis is placed under the flap during the first stage.

A neural coaptation is performed between the proximal recipient thoracodorsal nerve and the corresponding donor nerve if the axillary dissection is not too difficult (Table 22-2). An epifascicular epineural suture technique is used. Subjectively, in this small number of patients (three) there appears to be less muscle atrophy. It is postulated that capsular contraction and fibrosis will be minimized. The lengthy vascular pedicle is a great advantage, facilitating placement of the flap and performance of the vascular anastomoses.

End-to-end arterial and venous anastomoses to branches of the axillary artery and to one of the axillary venae comitantes are preferred (Table 22-3). However, if dissection is difficult because of excessive fibrosis, end-to-side anastomoses are performed. Usually this anastomotic technique necessitates total occlusion of the vessels to the limb for 1 to 1½ hours. Ten thousand units of heparin are administered intravenously before occlusion. We feel that the likelihood of thrombosis may be increased because of the combined effects of pro-

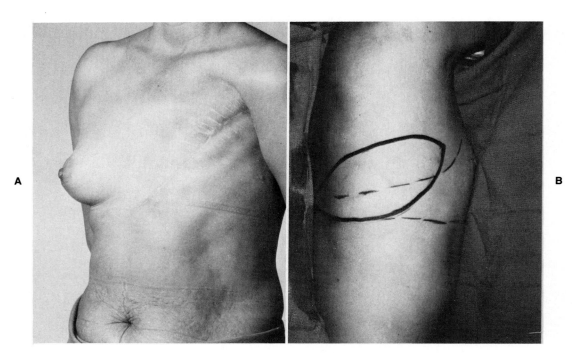

Fig. 22-5. A, Preoperative view demonstrating quantitative deficiency of skin following a left radical mastectomy. The thoracodorsal neurovascular pedicle was sacrificed during the original extirpative procedure. **B,** Intraoperative view demonstrating the donor contralateral latissimus dorsi musculocutaneous flap. The cutaneous portion of the flap is designed to provide maximal concealment of the donor scar in the brassiere line. (From Serafin, D., Voci, V.E., and Georgiade, N.G.: Microsurgical composite tissue transplantation: indications and technical considerations in breast reconstruction following mastectomy, Plast. Reconstr. Surg. **70:**24, 1982.)

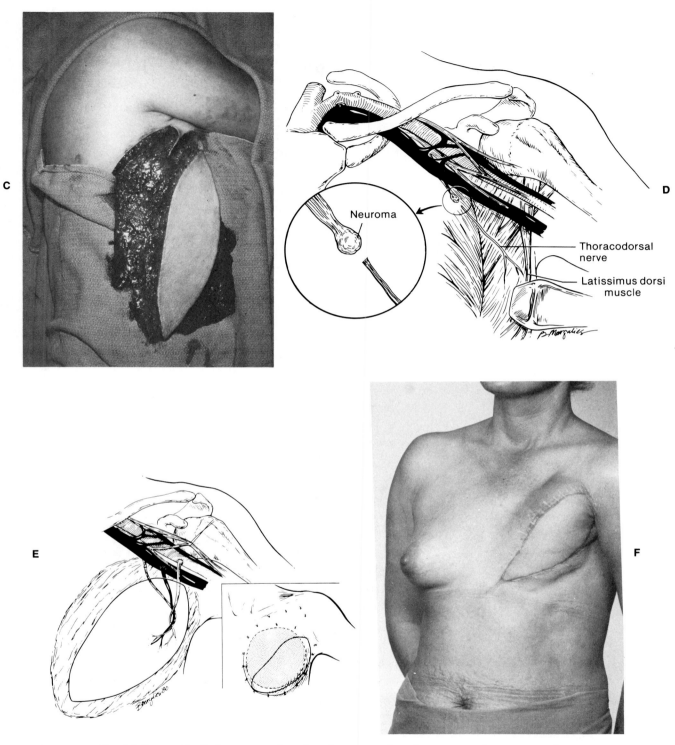

C

D

Neuroma

Thoracodorsal nerve

Latissimus dorsi muscle

E

F

Fig. 22-5, cont'd. C, Intraoperative view demonstrating donor musculocutaneous flap. Note that the entire latissimus dorsi muscle is employed to provide maximum coverage of the silicone prosthesis that will be put in place during the first stage of breast reconstruction. **D,** Intraoperative findings with neuroma of the thoracodorsal nerve. **E,** Neurovascular anastomoses. Note immediate placement of silicone prosthesis. Correction of the infraclavicular depression and reconstruction of the anterior axillary fold *(insert).* **F,** Postoperative result.

longed ischemia, intimal hyperplasia, and other morphologic and physiologic changes subsequent to irradiation and an arteriotomy.

A decreased range of shoulder motion, the presence of upper extremity edema, brachial plex-us neuropathy, and/or osteoradionecrosis of the clavicle should warn the reconstructive surgeon that a thorough axillary dissection to isolate the recipient vasculature would be hazardous. Recipient vasculature outside the area of irradiation should then be sought (Fig. 22-6, *A* to *F*).[15] The external carotid artery and a facial vein are good choices. End-to-end anastomoses are frequently performed (Table 22-3). The neurovascular pedicle is often of sufficient length to reach these more distant recipient vessels without an interpositional vein graft. A difficult axillary dissection can thus be avoided and the incidence of success will be increased.

Table 22-3. Technical considerations: selection of recipient vasculature

Recipient artery	
Axillary	15
Subscapular	5
Circumflex scapular	1
External carotid	
Superior thyroid	2
Lingual	1
Internal mammary	2
Recipient vein	
Axillary vena comitans	12
Axillary vein	3
Subscapular	4
Circumflex scapular	1
Lateral thoracic	1
Facial vein	1
External jugular	2
Internal mammary	2

From Serafin, D., Voci, V.E., and Georgiade, N.G.: Microsurgical composite tissue transplantation: indications and technical considerations in breast reconstruction following mastectomy, Plast. Reconstr. Surg. **70:**24, 1982.

Vascularized tensor fascia lata musculocutaneous flap

The tensor fascia lata musculocutaneous flap has had limited use by others in breast reconstruction.[16] This flap is most useful when its tough fascia lata can be used to stabilize large thoracic wall defects. Its lengthy vascular pedicle is a definite advantage. The donor defect can be closed primarily, but the resulting deformity is significant. The indications for this flap are rare.

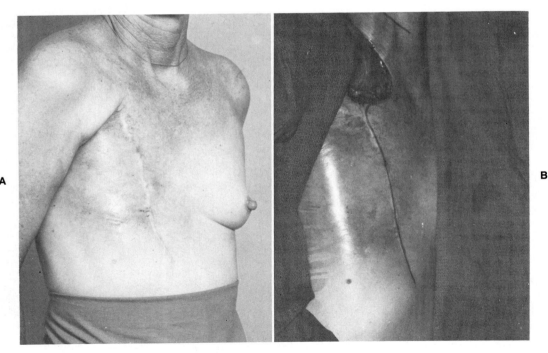

Fig. 22-6. A, Preoperative photograph following right radical mastectomy and extensive postoperative irradiation and secondary brachial plexus neurropathy. **B,** Intraoperative view demonstrating incisions for external brachial plexus neurolysis and exposure of recipient vasculature. (From Serafin, D., Voci, V.E., and Georgiade, N.G.: Microsurgical composite tissue transplantation: indications and technical considerations in breast reconstruction following mastectomy. Plast. Reconstr. Surg. **70:**24, 1982.)

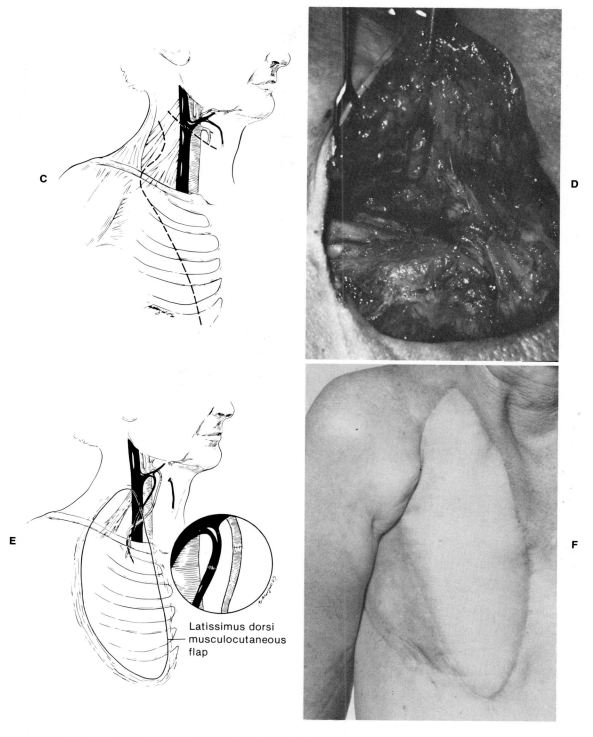

Fig. 22-6, cont'd. C, Operative incisions. **D,** Intraoperative view demonstrating external neurolysis C5, C6, and C7 of brachial plexus. **E,** Successful end-to-end anastomosis of recipient vasculature outside of the portals of irradiation in the neck with immediate coverage of the brachial plexus with vascularized composite tissue. **F,** Late postoperative result.

Vascularized gluteus maximus musculocutaneous flap

The first vascularized composite tissue used to reconstruct the breast was the gluteus maximus musculocutaneous flap.[3] Shaw has subsequently used this donor tissue in three patients.[16] It has several demonstrated advantages. The vascular pedicle is lengthy, facilitating anastomosis; the donor deformity is concealed within the pant line; and augmentation, particularly in moderately obese patients, may not be necessary because of adequate bulk already present in the flap.[16] Flap ischemia and operative times may be prolonged because of the inability to adequately expose the donor and recipient sites simultaneously. This is its single disadvantage.

SUMMARY

Twenty-six patients underwent microsurgical reconstruction of the breast and thorax following mastectomy in this series.

Indications for the use of microsurgical composite tissue transplantation in breast reconstruction following mastectomy include:

1. Conditions precluding an island latissimus dorsi musculocutaneous flap
2. Previous failure of an island latissimus dorsi musculocutaneous flap
3. The restoration of form and contour with minimal secondary donor deformity

Twelve patients underwent reconstruction with vascularized groin flaps and fourteen with a contralateral latissimus dorsi musculocutaneous flap. Success is reported in twenty-five of the twenty-six patients (96%).

The advantages and disadvantages of each are presented. These are contrasted to other vascularized donor tissues also employed in breast reconstruction following mastectomy. Technical considerations contributing to successful transplantation are detailed.

We wish to emphasize that microsurgical composite tissue transplantation is indicated in only a very small, carefully selected group of breast reconstruction patients—approximately 9%.

REFERENCES

1. Cannon, B., Lischer, C.E., and Brown, J.B.: Open jump flap repairs of the lower extremity, Surgery **22:**335, 1947.
2. Fisher, J., and Bostwick, J.: The latissimus dorsi flap: clinical and laboratory definition of the serratus collateral following thoracodorsal ligation. Presented at the Sixtieth Annual Meeting of the American Association of Plastic and Reconstructive Surgeons, May 10-13, 1981, Williamsburg, Va.
3. Fujino, T., Harashina, T., and Enomoto, K.: Primary breast reconstruction after a standard radical mastectomy by a free flap transfer, Plast. Reconstr. Surg. **58:**371, 1976.
4. Georgiade, N.G., Serafin, D., Riefkohl, R., Barwick, W., and Georgiade, G.: Unpublished data.
5. Harii, K.: Microvascular surgery and its clinical applications. Clin. Orthop. **133:**95, June, 1978.
6. Harii, K.: Microvascular free tissue transfers, World J. Surg. **3:**29, 1979.
7. Howland, W., Loffler, K., Starchaian, D., and Johnson, R.: Postirradiation atrophic changes of bone and related complications, Radiology **117:**677, 1955.
8. Jayes, P.H.: Cross-leg flaps: a review of sixty cases, Br. J. Plast. Surg. **3:**1, 1950.
9. Kim, J., et al.: Time dose factors in radiation induced osteitis, Am. J. Roentgenol. **120:**684, 1974.
10. Meyer, J.E.: Thoracic effects of therapeutic irradiation for breast carcinoma, Am. J. Roentgenol. **130:**877, 1978.
11. Serafin, D., Georgiade, N.G., and Given, K.S.: Transfer of free flaps to provide well-vascularized thick cover for breast reconstructions after radical mastectomy, Plast. Reconstr. Surg. **62:**527, 1978.
12. Serafin, D., Georgiade, N.G., and Smith, D.H.: Comparison of free flaps with pedicle flaps for coverage of defects of the leg or foot, Plast. Reconstr. Surg. **59:**492, 1977.
13. Serafin, D., Sabatier, R.E., Morris, R.L., and Georgiade, N.G.: Reconstruction of the lower extremity with vascularized composite tissue: improved tissue survival and specific indications, Plast. Reconstr. Surg. **66:**230, 1980.
14. Serafin, D., Voci, V.E., and Georgiade, N.G.: Microsurgical composite tissue transplantation: indications and technical considerations in breast reconstruction following mastectomy, Plast. Reconstr. Surg. **70:**24, 1982.
15. Serafin, D., et al.: Reconstruction with vascularized composite tissue in patients with excessive injury following surgery and irradiation, Ann. Plast. Surg. **8:**35, 1982.
16. Shaw, W.W.: Reconstruction by microsurgical means. Presented at the Symposium on Reconstruction of the Female Breast Following Mastectomy, sponsored by the Educational Foundation of the Association of Plastic and Reconstructive Surgeons, Oct. 30-Nov. 1, 1980, Piscataway, N.J.
17. Stranc, J.F., Sabandter, H., and Roy, A.: A review of 196 tubed pedicles, Br. J. Plast. Surg. **28:**54, 1975.
18. White, W.L., et al.: Evaluation of 114 cross leg flaps. In Skoog, T., and Ivy, R.H., editors: Transactions of the First Congress of the International Society of Plastic Surgeons, Baltimore, 1955, The Williams & Wilkins Co.

Chapter 23

Reconstruction of the breast by free myocutaneous gluteal flap

Toyomi Fujino

An ablated breast can create a significant emotional handicap for the patient, especially when she is of marriageable age. With earlier diagnosis life expectancy has been improved; reconstruction of the breast offers improved quality of life.

RECONSTRUCTION

No recent technique has satisfactorily dealt with the axillary-subclavian deformity; most efforts have been directed toward building only an acceptable breast mound. However, the aim of reconstruction of the breast is the restoration of volume, position, warmth, softness, mobility, and sensation, thereby returning the patient to her normal appearance and social life.[1-6]

Implants. Recent advances in the design of breast implants have been appreciated by patients and have been more acceptable clinically, but filling of the axillary-subclavian deformity is as yet unsatisfactory.

Free myocutaneous flap transfer

Donor site. The buttock provides a donor site with minimal scar formation and minimal deformity of the hip contour, even after sacrifice of the major gluteal muscle. (Some patients desire the removal of hip tissue for aesthetic improvement.) A large amount of fat and muscle tissue is available for transfer, and prosthetic implants are not needed. The elliptical incision permits easy primary closure (Fig. 23-1).

Operating techniques. Two teams work separately, one preparing the donor site, the other the recipient site.

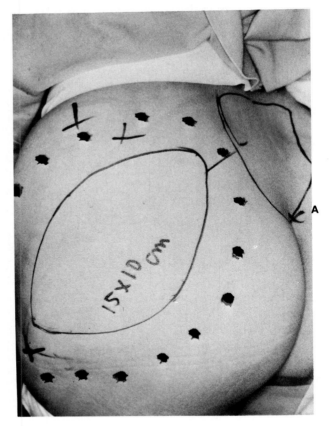

Fig. 23-1. Free myocutaneous gluteal flap. **A,** Preoperative design on hip. Skin incision corresponds to the size of skin incision of a standard radical mastectomy. Dotted line is an extension of the adipose tissue resection to fill the subcutaneous tissue defect after surgery.

Continued.

203

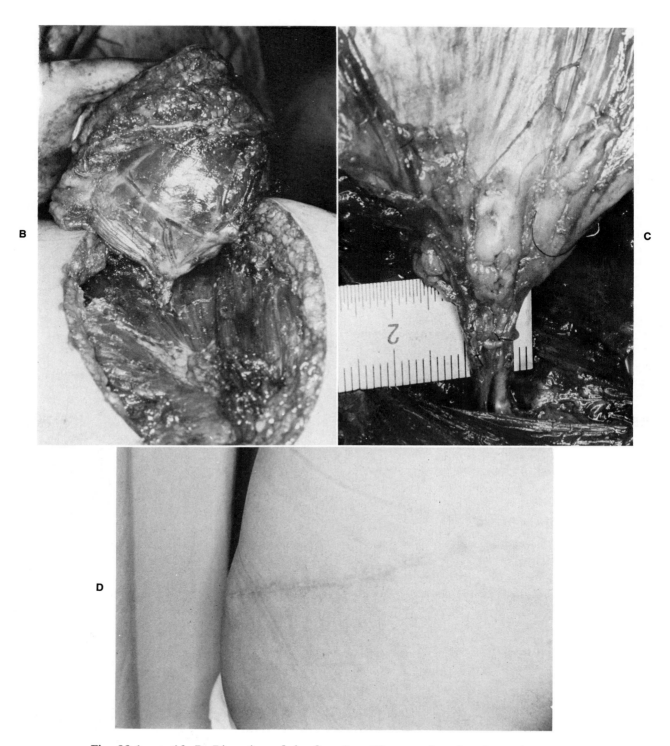

Fig. 23-1, cont'd. B, Dissection of the free flap. The superior gluteal vessels course through the proximal portion of the free flap under the gluteus maximus muscle; then, at the middle portion, they penetrate through the muscle layer, furnishing perforating vessels to the overlying skin and adipose tissue. **C,** The superior gluteal artery (2 mm) and vein (3 mm) are ready to be divided just between the gluteus medius and piriformis muscles. **D,** Appearance of the donor site 6 months postoperatively. (From Fujino, T.: Primary reconstruction of the breast by free myocutaneous gluteal flap, Int. Adv. Surg. Oncol. **4:**127, 1981.)

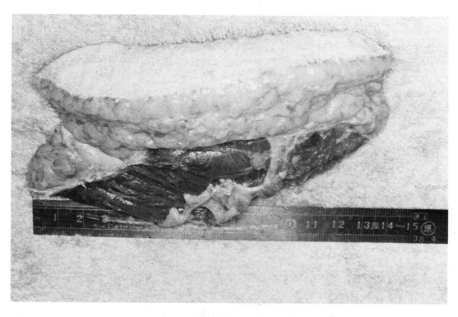

Fig. 23-2. A dermal fat segment is prepared by cutting off a thick split-thickness skin graft with a dermatome.

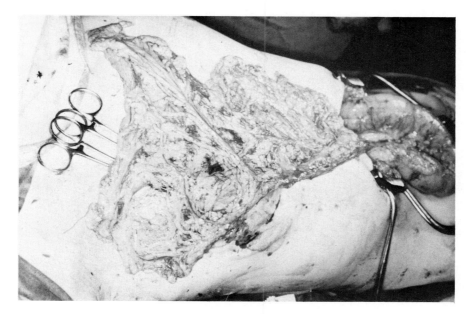

Fig. 23-3. A flap of omentum is transferred to the anterior chest through a subcutaneous tunnel to provide a substitute for the recipient vessels in the absence of satisfactory local vessels. (From Fujino, T.: Reconstruction of the breast following radical mastectomy by a free gluteal musculocutaneous flap and/or pedicled omental flap transfer. In Ely, J., editor: Transactions of the Seventh International Congress of Plastic and Reconstructive Surgeons, Sao Paulo, 1979, Cartigraf, p. 588).

Preparation of the donor site. With the patient in the lateral recumbent position, the entire chest and the ipsilateral hip region are prepared. One team outlines the donor flap with an elliptical incision from the upper sacrum to the greater trochanter region. Dissection is started from the upper edge of the ellipse, going to the upper border of the gluteus maximus muscle. We then separate the fibers of the gluteus maximus, mobilizing the upper third of the muscle. The insertion is then detached from the greater trochanter and is reflected toward the sacrum. The superior gluteal artery and vein are exposed between the gluteus medius and piriformis muscles, near the sacrum. The superior gluteal vessels are prepared (Fig. 23-1). A dermatome is used to deepithelialize the parts to be buried.

Immediately after dividing the vessels (Fig. 23-2), we immerse the flap in a chilled physiologic saline solution containing heparin (10 IU/ml), and the clots in the vessels are gently expressed. The donor site on the hip is closed directly.

Preparation of the recipient site

Congenital breast aplasia. A second team undermines the breast to above the intermuscular fascia, through lateral thoracic and inframammary incisions. The recipient vessels (thoracolateral artery and vein) are prepared.

Ablated breast (following mastectomy). If either the thoracoacromial or lateral thoracic vessels are too short to allow positioning of the free myocutaneous flap in a normal position, a pedicled flap of greater omentum is used as a substitute source of recipient vessels. After celiotomy the greater omental flap is mobilized on the right gastroepiploic vessels and transposed through a subcutaneous tunnel to the chest wall (Fig. 23-3).

Microneurovascular anastomoses. The microvascular anastomoses are then done, first the venous (average diameter 2 to 4 mm) and then the arterial (average diameter 1 to 3 mm), using 18-μm monofilament nylon sutures. Next the upper and lower portions of the flap are anchored to the muscle fascia (Fig. 23-3). The major gluteal muscle is used only for bulk; therefore a nerve anastomosis is not mandatory but is done if possible to prevent atrophy of the transplanted muscle.

Result. Typical cases are shown in Fig. 23-4. Patient I is a 22-year-old single female with congenital absence of the right breast and pectoral muscle. Patient II is a 36-year-old single female with a primary reconstruction after a Halstead radical mastectomy. Patient III is a 28-year-old female who had radical mastectomy with secondary reconstruction 1 year after surgery. All show complete survival of the free flap.

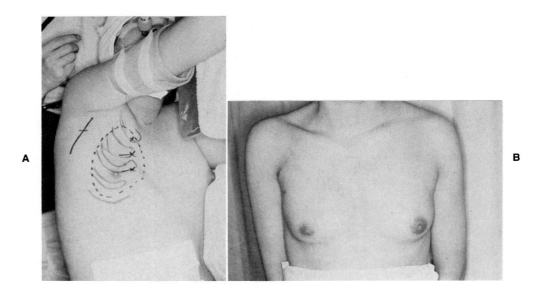

Fig. 23-4. A, Patient I. First successful transfer of a free myocutaneous gluteal flap. A 22-year-old single female with a congenital absence of the right breast and pectoral muscles (before surgery). **B,** Four years after surgery. (From Plast. Reconstr. Surg. **56:** 179, 1975.)

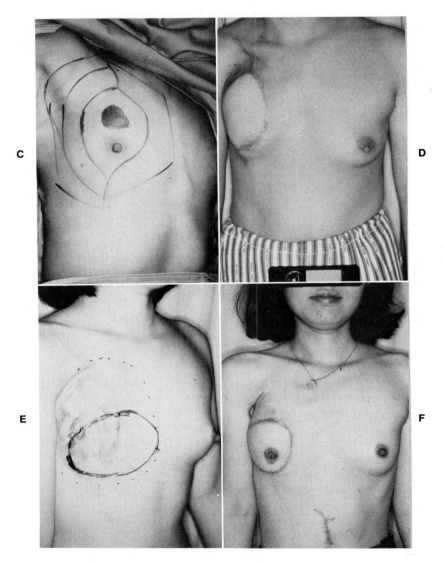

Fig. 23-4, cont'd. C, Patient II. Primary reconstruction of the breast in a 36-year-old single female. Preoperative design of a Halstead radical mastectomy. Dark spot indicates the location of the tumor. **D,** Postoperative appearance 3 months after transferring the free myocutaneous gluteal flap. **E,** Patient III. Secondary reconstruction of the breast in a 28-year-old single female. One year after standard radical mastectomy. Solid line is proposed position of the breast mound. Dotted line indicates the area to be filled subcutaneously. **F,** Patient 1½ years after reconstruction with a free myocutaneous gluteal flap and pedicled greater omental flap. (From Fujino, T.: Primary reconstruction of the breast by free myocutaneous gluteal flap, Int. Adv. Surg. Oncol. **4:**127, 1981.)

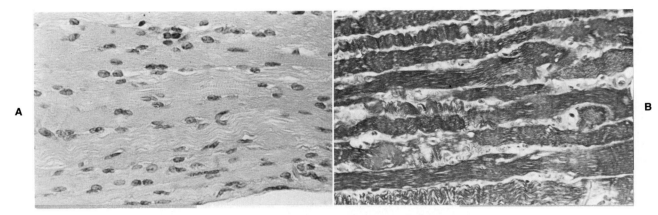

Fig. 23-5. Muscle biopsy 2 years after surgery. **A,** Slight atrophic change in the muscle fiber is noted (hematoxylin-eosin stain; ×400). **B,** Phosphotungstic acid–hematoxylin staining demonstrates the muscle stria very well. Some inactive atrophic changes are observed, but no degenerative changes are noted (×400).

DISCUSSION

Periodic xerograms were carried out to check for recurrences. The xerographic findings in our longest follow-up (2½ years) show no essential changes except for a fibrotic area at the site of the muscle biopsy. A muscle biopsy of the free myocutaneous gluteal flap is performed every 2 years after surgery. Initially a motor nerve anastomosis was not done, and there was a slight to moderate degree of muscle atrophy but no degenerative changes of the muscle (Fig. 23-5), and decrease in the breast volume did not prove to be significant. However, we now do microneurorrhapy.

The position of the reconstructed breast is determined with the patient in a sitting position when she is awake and in a semisitting position when she is anesthetized. The final position chosen is usually influenced by the length of the recipient and donor vessels. Short vessels are a major obstacle to satisfactory positioning. Greater length of the recipient vessels could perhaps be preserved by the oncologic surgeon, but the caliber of vessels becomes smaller with length.

The end-to-end microvascular anastomosis becomes difficult when the discrepancy in the diameters of vascular pairs is more than double. For easy microvascular anastomosis, it is advisable to preserve a vascular diameter greater than 1 to 2 mm at the distal end.

The donor vessels can be elongated by trimming the proximal portion of the fat and muscle layers of the free flap without injuring the perforating vascular trees within the layers. However, secondary trimming of the excess tissue is much preferred, because augmentation is much harder to accomplish than trimming. If the length of the recipient vessels is clearly inadequate as the result of scar tissue or radiation, omental vessels are a useful substitute. The greater omental flap also contributes to the volume of the breast and provides lymphatic drainage.

For ease in positioning of the free flap, we prefer the Stewart incision to the Halstead.

Warmth is a desirable quality in the reconstructed breast. Recently prosthetic implantation under a pedicled or free skin flap has been commonly used for breast reconstruction. Using thermography to compare breasts reconstructed with free myocutaneous gluteal flaps with breasts reconstructed by free groin flaps and mammary prostheses, we found a temperature difference of 10° or more. We therefore believe that the free autogenous myocutaneous gluteal flap is the better technique for breast reconstruction.

Softness returns to the free myocutaneous flap transfer within 2 to 3 months after surgery. Mobility of the breast reconstructed with a free myocutaneous flap is good, although mild fibrosis occurs under the flap. Restoration of sensation is also desirable in breast reconstruction. We have done no sensory nerve anastomoses, but there has been a considerable return of sensation in every case.

Our technique has been particularly effective in replacing the tissues of the anterior axillary fold after standard radical mastectomies.

From an aesthetic standpoint, breast symmetry is desirable. Our patients, however, have not wanted either reduction mammoplasties or subcutaneous mastectomies on the other breast. We have not recommended either procedure, since the incidence of cancer in the other breast is only about 1% as a primary site and 6% as a site of metastasis.

REFERENCES

1. Fujino, T.: Reconstruction of the breast following radical mastectomy by a free gluteal musculocutaneous flap and/or pedicled omental flap transfer. In Ely, J.F., editor: Transactions of the Seventh International Congress of Plastic and Reconstructive Surgeons, Sao Paulo, 1979, Cartigraf, p. 588.
2. Fujino, T.: Primary reconstruction of the breast by free myocutaneous gluteal flap, Int. Adv. Surg. Oncol. **4:**127, 1981.
3. Fujino, T., and Harashina, T.: Study of transplantation of free island flap with the aid of Inokuchi's microvascular stapler machine, Jpn. J. Plast. Reconstr. Surg. **11:**234, 1968.
4. Fujino, T., Harashina, T., and Aoyagi, F.: Reconstruction for aplasia of the breast pectoral region by microvascular transfer of a free flap from the buttock, Plast. Reconstr. Surg. **56:**178, 1975.
5. Fujino, T., Harashina, T., and Enomoto, K.: Primary breast reconstruction after a standard radical mastectomy by a free flap transfer, Plast. Reconstr. Surg. **58:**371, 1976.
6. Fujino, T., Harashina, T., and Mikata, A.: Autogenous en bloc transplantation of the mammary gland in dogs, using microsurgical technique, Plast. Reconstr. Surg. **50:**376, 1972.

Part VII

Reconstruction of the hand and upper limb

Chapter 24

Current techniques of limb reconstruction

Harold E. Kleinert
Carl H. Manstein

The battlegrounds of the Pacific were laboratories for reconstructive surgery of the upper limb and were a prologue to the use of magnification for operative repair. Loupe magnification gave precision to nerve and blood vessel repairs and aided in neurovascular island flaps.[9] The operating microscope gained popularity, and limb revascularization[7] and limb replantation[3,11] became realities. Finally blood vessels 1 mm in diameter were anastomosed.[1,6,8]

Often the most pressing problem in limb reconstruction is to provide skin and soft tissue coverage for large defects. Exposed joints, tendons, and nerves are not suitable surfaces for simple skin grafts. Local flaps are inadequate for large defects. Composite tissue transfers are often the best answer.

RECONSTRUCTIVE PROCEDURES
Groin flap

The groin flap, developed by McGregor, was an important advance in flap design.[10] The free groin flap, having been the first cutaneous free flap, is the standard to which all other free flaps are compared. This flap is based on the superficial circumflex iliac artery and vein. It provides extensive skin and subcutaneous tissue for coverage of bone, joints, and exposed tendons (Fig. 24-1). The donor site of non-hair-bearing skin may be closed primarily and easily hidden. Ilium may be included for reconstructing bone. However, patients may be dissatisfied with the poor color match of this flap, and the short vascular pedicle is a limiting feature.

Scapular flap

The scapular flap, useful for covering defects anywhere on the extremities, is based on the circumflex scapular vessels that exit through the triangular space formed by the teres major, teres minor, and long head of the triceps. It is easily harvested, with a pedicle as long as 8 to 9 cm. A large area of tissue can be transferred and the donor site can be closed primarily. Donor site problems are rare, but the scar may be conspicuous.

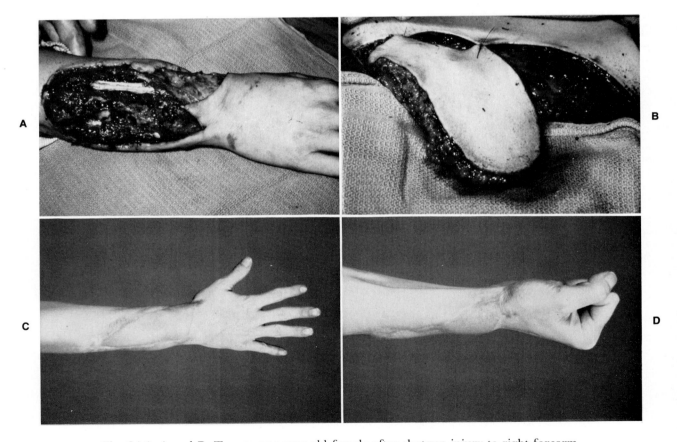

Fig. 24-1. A and **B,** Twenty-one-year-old female after shotgun injury to right forearm, with exposed tendons and fractured bone. Free groin flap transferred for cover and to allow further reconstruction. **C** and **D,** Function and appearance 20 months after reconstruction. (Courtesy T.M. Tsai.)

Latissimus dorsi flap

The latissimus dorsi flap may be transferred with or without the overlying skin. It receives its major vascular pedicle from the third portion of the axillary artery via the subscapular artery and the thoracodorsal artery. Because of its large muscle bulk, trimming and revisions are often required. It provides excellent soft tissue coverage for exposed bone, tendons, and neurovascular structures, particularly in areas exposed to shearing forces (Fig. 24-2).

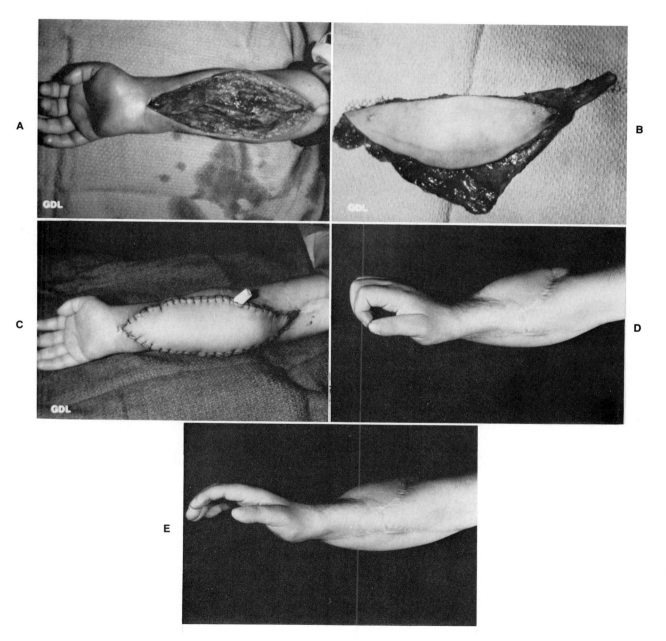

Fig. 24-2. A and **B,** Ischemic contracture of the forearm in a 5-year-old male (onset after a difficult delivery). Debridement of necrotic fibrotic muscle and replacement with a functional myocutaneous latissimus dorsi free flap to provide forearm flexor muscle. **C,** Immediate postoperative appearance. **D** and **E,** Extension and flexion 4 months after myocutaneous flap transfer. (Courtesy G. Lister.)

Vascularized bone graft

A vascularized bone graft allows the transfer of a large segment of cortical and cancellous bone. The iliac crest osteocutaneous flap[12] provides a solid piece of bone to bridge a defect and can incorporate a large amount of skin and soft tissue. The vascularized rib graft is technically difficult; it is probably most applicable in maxillofacial reconstruction. A free fibular transfer is useful when a growing epiphysis is needed in the young patient (Fig. 24-3).

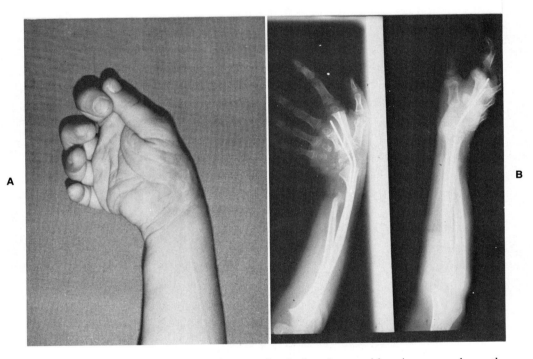

Fig. 24-3. A and **B,** Appearance of hand and wrist in a 5-year-old patient several months after a lawn mower avulsion of ulnar metacarpals and distal ulna.

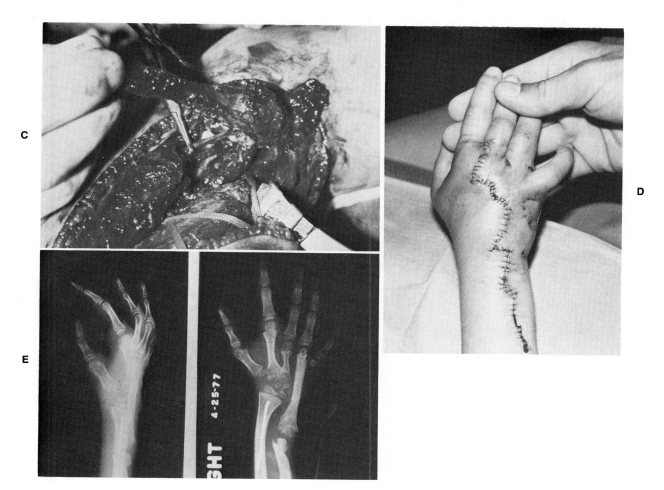

Fig. 24-3, cont'd. C, Removal of fibula with epiphysis on vascular peroneal and geniculate vessels to correct defect and provide epiphyseal growth. **D,** Immediate correction obtained at operation. **E,** Radiographic appearance of vascularized fibular bone graft with continued growth 2 years after the procedure. (**A, B,** and **E** from Weiland, A.J., et al.: Vascularized bone grafts in the upper extremity. In Serafin, D., and Buncke, H.J., editors: Microsurgical composite tissue transplantation, St. Louis, 1979, The C.V. Mosby Co., p. 605.)

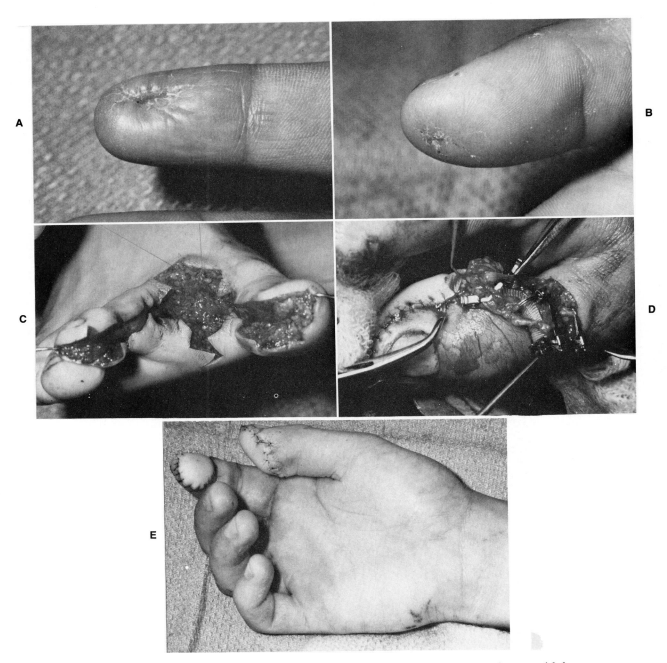

Fig. 24-4. A and **B,** Chronic ulceration and ischemia of thumb and index fingers with loss of sensation secondary to radiation injury. **C** to **E,** Small neurovascular skin flaps from the first and second toe pads to replace the thumb and index fingertip pads. (From Stern, P.J., et al.: Neurovascular cutaneous flaps for the management of radiation-induced fingertip dermal necrosis, J. Hand Surg. **8:**88, 1983.)

Neurosensory flap

Toe pads with or without the first web space of the foot can provide large sensate donor areas. The quality of the skin is much like that on the hand, and two-point discrimination closely approximates that of a normal fingertip (Fig. 24-4). Its blood supply originates from the dorsalis pedis and first dorsal metatarsal or first plantar metatarsal arteries. The nerve supply originates from the plantar digital and deep peroneal nerves.

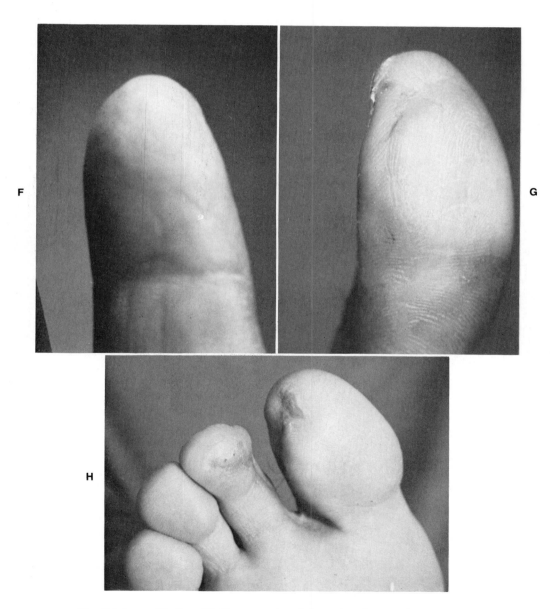

Fig. 24-4, cont'd. F to **H,** Donor and recipient sites 1 year after surgery.

Nerve repair and grafting

Severed nerves are repaired under magnification with precise alignment of corresponding fascicles or fascicular groups. Tension on the repair must be avoided, and the interposition of epineurium in the repair must be prevented. When the gap between the transected ends of an injured nerve is greater than 2 cm, an interposition nerve graft is usually needed. Interfascicular nerve grafting can produce recovery of useful function in 80% of the cases, which equals the results of primary nerve suture under ideal conditions; this is significantly better than the results of nerve repairs done under tension (Fig. 24-5).

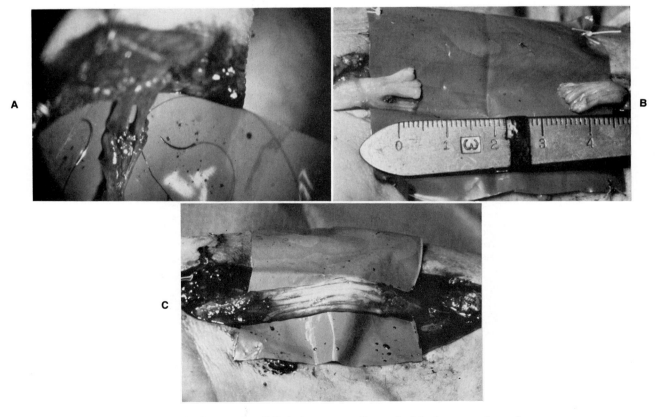

Fig. 24-5. A, Fascicular repair of digital nerve performed with the operating microscope; **B,** 3 cm gap in median nerve; **C,** insertion of five fascicular nerve grafts (donor sural nerve).

Brachial plexus reconstruction

Brachial plexus injuries usually occur in young males during the prime of life. The extremity is often a useless, painful hindrance to the patient. Reconstructive goals are restoration of elbow flexion, provision of some sensation, and amelioration of pain. The presence of Tinel's sign, even in complete plexus avulsion, indicates that some proximal nerve root fibers are available. If nerve roots are avulsed within the bony foramina, there is almost no potential for repair. The more nerve roots available for proximal nerve graft attachment, the more complete the restoration can be (Fig. 24-6).

Free muscle transfer

The pectoralis major, the gracilis,[5] and the latissimus dorsi muscles are the most common donor muscles for transfers to the forearm.

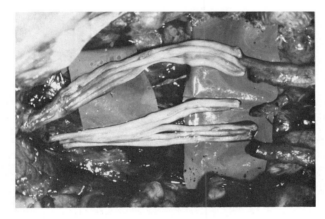

Fig. 24-6. Reconstruction of an avulsion injury to the brachial plexus with three roots remaining for nerve graft attachment.

Toe-to-hand transfer

The toe-to-hand transfer[2] is useful for reconstruction of an absent thumb or digits. It gives a mobile, stable, innervated, and cosmetically acceptable digit that functions as a motor unit. It is readily incorporated psychologically as a thumb (Fig. 24-7). The great toe produces a more powerful thumb than does the second toe.[4] The second toe gives better appearance and is preferred for thumb reconstruction in women or for replacement of digits other than the thumb.

Dissection of the vascular pedicle should be carried well proximal to allow anastomosis with the largest possible vessel. The entire second metatarsal can be taken without creating a problem in the foot. If the donor site is closed primarily, the foot is narrowed, but the patient can still wear regular shoes.

The contralateral second toe is preferred for digital reconstruction because it facilitates anastomosis of the first dorsal metatarsal artery in the hand (usually in the anatomic snuffbox or at the ulnar side of the first metacarpal).

If all the fingers have been amputated, the surgeon may use both the second and third toes as a composite transfer to the rays of the third and fourth fingers (Fig. 24-8). For the patient who is missing all the fingers and the thumb, bilateral second toe transplantation should be considered. Both the right and left second toes are transferred to the stump, carefully positioned, and provided with muscle power to oppose one another.

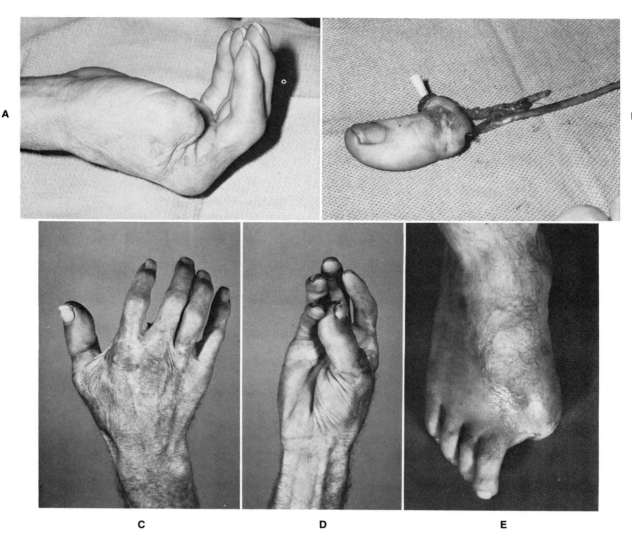

Fig. 24-7. A, Amputation of thumb just distal to the metacarpophalangeal joint. **B,** Transfer of the great toe. **C** and **D,** Extension and opposition 4 months after transfer. **E,** Donor site appearance.

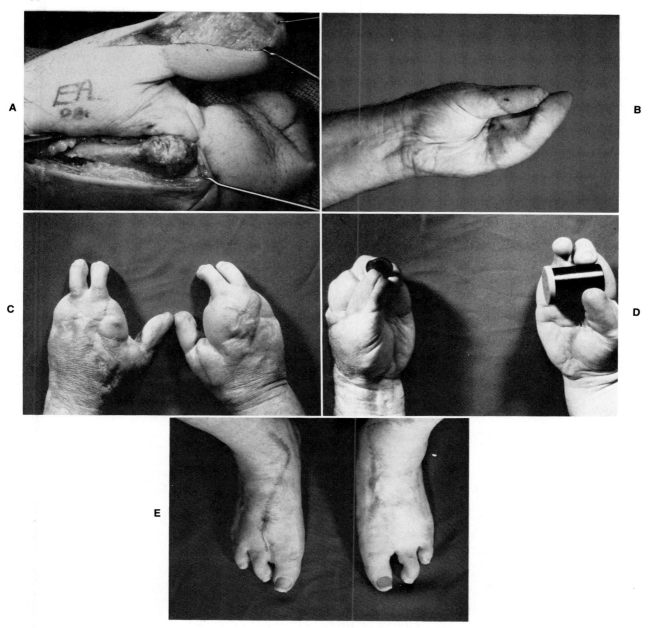

Fig. 24-8. Forty-three-year-old male who lost all fingers including partial thumb loss secondary to a frostbite injury. **A,** Right hand after groin flap to the thumb and finger position. The second metacarpal is used as a thumb bone graft. **B,** Left hand after flap coverage. **C** and **D,** Appearance and function 3 years after bilateral free neurovascular toe transfer for finger reconstruction. **E,** Donor sites after surgery; foot disturbance is minimal to none.

Free joint transfer

A vascularized, autogenous whole joint transfer is a suitable method for reconstruction of either the severely traumatized or congenitally deficient joint (Fig. 24-9)

The surgical approach is similar to that of a free toe transfer. The dorsalis pedis and first dorsal metatarsal arteries are identified, along with the dorsal venous arch. A small skin island over the dorsal aspect of the proximal interphalangeal joint of the second toe is preserved and transferred along with the joint as a visible monitor of the un-derlying circulation. The joint is exposed by disarticulation through the distal interphalangeal joint and by osteotomy through the proximal phalanx. Sufficient tendon, usually the extensor, is included for tendon reconstruction. After transfer the toe joint is stabiized with intraosseous wiring or Kirschner wires. Tendons are repaired and vascular anastomoses completed. The osseous donor site in the foot is arthrodesed with a bone peg and the toe is left intact. With immediate revascularization of transplanted whole joints, bony union is achieved and articular cartilage preserved.

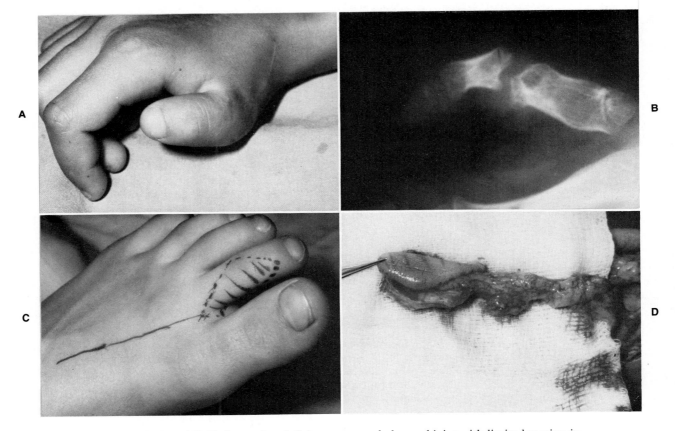

Fig. 24-9. A and **B,** Deformed, painful metacarpophalangeal joint with limited motion in a 6-year-old male. **C** and **D,** Outline of skin island over donor proximal interphalangeal joint to be transferred on its vascular pedicle. (**A, B,** and **H** from Tsai, T.M., et al.: Vascularized autogenous whole joint transfer in the hand—a clinical study, J. Hand Surg. 7:335, 1982.)

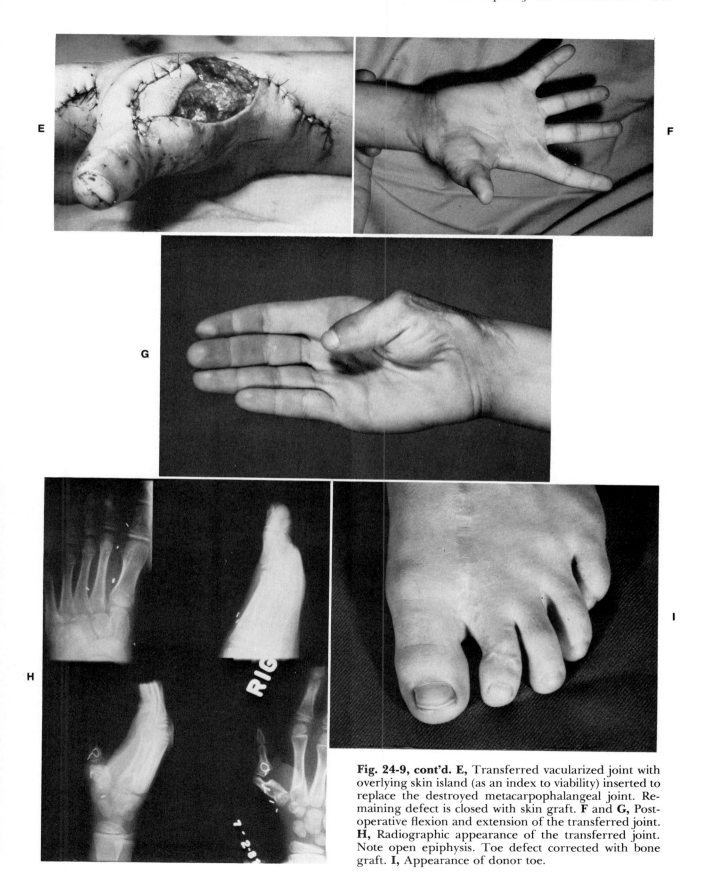

Fig. 24-9, cont'd. E, Transferred vacularized joint with overlying skin island (as an index to viability) inserted to replace the destroyed metacarpophalangeal joint. Remaining defect is closed with skin graft. **F** and **G,** Postoperative flexion and extension of the transferred joint. **H,** Radiographic appearance of the transferred joint. Note open epiphysis. Toe defect corrected with bone graft. **I,** Appearance of donor toe.

SUMMARY

Free microvascular tissue transfer for upper extremity reconstruction has allowed reconstruction for patients previously considered hopeless.

REFERENCES

1. Buncke, H.J., and Schulz, W.P.: Total ear replantation in rabbits utilizing microminiature vascular anastomoses, Br. J. Plast. Surg. **19:**15, 1966.
2. Buncke, H.J., Buncke, C.M., and Schulz, W.P.: Immediate Nicolandoni procedure in rhesus monkey, or hallux-to-hand transplantation utilizing vascular anastomosis, Br. J. Plast. Surg. **19:**332, 1966.
3. Chen, C.W., and Yun-Ching, C.: Case report, Shanghai, 1963, Department of Surgery, Sixth People's Hospital.
4. Cobbett, J.R.: Free digital transfer: report of a case of transfer of a great toe to replace an amputated thumb, J. Bone Joint Surg. **51B:**677, 1969.
5. Harii, K., Ohmori, K., and Torii, S.: Free gracilis muscle transplantation with microneurovascular anastomoses for the treatment of facial paralysis, Plast. Reconstr. Surg. **57:**133, 1976.
6. Jacobson, H.J., and Suarez, E.L.: Microsurgery in anastomosis of small vessels, Surg. Forum **11:**243, 1960.
7. Kleinert, H.E., and Kasdan, M.L.: Salvage of devascularized upper extremities including studies on small vessel anastomosis, Clin. Orthop. **29:**29, 1963.
8. Kleinert, H.E., and Kasdan, M.L.: Anastomosis of digital vessels, J. Ky. Med. Assoc. **63:**106, 1965.
9. Littler, J.W.: Neurovascular pedicle transfer of tissue in reconstructive surgery of the hand, J. Bone Joint Surg. **38:**917, 1956.
10. McGregor, I.A., and Jackson, I.T.: The groin flap, Br. J. Plast. Surg. **25:**3, 1972.
11. Snyder, C.C., Knowles, R.P., Mayer, P.N., and Hobbs, J.C.: Extremity replantation, Plast. Reconstr. Surg. **26:**251, 1960.
12. Taylor, G.I., and Watson, N.: One-stage repair of compound leg defects with free revascularized flaps of groin skin and iliac bone, Plast. Reconstr. Surg. **61:**494, 1978.
13. Tsai, T.M., et al.: Vascularized autogenous whole joint transfer in the hand—a clinical study, J. Hand Surg. **7:**335, 1982.
14. Weiland, A.J., et al.: Vascularized bone grafts in the upper extremity. In Serafin, D., and Buncke, H.J., editors: Microsurgical composite tissue transplantation, St. Louis, 1979, The C.V. Mosby Co., p. 605.

Chapter 25

Reconstruction of the hand with two-toe block transfer and neurovascular flaps from the foot

Edgar Biemer

With the advent of microvascular free flaps, many new methods have been established for reconstruction of defects of the hand.

The foot has become a most important donor site for reconstruction of the hand because of its anatomic similarity and its ideal vascular and nerve patterns.

DONOR AREA—ANATOMY OF THE FOOT

Anatomically the foot and the hand are very similar. The tarsus, the metatarsus, and the toes are comparable to the carpus, the metacarpus, and the fingers, respectively. The foot has both a plantar and a dorsal arterial system. Although the plantar system is very similar to the palmar arterial system, it is much less important in tissue transfer than is the dorsal system.

The dorsal arterial system of the foot is fed by the dorsalis pedis artery. At the proximal end of the metatarsus this artery divides to form the arcuate artery, the first dorsal metatarsal artery, and a perforating artery that passes into the depths of the foot to anastomose with the plantar arterial system. This point of division (point X) is of great importance. The dorsalis pedis artery has a number of variants, and in about 15% of cases it is completely absent.[5] The presence of the dorsalis pedis artery is determined by palpation or by a Doppler apparatus. All of the structures on the dorsum of the foot and the first, second, and third toes are nourished by this arterial system. In addition, it furnishes blood supply to the metatarsus and to the tendons and intrinsic muscles. Along with the artery run sensory branches of the perineal nerve; the superficial branches go to the dorsum of the foot and the deep branch goes to the dorsum of the first and second toes, including the web space. The deep branch lies very close to the artery.

The artery lies between two venae comitantes. Another venous system lies directly beneath the skin. This is composed of a venous arch that is drained medially by the long saphenous vein and laterally by the short saphenous vein; the veins are relatively large. Even in overweight individuals this tissue is always thin with good skin texture.

The major disadvantage of this donor site is that only very small defects can be closed primarily. The defects from flaps greater than 2 cm need to be resurfaced with split skin grafts. Aesthetically and functionally this repair has disadvantages. An advantage of this site is that regardless of the type of defect, the flap must usually be elevated by the same technique. This leads to great familiarity with the anatomy, making this part of the operation quick and safe.

SKIN FLAPS
Dorsalis pedis flap

If bare bone or bare tendon are exposed in a skin–soft tissue defect of the hand, skin flap coverage is required. If a large area of coverage is needed, it is possible to raise a flap that includes the skin of the entire dorsum of the foot. The proximal limit of a free flap is the level of the malleoli, and the distal limit is the level of the metatarsal-phalangeal joints; the medial and lateral limits are the junction between the dorsal and plantar surfaces. If necessary the flap can be extended into the first web space, or it can include skin from the lateral aspects of the big toe or from the medial aspect of the second toe (or the entire dorsal integument can be taken from both of these toes). If a smaller flap is desired, it must be raised distally as it is nourished by the metatarsal artery at point X; the tissue proximal to this point is nourished in a random pattern. An advantage to the dorsalis pedis flap is that the arterial stump can be lengthened simply by including part of the anterior tibial artery.

Inasmuch as the sensory nerves supplying sensation to the flap are included with the dissection, this flap has the potential for sensory restoration. This feature is of great value in the hand. When a dorsalis pedis flap is elevated, a superficial vein should be included with the flap to augment the venous drainage from the venae comitantes.

The first step in raising this flap is to identify and dissect the dorsalis pedis artery and veins, the deep branch of the perineal nerve (if required), and, more medially, the superficial branch of the perineal nerve. Dissection then proceeds along the medial aspect of the flap, passing over the extensor hallucis longus tendon into the first web space, where the dorsal metatarsal artery at point X is identified. The synovial sheath should always be preserved on the tendons to provide a bed for split skin grafting.

In the distal tarsal area the vessels are intimately related to the periosteum; branches pass proximally to the ankle joint and distally to the lateral aspect of the dorsum of the foot. The flap is elevated off of the periosteum and then dissection is continued, elevating the lateral border of the flap, progressing to the first metatarsal space. The tendon of the extensor hallucis brevis muscle invariably passes over the vessels and must therefore be divided. The muscle belly is always preserved because it is useful for covering defects in the tendon sheaths in preparation for skin grafts.

The flap is then elevated on all sides, progressing toward point X. By centering the dissection on point X, the exact position and depth of the main dorsal metatarsal artery are ascertained. In this way the flap is raised, connected only by the vasculature at point X. Once the vascular attachments are divided and ligated, the flap is ready for transfer. The structures in the flap are carefully marked by sutures and by different types of clips for easy identification.

Elevation should always be done with a tourniquet in situ. To outline the vascular pattern, we first render the limb bloodless with a rubber bandage. The tourniquet is then released briefly to allow some blood to outline the vessels, and then the tourniquet is reinflated. A split skin graft is applied to the defect on the dorsum of the foot after first releasing the tourniquet and obtaining hemostasis.

Large dorsalis pedis flaps are often needed for reconstruction of defects of the palm or dorsum of the hand or to open up the first web space. The dorsalis pedis flap is especially suitable for the latter, inasmuch as the flap can be planned exactly to fit the size and shape of the defect.

CASE REPORT

An 18-year-old male had an ischemic contracture of the hand. His thumb was severely adducted and immobile. An effort to correct the adduction contracture with a conventional pedicle had failed.

The first web space was incised and released. The radial artery, two veins, and a branch of the radial nerve were identified. A 13 by 4 cm flap was transferred from the dorsum of the foot to the defect and anastomoses and repairs were carried out. The flap survived completely. Postoperatively tenolysis and capsulotomies were carried out, after which reasonable function was achieved.

PULP FLAPS

If restoration of sensation at the fingertips or elsewhere is needed, a small pulp flap, usually taken from the lateral aspect of the great toe, is useful in carrying out the reconstruction. The dorsalis pedis artery is included to obtain a long vascular pedicle.

CASE REPORT (Fig. 25-1)

A 35-year-old male sustained a degloving injury of the second, third, and fourth fingers. Satisfactory coverage was obtained with a groin flap. However, the patient developed recurrent ulcerations because of his sensory deficit, especially on the palmar aspect of the index finger. A small pulp flap was transferred from the lateral aspect of the great toe to the volar surface of the index finger. Digital nerve repair was made.

The flap survived completely, and within a year two-point discrimination was less than 10 mm. No further ulceration has occurred in the index finger during the 3 years of postoperative follow-up care. However, ulceration has occurred in the middle finger, and another pulp flap is planned to correct this problem.

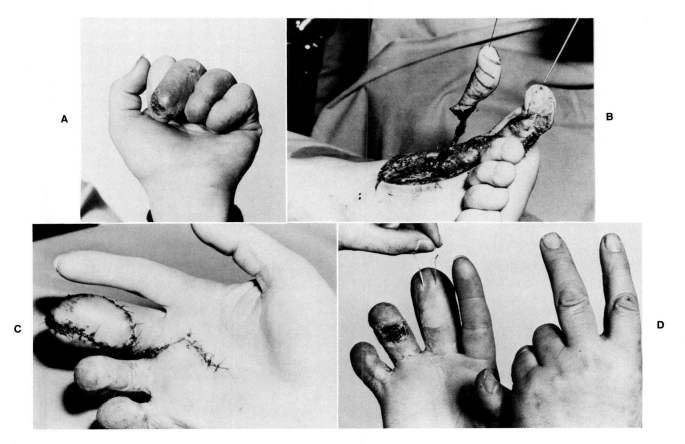

Fig. 25-1. A, Degloving injury of the third, fourth, and fifth fingers, with coverage by a groin flap. Lack of sensation resulted in chronic ulceration, primarily of the third finger. **B,** Elevation of a pulp flap on a neurovascular pedicle. **C,** Pulp flap in place. **D,** Twelve months postoperatively two-point discrimination is 8 mm. Ulceration of the ring finger is now present.

RECONSTRUCTION WITH COMBINED TISSUE TRANSFER
Flap with bone

The second metatarsal is supplied by branches of the dorsalis pedis and first metatarsal arteries. It is therefore possible to raise a dorsalis pedis flap of any size along with the second metatarsal bone and the tendons of the extensor hallucis brevis and the extensors digitorum longus and brevis to the second toe.

CASE REPORT (Fig. 25-2)

The patient was initially seen with traumatic loss of the first metacarpal bone and the overlying skin. This defect was reconstructed by means of an osteocutaneous dorsalis pedis flap that included the second metatarsal bone and the extensor digitorum longus and extensor hallucis brevis tendons to the second toe. These tendons were used to replace the extensor and adductor tendons of the thumb. The bone healed well, and the Kirschner wire was removed after 6 weeks. The result was good, although function was limited by an arthrodesis of the metatarsophalangeal joint.

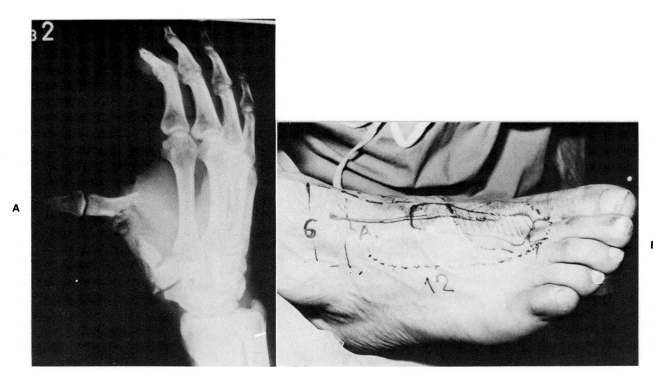

Fig. 25-2. A, Radiograph showing traumatic loss of the first metacarpal bone, including the overlying skin. **B,** Composite transplant incorporating second metatarsal bone, the short extensor tendon of the great toe, the long extensor tendon of the second toe, and a dorsalis pedis flap are outlined on the donor foot.

C 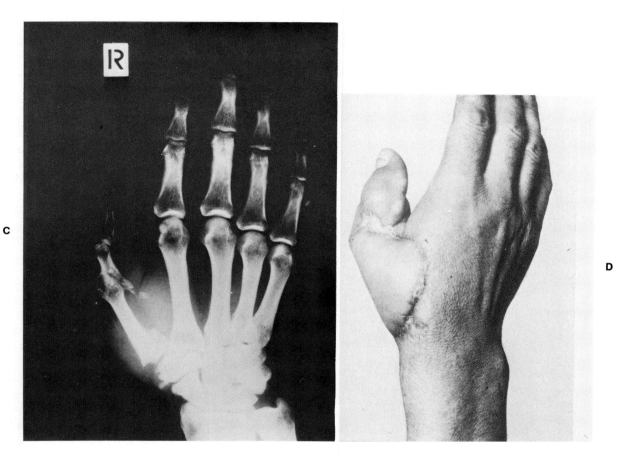 D

Fig. 25-2, cont'd. C, Radiograph at 8 weeks shows good bone healing. **D,** Complete healing of the dorsalis pedis flap is seen.

Flap with joint

It is also possible to include the metatarsophalangeal joint of the second toe as part of the flap.

CASE REPORT

A 22-year-old male sustained an explosion injury with loss of the first metacarpophalangeal joint and with subsequent adduction and flexion contracture of the thumb. The palmar surface of the thumb was devoid of sensation. A conventional Littler flap had resulted only in additional scarring. To release the first web space, restore sensation, and replace the metacarpophalangeal joint for provision of flexion and extension, a composite dorsalis pedis flap was transferred. This flap included the metatarsophalangeal joint of the second toe and a pulp flap from the lateral aspect of the great toe.

After the second metatarsophalangeal joint had been secured in its recipient site, the pulp flap had to be rotated through 90 degrees to reach the palmar aspect of the thumb. This maneuver caused the distal part of the pulp flap to blanch; therefore the flap was sutured to the wrist instead of the thumb. After healing the flap was elevated again and rotated to the palmar aspect of the thumb. Two-point discrimination was 12 mm after 12 months and movement at the new carpometacarpal joint was 25 degrees.

Toe flap with nail (wraparound technique)

It is possible to transplant skin and subcutaneous tissues, including the nail of the great toe or second toe. These flaps are ideal to cover degloved fingers or thumbs.

CASE REPORT

A 34-year-old male sustained a degloving injury to his right index finger, a finger that was essential for his work as a printer. The defect was repaired by degloving the distal two thirds and the tip of the second toe, including the nail. A long vascular pedicle was tunneled along the radial side of the index finger, and anastomosis was carried out in the anatomic snuffbox. The vein thrombosed because of compression within the narrow tunnel. The skin over the anastomosis was opened, a thrombectomy was performed, and the transplant survived completely, giving good functional and cosmetic results.

At the donor site the skin of the lateral aspect of the second toe was rotated to the plantar surface, and the remaining defect was covered with a split skin graft. The donor toe is now slightly disfigured, but it is retained to prevent the onset of hallux valgus.

Replacement of long fingers by toe transfer

Where an entire finger has been lost, it can be replaced by a toe transfer. This is particularly useful where the remaining fingers are severely damaged or limited in function.

CASE REPORT (Fig. 25-3)

A 19-year-old male had a normal thumb but had no satisfactory finger for opposition; his middle finger was missing. There was an unstable fracture of the proximal phalanx of the third finger, and the index and fourth fingers were deformed by unstable scar tissue.

A transplant of the second toe and the pulp from the lateral aspect of the great toe was performed. This achieved good function in the middle finger and significant improvement in the third finger.

Replacement of the thumb by toe transfer

In the early days of toe transfer (which dates back to Nicoladoni, 1897) the great toe was usually used.[2,3] In most cases, however, the great toe is too big to imitate a normal thumb, and the functional and cosmetic disability of the foot is significant; therefore we usually prefer to use the second toe for such transplantations.

The dorsalis pedis artery is anastomosed to the radial artery in the anatomic snuffbox in these cases. The thumb is opened with a fish-mouth incision. The flexor and extensor tendons are elevated, and the digital nerves are identified. The anatomic snuffbox is opened with an S-shaped incision, and the significant structures are identified and marked. Simultaneously the second toe, including the metatarsophalangeal joint, is elevated by a second team. Bone fixation is performed with a Kirschner wire and two transosseous wire sutures. This enables removal of the Kirschner wire after 10 to 12 days and permits early movement of all the joints. The toe is fixed in an exaggerated position of opposition, because this provides a better pinch grip. In this way aesthetically satisfactory thumbs with nearly normal function can be reconstructed.

If necessary, a dorsalis pedis flap can be included with the toe transfer. Occasionally the radial and ulnar sides of the new thumb around the metacarpophalangeal joint can be difficult to cover with skin.

The defect in the donor area is usually closed by approximating the first and third metatarsal heads. This gives a satisfactory cosmetic result, and normal shoes can be worn without difficulty.

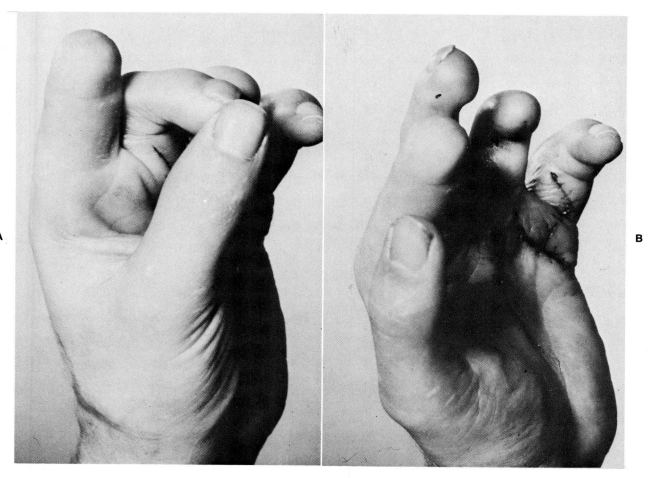

Fig. 25-3. A and **B,** Postoperative result following replacement of the third finger with the second toe in a hand in which only the thumb was functioning normally.

Two-toe en-bloc transplantation

In severely damaged hands with only a single remaining digit, satisfactory reconstruction can be performed by transplanting the second and third toes as a single block of tissue. The single remaining finger is used as a thumb. Generally such fingers give a better cosmetic and functional result than single toe transfers, which produce the appearance of a "lobster" hand. Inclusion of the third toe allows the patient to stabilize larger instruments in his hand.

CASE REPORT (Fig. 25-4)

A 16-year-old male sustained an explosion injury of his hand, and only his thumb could be saved. Reconstruction with a two-toe transplant and a large dorsalis pedis flap gave a reasonably functional hand.

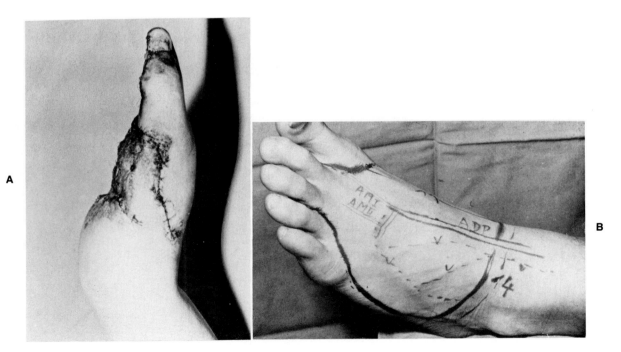

Fig. 25-4. A, Explosion injury of the right hand in a 16-year-old male. Only the thumb was preserved, which had sustained partial damage of the carpal-metacarpal joint and the pulp. **B,** Large dorsalis pedis flap is outlined on the donor foot, incorporating two toes and half of the two metatarsal bones.

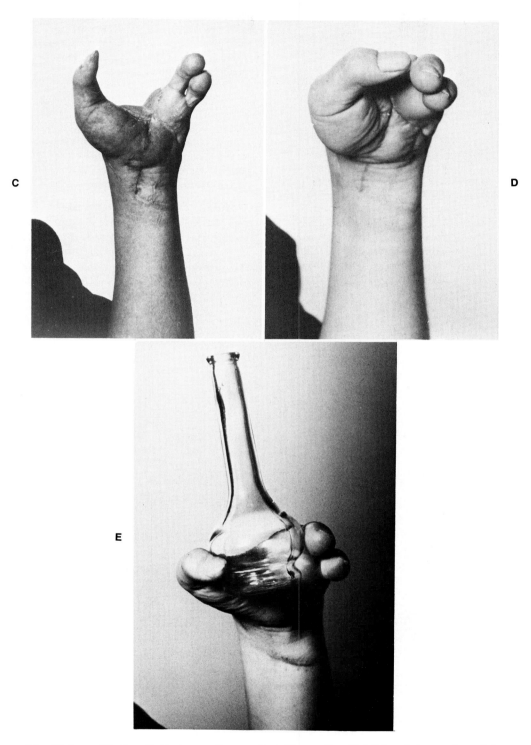

Fig. 25-4 cont'd. C to **E,** Postoperative result at 12 months. (Additional shortening of the thumb was carried out.)

Total hand reconstruction

In cases in which the entire hand is amputated, it is possible to construct a hand by combined transfer of a single second toe as a thumb and a two-toe en-block transfer from the opposite foot to serve as fingers. Large skin flaps must also be transferred to provide cover for the transplanted metatarsals.

CASE REPORT (Fig. 25-5)

A 28-year-old male lost both hands in an explosion. He refused to go through with the initial reconstructive plan consisting of a Krukenberg procedure on one arm and myoelectric procedures on the other arm. A hand was successfully reconstructed by transfer of a single second toe from one foot and a two-toe en-bloc unit from the other foot. To furnish a first web space on the reconstructed hand, pulp flaps were taken from the lateral aspects of both great toes and were placed parallel to each other in the new web space.

Flexor and extensor tendons of the donor digits were sutured to corresponding recipient tendons; the digital nerves of the toes were sutured to corresponding branches of the median nerve, and branches of the superficial perineal nerve were sutured to branches of the radial nerve. The dorsalis pedis artery was anastomosed to the radial artery.

In the early postoperative period, flexion was unsatisfactory. A tenolysis at 5 months brought about a better result with a good pinch grip and a reasonable span grip. Inclusion of the third toe in the reconstruction furnished sufficient stability for lifting a telephone receiver or using a spoon. Eight months after the operation the patient could open buttons, manipulate zippers, and perform other fine movements.

The two-toe transfer produces a significant defect of the foot. If healing is lengthy, the transverse arch of the foot is disrupted; the patients are therefore given special support inlays for their shoes. However, in the first patient, sufficient stability of the foot was achieved so that after 2 years the inlay could be discarded.

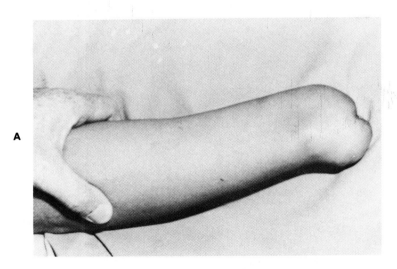

Fig. 25-5. A, Complete amputation of the hand. (The patient was a bilateral hand amputee.)

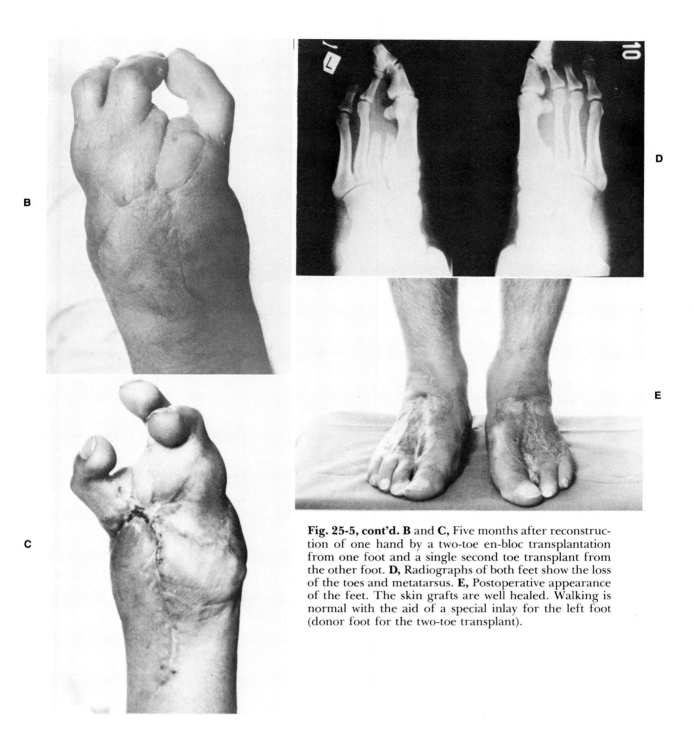

Fig. 25-5, cont'd. B and **C,** Five months after reconstruction of one hand by a two-toe en-bloc transplantation from one foot and a single second toe transplant from the other foot. **D,** Radiographs of both feet show the loss of the toes and metatarsus. **E,** Postoperative appearance of the feet. The skin grafts are well healed. Walking is normal with the aid of a special inlay for the left foot (donor foot for the two-toe transplant).

DISCUSSION

This procedure is comparatively safe to perform because of the long vascular pedicle and relatively easy anastomosis. The most difficult step in these operations is the planning and preparation.

An interesting feature is that, 2 years postoperatively in the cases cited, the two-point discrimination in the toe transplants and in the pulp flaps was comparable to the normal finger, having exceeded the accuracy of the untransferred "control" toes. The toes' recovery to beyond the level of normal indicates that two-point discrimination depends not only on the density of the sensory receptors or the number of ingrowing axons but also on the intelligence of the patient and the training he receives. This finding is supported by a study of children born without arms who use their feet in writing, painting, and eating. Two-point discrimination in these children, even those under the age of 10, was comparable to that of a normal hand.

The major disadvantage of this donor area is the unsatisfactory secondary defect. Ulceration of the foot or hyperkeratosis of the skin grafts can result.

The defect after a one-toe transplantation can be neglected. With two-toe transfers, morbidity is low initially and negligible after the first 2 years.

All of our patients have been satisfied with their results and have effectively used the constructed parts in their normal hand function. Patient selection is important, and an intelligent, cooperative patient is necessary if maximum function is to be obtained.

SUMMARY

The development of the free tissue transfer has made possible the reconstruction of severely damaged hands and the replacement of fingers and thumbs. In this context the foot has become very important as a donor area. Because of its anatomic similarity and the ideal situation of the dorsalis pedis artery, a great variety of transplants can be carried out. The cases discussed illustrate the pos-

Table 25-1. Results of transplantations from the foot

Procedure	Number	Success	Other effects
Dorsalis pedis flap	26	24	1 Partial necrosis
Pulp flaps	5	5	
Web space flaps	2	2	
Combined transplants with nail, bone, tendon, joints	5	5	
Two-toe	21	19	1 Partial necrosis
Two-toe en-bloc	4	4	
TOTAL	63	59 = 93.7%	

sibilities of providing skin cover with sensibility and of reconstruction by combined tissue transfer such as skin–subcutaneous tissue–bone, or skin–subcutaneous tissue–tendon, or toe transfer, or two-toe en-block transplantation. The operation is comparatively safe. In the series of 63 cases represented in Table 25-1, the success rate was 93.7%. Functional and cosmetic results are good. The secondary defect of the foot presents problems that for the most part can be acceptably solved.

REFERENCES

1. Biemer, E.: Two-toe transfer for thumb and finger replacement, microsurgery, Proceedings of the Fifth International Congress of the International Microsurgical Society, Bonn, (October, 1978) **7:**17, 1979.
2. Biemer, E., Stock, W., Herndl, E., and Duspiva, W.: Reconstruction of the hand by free tissue transfer, Int. J. Microsurg. **2:**159, 1980.
3. Buncke, H.J.: Toe digital transfer, Clin. Plast. Surg. **3:**49, 1976.
4. Buncke, H.J., et al.: Thumb replacement: great toe transplantation by microvascular anastomosis, Br. J. Plast. Surg. **26:**194, 1973.
5. Lanz, T., and Wachsmuth, W.: Praktische anatomie, Bank 1, Berlin, 1972, Springer-Verlag.
6. O'Brien, B.M., et al.: Hallus-to-hand transfer, Hand **7:**128, 1975.
7. Serafin, D., and Buncke, H.J.: Microsurgical composite tissue transplantation, St. Louis, 1979, The C.V. Mosby Co.

Chapter 26

Great toe–to–thumb transfer: indications and results in forty-one cases

Leonard Gordon

Harry J. Buncke

Bernard S. Alpert

Norman K. Poppen

Tom R. Norris

Nicoladoni performed a staged pedicle transfer of a toe to the hand in 1898.[17] Seventy years elapsed before this operation was accomplished in a single stage on a rhesus monkey by anastomosing the digital vessels.[4] Clinical refinements over the past 10 years have established great toe–to–hand transfer as a reliable and useful method of thumb reconstruction.*

INDICATIONS AND PATIENT SELECTION

Opposition, large object grasp, power, pinch, and fine pinch are all compromised if all or part of the thumb is absent. Many methods are available to restore these functions and improve the appearance of the hand.† This chapter provides an analysis of function after great toe transfer, including comparison with other methods.

In most thumb amputations from the base of the metacarpal to the interphalangeal joint, great toe transfer provides an excellent method of reconstruction with respect to both function and appearance (Fig. 26-1). In some cases pollicization remains the procedure of choice in thumb reconstruction. Congenital deformities representing longitudinal arrest of development are seldom amenable to toe-to-hand transfer, because this

---

*References 2, 3, 5, 8, 15, 16, 18.
†References 1, 6, 7, 11, 13, 14, 20.

procedure requires the presence of normal recipient vessels and nerves in the first ray of the hand. Also, traumatic cases with loss of the entire first metacarpal are often best treated by other methods of reconstruction, such as pollicization or second toe–to–hand transfer because of problems with weight-bearing if the entire first metatarsal is removed from the foot.

Toe-to-thumb transfer is particularly indicated in hands with multiple injuries or several missing digits and will effectively provide an opposable thumb for the remaining digits. If no opposable digits remain, then metacarpal lengthening can lengthen a digit for opposition with the transferred thumb. In some cases the second toe from the opposite foot may be transferred to oppose the thumb. We have performed simultaneous double toe-to-hand transfers in five cases. In these cases three surgical teams work independently, one on each foot and the third on the hand, so that the operative time is not unduly lengthened (Fig. 26-2, A to C). These five cases are not included in the results of this series. Amputations distal to the interphalangeal joint that produce a significant functional deficit may be amenable to metacarpal lengthening.

Transfer of various parts of the great toe is also possible and adds further versatility to thumb reconstruction. The transfers of the metatarsophalangeal joint alone for joint and bone loss, digital

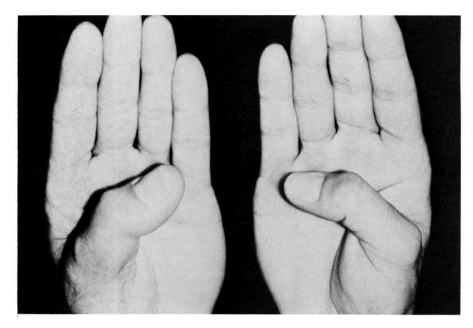

Fig. 26-1. Great toe transfer with excellent appearance and function.

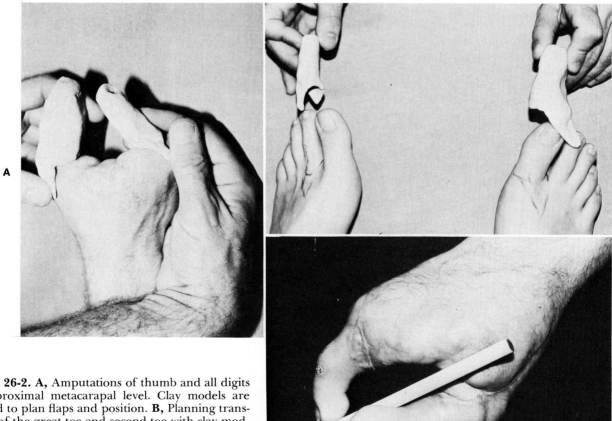

Fig. 26-2. A, Amputations of thumb and all digits at proximal metacarapal level. Clay models are used to plan flaps and position. **B,** Planning transfer of the great toe and second toe with clay models. **C,** Functional result 3 months later.

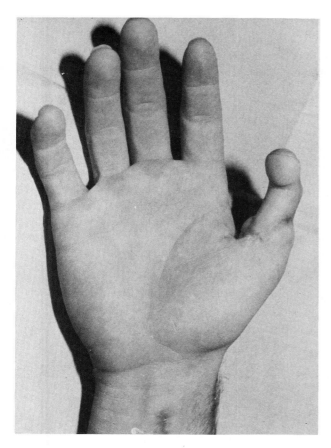

Fig. 26-3. The second toe is narrower and smaller than the thumb.

Table 26-1. Cause of initial problem

Congenital	1
Burn	1
Frostbite	1
Snakebite	1
Saw injury	3
Crush	3
Avulsion	8
Explosion	3
TOTAL	21

PATIENT POPULATION

Forty-one great toe–to–thumb transfers were performed at the Ralph K. Davies Medical Center in San Francisco from 1974 to 1981. Of these, ten patients were from other parts of the country and detailed follow-up examinations could not be carried out. Twenty-one patients who were followed for at least 18 months were examined in detail and are included in this report.

The cause of the initial problem for these patients is listed in Table 26-1. There were eleven male and ten female patients; the dominant hand was involved in eleven cases. The age distribution is reflected in Fig. 26-4. Most patients were between 20 and 30 years old; the oldest patient in this series was 34 years old. Subsequent toe-to-thumb transfers have been performed in patients over 60 years old, and age itself does not appear to be a contraindication unless severe vascular disease is present. The two youngest patients in this series had open epiphyses, which continued to grow postoperatively. No transfers were done at the time of the initial injury. The earliest reconstruction was carried out once all wounds were healed, 3 months after the initial injury (Fig. 26-5).

METHOD
Planning

Adequate skin cover in the area that is to become the first web space is important, especially in the hand with several digits missing (Fig. 26-6). In three cases a preliminary groin flap was performed to provide such cover before toe-to-hand transfer. If only a limited amount of skin is required, this may be included with the toe as a dorsalis pedis flap. This was done in three cases.

Clay models of the great toe and skin flaps are extremely helpful in planning the skin incisions (Fig. 26-6, *B*). In most cases the ipsilateral toe is preferred. Using the contralateral toe with a larger amount of medial skin can occasionally provide better cover in the first web space. This was preferable in only two cases; the choice depends on the flap design and orientation.

pulp for neurovascular skin cover, or skin from the first web space for soft tissue contractures have proved to be useful techniques.[16,21]

The patient's occupational requirements, age, motivation, and donor site preferences should be carefully considered. In patients reluctant to lose their great toe, the second toe may be used.[19] This may result in better appearance of the donor foot, and in addition, the entire second metacarpal may be included so that reconstruction can be accomplished in cases in which the amputation is at the base of the metacarpal. The second toe is significantly narrower and shorter than the thumb, and the appearance and function of the hand are compromised (Fig. 26-3). In patients who consider appearance of the foot of primary concern, use of the second toe is often an acceptable alternative.

Preoperative evaluation of the hand is often useful to clarify specific functional problems, and an orthotic thumb post may assist patients in deciding whether or not they desire surgery.

The surgeon maps out the arterial supply in the wrist and hand, using a Doppler probe. In cases with extensive tissue loss in the hand, an arteriogram is useful to confirm the presence, position, and quality of the recipient vessels. Similarly the Doppler probe is used to follow the dorsalis pedis artery distally and to identify the course of the first metatarsal artery. Experience with the Doppler often allows the surgeon to differentiate between dorsal and volar metatarsal vessels. If a question remains as to the anatomy of these vessels, an arteriogram provides useful information about the variable arterial supply to the first metatarsal area. Lateral and oblique views of the foot are necessary to distinguish between volar and dorsal metatarsal vessels within the first metatarsal space.

Operating technique

Once the skin flaps have been raised, the first part of the dissection is directed at the vascular pedicles. Large superficial veins on the medial aspect of the first metatarsal are constant and can be dissected without difficulty. The abundant greater saphenous venous system allows as long a pedicle to be taken as is required for the hand. Extra venous length can be used for vascular cuffs around the anastomosis or vein grafts on the arterial side if needed. The arterial supply to the great toe and first metatarsal space has been well described in the literature.[9,10,21] Either dorsal or plantar first metatarsal arteries may represent the dominant supply to the great toe. In this series a high proportion (approximately 50%) of predominantly plantar

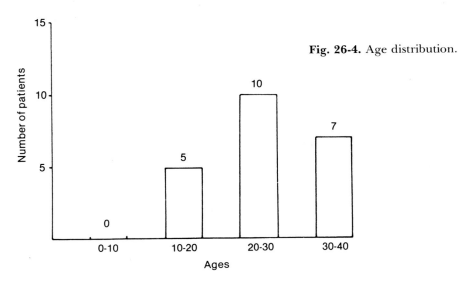

Fig. 26-4. Age distribution.

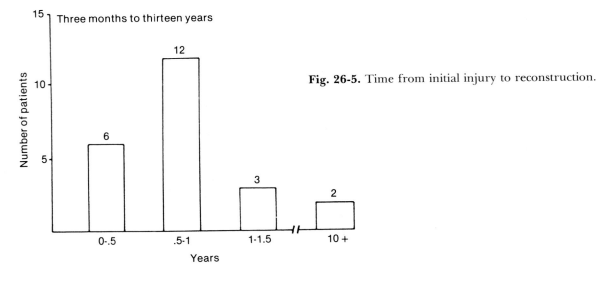

Fig. 26-5. Time from initial injury to reconstruction.

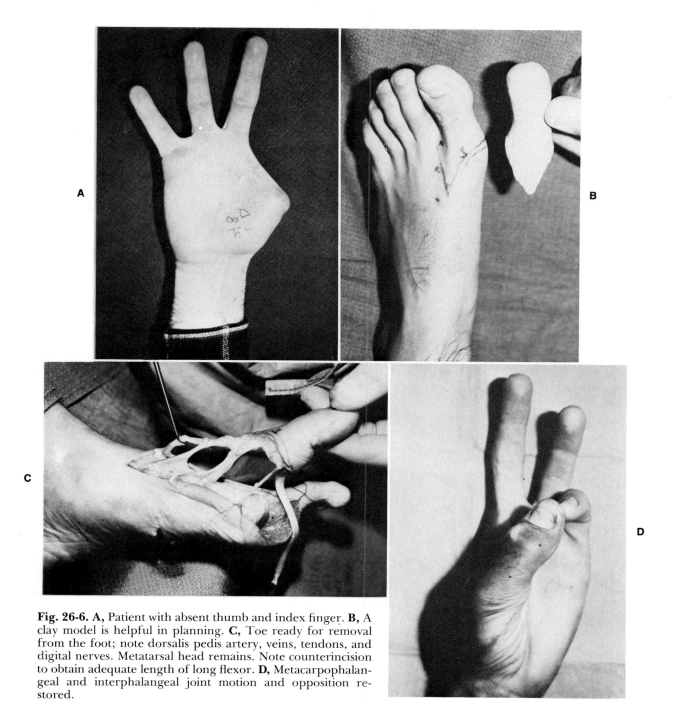

Fig. 26-6. A, Patient with absent thumb and index finger. **B,** A clay model is helpful in planning. **C,** Toe ready for removal from the foot; note dorsalis pedis artery, veins, tendons, and digital nerves. Metatarsal head remains. Note counterincision to obtain adequate length of long flexor. **D,** Metacarpophalangeal and interphalangeal joint motion and opposition restored.

vessels was found. In these cases in which the dominant vessel passes plantar to the transverse metatarsal ligament, it is helpful to dissect this vessel from the first web space in a proximal direction. This vessel lies in close relation to the metatarsal head. When the dorsal vessel is larger, the dissection may be more easily carried out from the dorsalis pedis vessel and then directed distally. Unless the dominant supply can be definitely identified by Doppler examination or arteriography as being dorsal, we begin the dissection in the first web space. Here the digital vessels to the great toe and second toe are dissected and the vessel to the second toe is ligated and divided. The great toe vessel can then be dissected proximally and either volarly or dorsally, as the case may be. In dissecting the volar vessel one must divide the transverse metatarsal ligament; a plantar incision a few inches long is often helpful. The dorsal vessel can usually be found without difficulty deep to the extensor hallucis brevis, which is divided and elevated, thereby exposing the neurovascular structures. The deep peroneal nerve can be found just lateral to the dorsalis pedis vessel on the dorsum of the foot, and if a recipient nerve is present on the dorsal aspect of the thumb metacarpal, this nerve should be sutured to provide dorsal sensation.

The great toe digital nerve on the lateral side should be separated from the nerve supplying the second toe. The digital nerves are sectioned on either side of the great toe. These nerves and the flexor tendon are measured and divided at a level determined by the length required in the hand (Fig. 26-4, *C*). Tendon suture by the Pulvertaft weave technique carried out at the wrist level is optimal, but can also be carried out in the palm or base of the thumb. A transverse counterincision in the sole of the foot is often required to gain greater length of the flexor tendon. Tendinous junctions between the flexor hallucis and flexor digitorum prevent obtaining the tendon through an incision at the ankle.

Next the site of joint or bone division must be considered. Our biomechanical studies indicate that the first metatarsal head should be retained for weight-bearing and gait. The joint capsule may be removed at its metatarsal attachment and a new metacarpophalangeal joint reconstructed on the thumb if the metacarpal head remains. Otherwise disarticulation at the metatarsophalangeal level is appropriate, with osteosynthesis of the proximal toe phalanx to the remaining proximal phalanx or metacarpal of the thumb. In cases in which only part of the proximal metacarpal remains, part of the metatarsal may be removed by using an oblique osteotomy, starting distally on the plantar surface and ending proximally and dorsally. This retains the weight-bearing portion of the first metatarsal head and the sesamoid bone.

Osteosynthesis may be accomplished by a number of techniques. Fashioning the thumb phalanx into a peg and hollowing out the toe phalanx provides an excellent fit with a large area of bony contact. Often no internal fixation is necessary. This method was used in many cases, while in others interosseous wires or cross-Kirschner wires were used. A metacarpophalangeal joint comprising the thumb metacarpal and the great toe phalanx was reconstructed in six cases.

If possible the great toe artery is anastomosed end to side or end to end to the radial artery between the first and second metacarpals. When this artery has been damaged or is unavailable, the radial artery at the wrist may be used by end-to-side anastomosis. Occasionally the digital vessels of the remaining thumb stump can be used when these are of adequate caliber and quality. The vein is then anastomosed to a large vein on the dorsum of the hand and the toe nerves to the respective digital and dorsal radial nerves. Skin grafts in the hand, especially on the dorsal surface, heal well and do not require prolonged periods of bed rest as they do on the foot. For this reason skin grafts on the hand are preferred.

Postoperative care

The hand is kept elevated in a loose palmar plaster splint for the first week. The patient receives 30 to 55 ml/hr of low molecular weight dextran for 3 days. Smaller doses of dextran should be used in children. The patient is given isoxsuprine if there is any evidence of vascular spasm and is maintained on 1,200 mg of aspirin for 2 to 3 weeks postoperatively. A series of patients received isoxsuprine, 10 mg, 3 times a day for 2 weeks before surgery.

After a hospital stay of 7 to 10 days, the patient is again seen 3 weeks after surgery, when hand therapy is begun with gentle, active, assisted exercises. Therapy progresses slowly through a graded program lasting approximately 2 months. The donor site should be kept elevated continuously for approximately 2 weeks. If healing appears good at that stage, very slow mobilization is commenced, with supportive elastic bandages or stockings for 3 months.

RESULTS
Survival

Of forty-one cases, one thumb failed to survive. A second had partial loss, requiring a neurovascular island flap for coverage of the ulnar aspect of the thumb. Four patients were taken back to surgery for reexploration because of vascular problems. In these cases vein grafts were inserted, and vascularity was restored in three cases.

Function

Sensation in the thumb was compared with that of the opposite thumb and opposite toe (Fig. 26-7). All the opposite thumbs had a two-point discrimination under 5 mm, while most of the opposite toes were between 5 and 10 mm. All cases displayed useful sensation; these values are represented in the histogram in Fig. 26-7. In no case was the two-point discrimination over 2 cm on either the radial or ulnar sides.

Although we realized that a comparison was being made between dominant and nondominant hands, accounting for some values at both ends of the spectrum, the pinch and grip strengths in the recipient hands were compared with those of the opposite hands. As can be seen in Fig. 26-8, most patients achieved between 40% and 80% of both pinch and grip strength compared to the opposite side.

In this series of patients fourteen out of twenty-one had major injuries to the recipient hand. For this reason a measure of dexterity and fine manipulative skills was not a reliable parameter of the functional result. In all cases with three or four normal remaining digits, dexterity and find manipulation were excellent, and it was these cases that represented the favorable end of the spectrum when grip strength and pinch were considered.

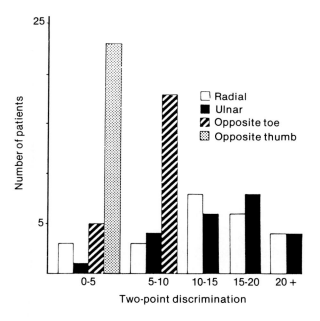

Fig. 26-7. Sensation after toe-to-hand transfer.

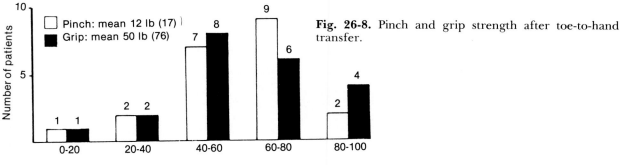

Fig. 26-8. Pinch and grip strength after toe-to-hand transfer.

Appearance

All patients were satisfied with the appearance of the thumb. Despite the fact that the great toe is slightly larger than the thumb, it tended to atrophy following the transfer and 18 months later closely resembled the opposite side (Fig. 26-1). Callosities present on the plantar surface decreased during this period. The patients subjectively felt that the toe "became a thumb" at an average of 4 months after the transfer.

Motion at the interphalangeal joint level averaged 20 degrees and at the metacarpophalangeal joint 15 degrees (Fig. 26-6, *D*). In all of these cases the carpometacarpal joint was normal. Those cases with reconstituted metacarpophalangeal joints using the toe phalanx and hand metacarpal had a similar average range of motion.

Donor site

In most cases the donor site healed within the first 3 weeks but on occasion took as much as 2 months. A mandatory 2-week period of elevation was found to improve results. All cases ultimately healed well. Subsequent biomechanical studies have demonstrated no significant gait abnormalities as a result of the loss of the great toe, and no patients have limited their sporting or other activities.[12]

SUMMARY

Survival following great toe transfer is predictable, and both sensory and motor return are gratifying. The obvious disadvantage of the loss of a great toe does not appear to represent a significant functional deficit, but compromises appearance. When used in conjunction with metacarpal lengthening, first web deepening, pollicization, and other techniques, toe-to-hand transfer constitutes a useful and indispensable alternative in thumb reconstruction.

REFERENCES

1. Buck-Gramcko, D.: Pollicization of the index finger, J. Bone Joint Surg. **53B:**1605, 1971.
2. Buncke, H.J.: Toe to hand transplantation by microvascular anastomosis, Sixth International Congress of Plastic Surgeons, Paris, 1975, p. 69.
3. Buncke, H.J.: Toe digital transfer, Clin. Plast. Surg. **3:**49, 1976.
4. Buncke, H.J., and Schultz, W.P.: Immediate Nicoladoni procedure in the rhesus monkey, Br. J. Plast. Surg. **19:**332, 1966.
5. Buncke, H.J., et al.: Thumb replacement: great toe transposition in microvascular anastomosis, Br. J. Plast. Surg. **26:**194, 1973.
6. Bunnell, S.: Reconstruction of the thumb, Am. J. Surg. **95:**168, 1958.
7. Chase, R.A.: An alternative to pollicization in subtotal thumb reconstruction, Plast. Reconstr. Surg. **44:**421, 1969.
8. Cobbett, J.R.: Free digital transfer: report of a case of transfer of a great toe to replace an amputated thumb, J. Bone Joint Surg. **51B:**677, 1969.
9. Edwards, E.A.: Anatomy of the small arteries of the foot and toes, Acta Anat. **41:**81, 1960.
10. Edwards, E.A.: Organization of the small arteries of the hand and digits, Am. J. Surg. **99:**837, 1960.
11. Gosset, J.: Reconstruction of an amputated thumb. In Reid, D.A.C., and Gosset, J., editors: Mutilating injuries of the hand, Edinburgh, 1979, Churchill Livingstone.
12. Hmura, M.S., and Buncke, H.J.: Biomechanical analysis of toe-to-thumb transplants: a look at both sides, J. Hand Surg. **1:**81, 1976.
13. Littler, J.W.: Neurovascular pedicle method of digital transposition for reconstruction of the thumb, Plast. Reconstr. Surg. **12:**203, 1953.
14. Littler, J.W.: On making a thumb: one hundred years of surgical effort, J. Hand Surg. **1:**35, 1976.
15. May, J.W., and Daniel, R.K.: Great toe–to–hand free tissue transfer, Clin. Orthop. **133:**140, 1978.
16. Morrison, W.A., O'Brien, B.M., and Hamilton, R.B.: Neurovascular free foot flaps in reconstruction of the mutilated hand, Clin. Plast. Surg. **5:**265, 1978.
17. Nicoladoni, C.: Daumenplastik und organischer ersutz de finger-spitze (anticheiroplastik und dactyloplastik) Arch. Klin. Chir. **61:**605, 1900.
18. O'Brien, B.M., MacLeod, A.M., Sykes, P.J., and Donahue, S.: Hallux-to-hand transfer, **7:**128, 1975.
19. O'Brien, B.M., et al.: Microvascular second toe transfer for digital reconstruction, J. Hand Surg. **3:**123, 1978.
20. Smith, R.J., and Dworecka, F.: Treatment of the one-digit hand, J. Bone Joint Surg. **55A:**113, 1973.
21. Strauch, B., and Shafiroff, B.B.: The foot: a versatile source of donor tissue. In Serafin, D., and Buncke, H.J.: Microsurgical composite tissue transplantation, St. Louis, 1979, The C.V. Mosby Co.

Part VIII

Lower limb reconstruction

Chapter 27

Reconstruction of the lower leg

Kiyonori Harii

Defects of the lower one third of the leg often present problems because of the scarcity of local tissues for reconstruction. Microvascular free tissue transfers are an ideal solution because they permit direct transplantation of the various tissues available for reconstruction.[2] Nonetheless there is some question as to whether or not the overall success rate of free flaps to the leg is as good as that of other flaps.[3,6,7] We will summarize our data on free tissue transfers for leg defects and discuss the scope of free tissue transfers in reconstruction of these troublesome defects.

CLINICAL DATA
Applications (Table 27-1)

A total of eighty-four free flaps were transferred to the legs of eighty-one patients from May 1973 to April 1981 at the Tokyo Metropolitan Police Hospital, the University of Tokyo Hospital, and related hospitals. The diagnoses are categorized in Table 27-1. Trauma accounted for 64%. Two free flap transfers, each to a different leg, were performed in two patients, and both transfers to a single leg were performed in one patient.

Table 27-1. Clinical cases treated (May 1973 to April 1981)

Cause of recipient defect	Number of cases
Scar contracture or skin defect resulting from trauma	34
Scar contracture or ulcer resulting from burns (including electric burns and frostbite)	11
Chronic leg ulcer	16
Nonunion of fractured bone, osteomyelitis	18
Others (tumor, malformation)	2
TOTAL	81

Types of tissue employed (Table 27-2)

The selection of the donor flap is influenced by the type of defect, the patient's age, obesity, and other individual characteristics. The groin flap is adequate for closure of numerous defects and results in minimal donor site deformity. During the first 4 years of this series (May 1973 to October 1977), forty-eight of a total of fifty-two flaps were from the groin. The remaining four flaps included a compound gracilis flap, a dorsalis pedis flap, and two omental flaps with split-thickness skin grafts. Five of the groin flaps were iliac osteocutaneous flaps nourished by the superficial circumflex iliac vessels.[4]

During the last 4 years of the series (November 1977 to April 1981), only sixteen of thirty-two flaps transferred were obtained from the groin region. Four of these sixteen were free osteocutaneous

Table 27-2. Donor flaps employed (May 1973 to April 1981)

Donor flaps	Number of flaps
Groin skin flap	55
Groin osteocutaneous flap	
SCIA—bone graft*	5
DCIA—bone graft†	4
Latissimus dorsi flap	
Musculocutaneous flap	10
Muscle flap with skin graft	1
With serratus anterior flap	1
With ribs	1
Gracilis musculocutaneous flap	2
Dorsalis pedis flap	2
Tensor fascia lata flap	1
Omental flap	2
TOTAL	84

*SCIA—bone graft: iliac osteocutaneous flap nourished by superficial circumflex iliac vessels.
†DCIA—bone graft: iliac osteocutaneous flap nourished by deep circumflex iliac vessels.

flaps nourished by the deep circumflex iliac vessels. The sixteen other flaps included thirteen latissimus dorsi musculocutaneous flaps, which included one muscle flap with free skin grafts for the treatment of a chronic leg ulcer, one osteocutaneous flap with two ribs (for tibial nonunion), and one latissimus dorsi–serratus anterior flap. The remaining three included a gracilis musculocutaneous flap, a dorsalis pedis flap, and a tensor fascia lata flap.

Recipient vessels (Table 27-3)

One of the more important factors for successful flap transfer is the suitability of the recipient vessels. The artery should have good perfusion pressure and as little degeneration of the vascular wall as possible. Preoperative angiography offers valuable information in cases in which there is extensive injury. In this series preoperative angiography was performed in fifteen patients to assess the proposed recipient artery.

Of the eighty-four free flap transfers, the anterior tibial system (anterior tibial artery and dorsalis pedis artery) was used in seventy-three cases (87%), whereas the posterior tibial artery was used in only nine cases. Other vessels were used in the remaining two cases. Most of the anastomoses were end to end; end-to-side anastomoses were employed in only two transfers. No significant circulatory problems occurred in the leg after ligation of the anterior tibial vessels when the posterior tibial artery and the peroneal artery were patent. If one of the major branches—either the anterior tibial artery or the posterior tibial artery—had been damaged, a ligated arterial stump was selected for the anastomosis.

Complications and survival of flaps (Tables 27-4 and 27-5)

The principal complications were of vascular origin. Acute arterial thrombosis occurred within 24 hours after the transfer in thirteen flaps, while

Table 27-3. Recipient vessels used in transfer

Recipient vasculature	Number of flaps
Anterior tibial artery and venae comitantes	62
Dorsalis pedis artery and cutaneous veins or venae comitantes	11
Posterior tibial artery and venae comitantes	9
Others	2
TOTAL	84

Table 27-4. Survival of transferred flaps to legs (May 1973 to April 1981)

Result	Number of flaps	Percentage
Complete survival	60	71.4
Necrosis		
Epidermal	3	3.6
Dermal	3	3.6
Partial	11	13.1
Complete	6	7.1
FTSG*	1	1.2
TOTAL	84	100

*Flap shaved of its fatty tissues to be used as free skin graft.

Table 27-5. Analysis of flap necrosis (May 1973 to April 1981)

Type of necrosis	Causes	Number of flaps
Total necrosis	Thrombosis	
	Acute arterial	4 (two flaps after thrombectomy)
	Late arterial	2
		6 flaps—7.1%
Partial necrosis	Thrombosis	
	Acute arterial	2 (after thrombectomy)
	Late venous	1
	Problems in flap vascularity	8
		11 flaps—13.1%
Superficial necrosis		
Dermal	Thrombosis	
	Late arterial	2
	Late venous	1
		3 flaps—3.6%
Epidermal	Thrombosis	
	Acute arterial	2 (after thrombectomy)
	Late venous	1
		3 flaps—3.6%
TOTAL		23 flaps of 84 flaps—27.3%

no venous thromboses were seen in this period. Ten of the thirteen flaps were promptly reexplored, and reanastomosis was carried out after thrombectomy. Five of the ten flaps were completely salvaged (three with complete survival and two with superficial epidermal necrosis, which healed spontaneously), but complete necrosis occurred in two flaps and partial necrosis occurred in two others. The fatty tissues of one flap were trimmed away, and the skin was replaced as a free full-thickness skin graft that survived completely. Prompt thrombectomy was not possible in three flaps, and total necrosis occurred in each of these.

Late arterial thrombosis, occurring more than 24 hours after surgery, was encountered in three of the eighty-four flap transfers—one deep circumflex iliac osteocutaneous flap, one latissimus dorsi flap, and one groin skin flap. Complete necrosis occurred in two of the flaps and dermal necrosis occurred in the other. Late venous occlusion, however, was seen in three flaps, but the losses were minor. (Even without thrombectomies there was only one dermal necrosis, one epidermal necrosis, and one small partial necrosis.)

Table 27-4 lists the survival statistics for this series. Sixty of the eighty-four flaps achieved complete survival, whereas three skin flaps underwent superficial epidermal necrosis with subsequent spontaneous epithelialization. In other words, sixty-three of the eighty-four flaps achieved complete survival.

Eleven flaps, eight of which were groin flaps, underwent partial necrosis. Seven of the eight showed distal necrosis resulting from poor vascularity, and one had an arterial thrombosis treated with thrombectomy. One gracilis flap and two latissimus dorsi musculocutaneous flaps also showed partial necrosis. All eleven flaps required additional minor surgery such as free skin grafts or local

flaps. No distant flaps were needed in the secondary repairs.

Arterial thrombosis was responsible in each of the six flaps (six patients) that underwent complete necrosis. Amputation was necessary in two patients, while the other cases were salvaged with a crossleg flap in one case and split-thickness skin grafts in the other three. The three patients with dermal necrosis of the flap required coverage with split-thickness skin grafts on the surviving subcutaneous tissues.

In summary, the essential goal of the operation was achieved in sixty flaps with total survival. In addition, three flaps with epidermal necrosis, nine with partial necrosis, and two with dermal necrosis were easily repaired with small skin grafts. The overall success rate was 88%, or seventy-four successful transfers in a total of eighty-four flaps. We consider this quite satisfactory in view of the special problems presented by defects of the lower extremities.

Additional complications. Although vascular complications were our basic problem, a few other complications were encountered. Five of nine surviving osteocutaneous flaps (nine patients) showed nonunion and required secondary free bone grafts (one fibular graft and four iliac bone chip grafts). All but one of these cases finally acquired solid union.

Edema was noticed in two flaps, but this subsided spontaneously. Hematomas and infections were not special problems. Donor site problems were rare, but one case of persistent meralgia paraesthetica occurred. Recurrence of the original disease was seen in three cases of chronic stasis leg ulcer; these required additional treatment. There were no recurrences of chronic osteomyelitis after successful free flap transfer.

CASE REPORTS
Patient I

A 2-year-old female suffered an avulsion injury with skin sloughover of the dorsum of her left foot. The ankle and intertarsal and metatarsophalangeal joints of the third, fourth, and fifth toes were exposed. After debridement, a 5 by 13 cm free groin flap was transferred to cover the defect. The flap vessels (superficial epigastric artery and cutaneous vein) were joined to the anterior tibial artery and the vena comitans proximal to the ankle region. Part of the defect was covered with a split-thickness skin graft (Fig. 27-1).

Patient II

An 8-year-old male suffered an avulsion injury of the lower areas of both legs when he was run over by a vehicle. His right tarsal bones and ankle joint were fractured and exposed, with extensive skin loss. The skin on the medial surface of the left leg was lost, exposing the medial malleolus. After extensive debridement, the exposed tarsal bones and ankle joint of the right leg were covered with an 8 by 13 cm latissimus dorsi musculocutaneous flap.

The flap was isolated with a pedicle of thoracodorsal vessels and nerve in the right lateral thoracic region. The anterior tibial vessels, which had initially been damaged and ligated at the ankle, were exposed proximal to the damaged area, and the anterior tibial nerve was preserved. The flap was then transferred to the defect. The proximal portion of the latissimus dorsi muscle was sutured to the avulsed stumps of the extensor digitorum muscles, while the distal portion was sutured to the remnants of the avulsed extensor digitorum tendons to restore dorsiflexion. The anterior tibial vessels and nerve were joined to the neurovascular pedicle of the latissimus dorsi muscle.

Simultaneously the exposed medial malleolus of the left foot was covered with a dorsalis pedis island flap from the dorsum of the foot. Both flaps survived completely, and 10 months later the patient had active flexion of the right ankle (Fig. 27-2).

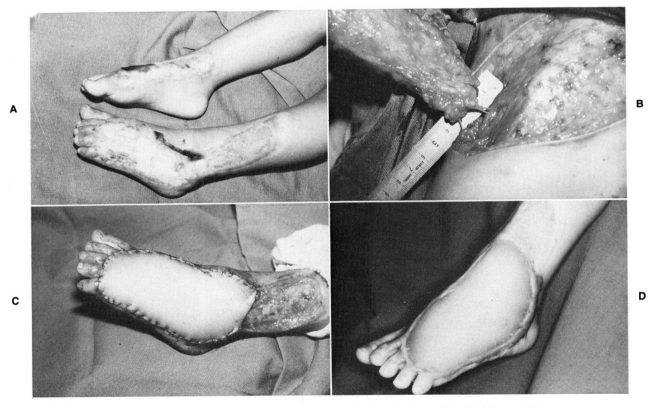

Fig. 27-1. Patient I. A 2-year-old female with an avulsion injury of the left foot. **A,** Preoperative view. **B,** Elevation of a 5.5 by 13 cm groin island flap. **C,** The flap immediately after revascularization. **D,** Two months after surgery. (From Iwaya, T., Harii, K., and Yamada, A.: Microvascular free flap treatment of avulsion injuries of the feet in children, J. Trauma **22**(1):15, © 1982 The Williams & Wilkins Co., Baltimore.)

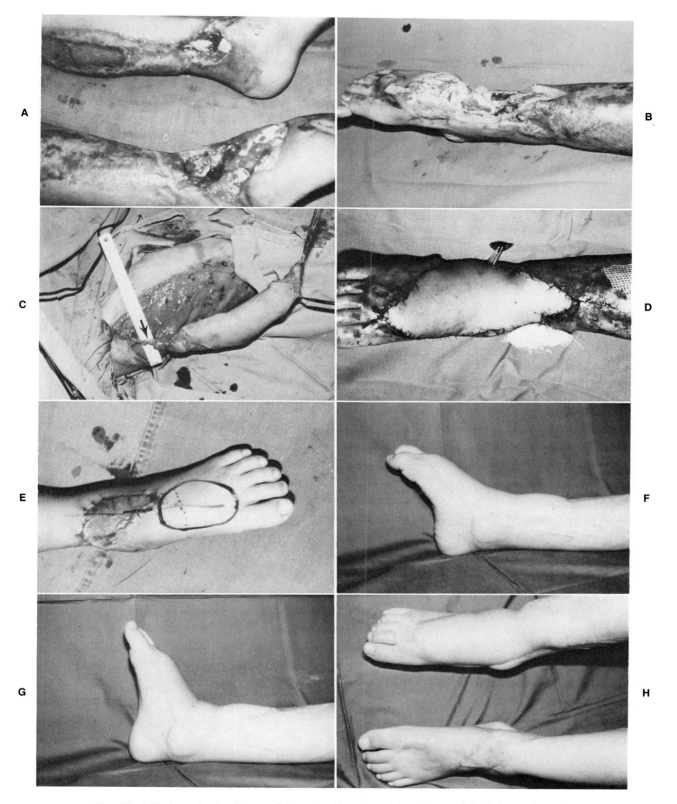

Fig. 27-2. Patient II. An 8-year-old male with an avulsion injury of both lower legs. **A,** Preoperative view. **B,** Defect of the right foot after debridement. **C,** Elevated latissimus dorsi musculocutaneous flap. Note thoracodorsal vessels and nerve *(arrow)*. **D,** Latissimus flap after revascularization. **E,** Design of dorsalis pedis island flap on the dorsum of the left foot for coverage of the medial malleolus skin defect. **F** and **G,** Ten months after transfer, active flexion of the right ankle has been obtained, with functional contraction of the transferred latissimus dorsi muscle. **H,** Both legs 10 months after surgery.

Patient III

A 45-year-old male developed a severe scar contracture of the right ankle after deep burns to both lower extremities; he was referred for treatment of the resulting ankylosis. (The left leg had previously been amputated.) After repositioning the ankle by lengthening the contracted Achilles tendon, the resultant raw surface was covered by a 17 by 27 cm free latissimus dorsi flap.

End-to-end anastomoses were carried out between the anterior tibial and thoracodorsal vessels. Satisfactory revascularization of the flap was achieved, but 20 hours after surgery the flap was pale, with no dermal bleeding. At exploration a thrombosed arterial anastomosis was resected and a new anastomosis performed. Revascularization of the flap was successful, with only a small area of partial necrosis at the distal margin (Fig. 27-3).

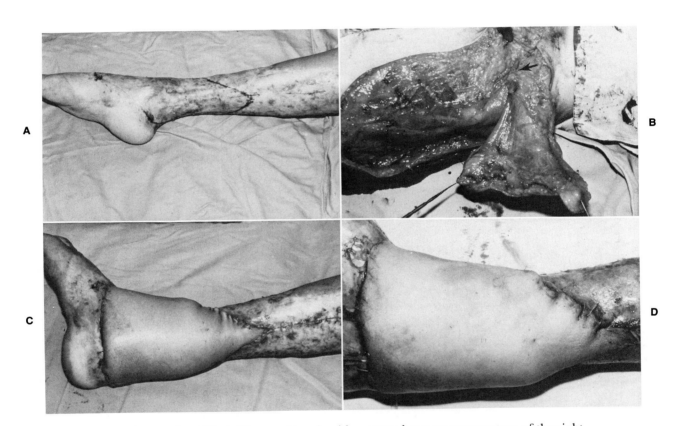

Fig. 27-3. Patient III. A 45-year-old male with a severe burn scar contracture of the right ankle. **A,** Preoperative view. **B,** Elevated latissimus dorsi flap. Note thoracodorsal vessels *(arrow).* **C,** Flap immediately after revascularization. **D,** Pale flap 20 hours after transfer. (**A** to **G** from Harii, K., Free flap transfer for reconstruction of the lower extremity, Jpn. J. Plast. Reconstr. Surg., **25**(2):121, Kokuseido Co., Tokyo, 1982.)

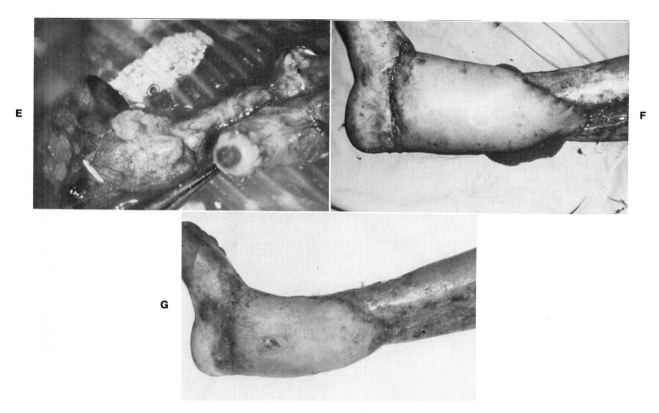

Fig. 27-3, cont'd. E, Arterial thrombosis observed under microscope. **F,** Revascularized flap with good capillary refill. **G,** Two months later, the flap has survived well with small partial necrosis at the distal margin.

Patient IV

A 25-year-old male had a 7 cm bony defect of the right distal tibia as the result of an automobile accident. An osteocutaneous flap composed of a 5 by 10 cm skin flap and 2.5 by 10 cm of iliac bone was isolated in the left groin region with a pedicle of the superficial circumflex iliac artery and cutaneous vein. The iliac bone was fixed into the stumps of the tibia with Kirschner wires, and the skin flap was placed to cover a skin defect in the anterior tibial region. The vessels to the osteocutaneous flap were then joined end to end with the anterior tibial vessels.

The distal junction of the bone graft united completely, but proximal union was delayed, requiring secondary cancellous bone chip grafts 3 months later. Complete bony union was finally obtained, and survival of the vascularized bone graft was complete (Fig. 27-4).

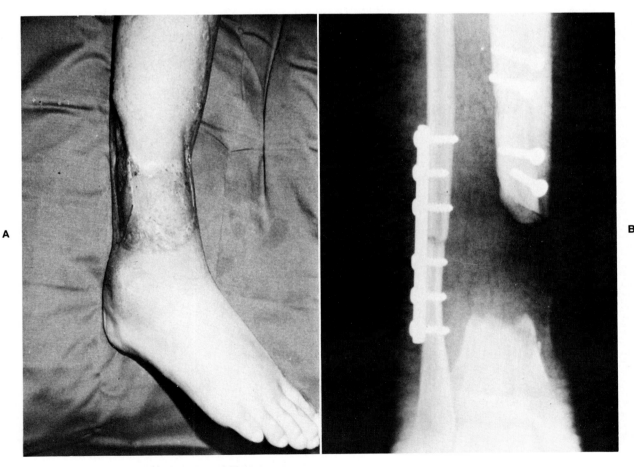

Fig. 27-4. Patient IV. A 25-year-old male with nonunion of the right tibia after an automobile accident. **A,** Preoperative view; **B,** radiographic view. (**A** to **E** from Harii, K.: Microvascular tissue transfer—fundamental techniques and clinical applications, Tokyo, 1983, Igaku-shoin, p. 173.)

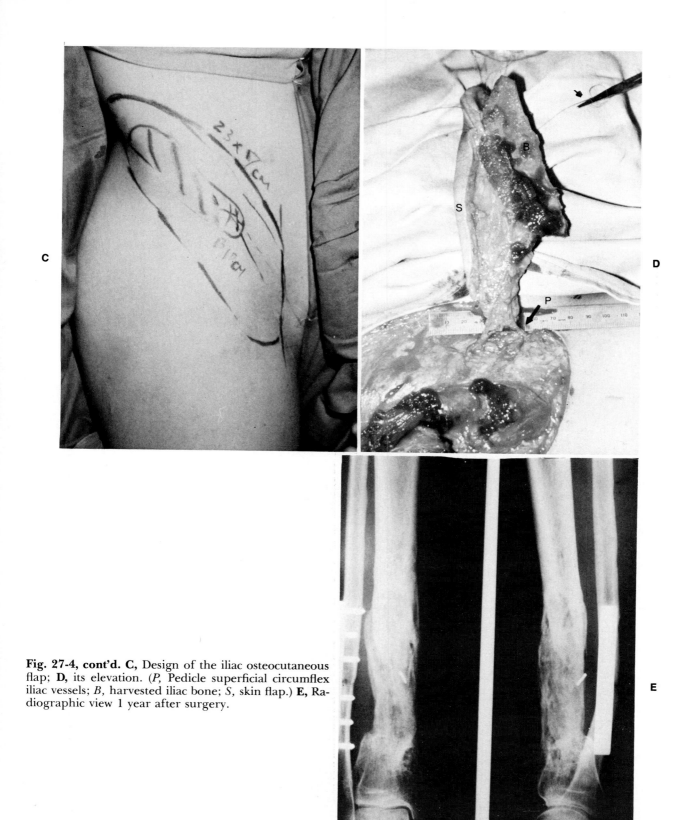

Fig. 27-4, cont'd. C, Design of the iliac osteocutaneous flap; **D,** its elevation. (*P,* Pedicle superficial circumflex iliac vessels; *B,* harvested iliac bone; *S,* skin flap.) **E,** Radiographic view 1 year after surgery.

Patient V

An 18-year-old male sustained a severe crush injury to the lower part of his right leg as the result of an automobile accident. Initial treatment included debridement, repositioning of the bony fragments, and application of skeletal traction at an emergency hospital. Two months after the injury, plate fixation and free bone grafts were employed to treat a nonunited tibia, but infection resulted. He was then referred to us for treatment of a nonunion and osteomyelitis of the tibia.

First the plate and screws were removed, the sequestra were excised, and continuous closed irrigation was carried out for treatment of the osteomyelitis. Ultimately the patient had a large defect in the lower part of the tibia, with extensive scarring and draining sinuses of the skin. After complete resection of the scar and the infected bone, arthrodesis of the talocrural joint and coverage of the skin defect was carried out with a free iliac osteocutaneous flap nourished by the deep circumflex iliac vessels. The anterior tibial vessels in the vicinity of the ankle were turned proximally to join with the deep circumflex iliac vessels that nourished a 6 by 13 cm skin flap and a 3 by 11 cm segment of iliac bone. The bone was fixed into the gap between the lower part of the tibia and the talus with Kirschner wires.

Bony union proceeded uneventfully. Partial weight bearing and full weight bearing were achieved at 10 months and 12 months, respectively (Fig. 27-5).

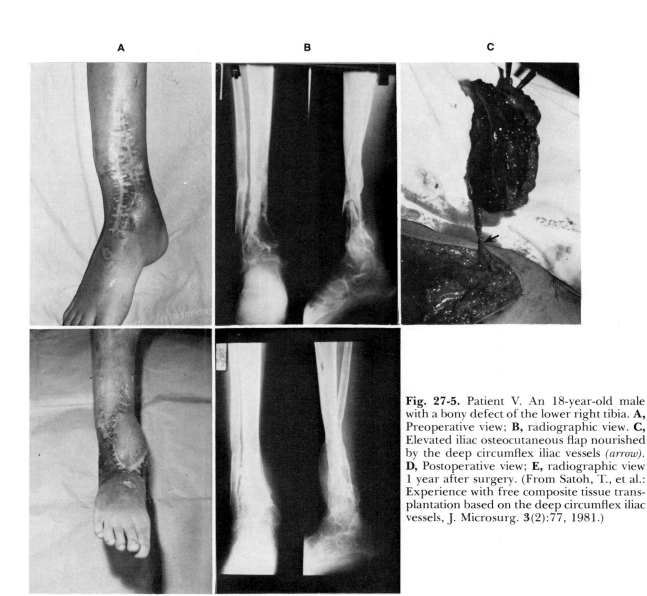

Fig. 27-5. Patient V. An 18-year-old male with a bony defect of the lower right tibia. **A,** Preoperative view; **B,** radiographic view. **C,** Elevated iliac osteocutaneous flap nourished by the deep circumflex iliac vessels *(arrow).* **D,** Postoperative view; **E,** radiographic view 1 year after surgery. (From Satoh, T., et al.: Experience with free composite tissue transplantation based on the deep circumflex iliac vessels, J. Microsurg. **3**(2):77, 1981.)

DISCUSSION

Although free flaps are now widely done, there are few reports of free flaps done for reconstruction of the lower extremities. Serafin et al.[3] compared their results with free groin flaps to the lower extremities with conventional distant flaps such as crossleg flaps and jump flaps; they found that free flaps were superior in a number of ways, such as time of immobilization, hospitalization, morbidity, and cost. However, the success rate of the free flap was lower than that of the crossleg flap. They noted complete necrosis in four of seventeen free flaps but in only one of eighteen crossleg flaps. This higher failure rate could have been caused by inexperience during their initial period or the use of a free groin flap with its small, short vascular pedicle. Godina[1] also reported a high failure rate during his early experience with free groin flaps and then a 100% success rate after initiating the use of end-to-side anastomoses. He therefore strongly recommended end-to-side anastomoses because they preserved distal circulation of the limb, provided easier planning, prevented retraction and subsequent spasm of the recipient artery, and avoided serious disturbances of the flow. Indeed, we agree that end-to-side anastomosis is essential in special cases but consider it unwarranted in all lower leg flaps.

As noted by Godina, the latissimus dorsi flap has a far longer and larger stalk than does the groin flap, and this is one of the reasons for improved success. Although the latissimus dorsi flap facilitates end-to-side anastomosis, it also improved our results when end-to-end anastomoses were used. All six cases of total necrosis in our present series involved groin flaps, and partial necrosis was also observed in many free groin flaps, while the latissimus dorsi flap with end-to-end anastomosis achieved a high rate of success. For closure of extensive skin defects, we now prefer to use the latissimus dorsi flap, although the specific advantages of the free groin flap cannot be overlooked.

Selection of the recipient artery is important in achieving successful transfer. In cases of extensive trauma, vascular spasm of the exposed artery frequently presents problems. A site for anastomosis should, therefore, be selected away from the injury and should be exposed with minimal trauma. Local administration of 2% lidocaine (Xylocaine) helps relieve arterial spasm, while intravenous prostaglandin E_1 may increase the peripheral arterial flow. In most of our cases the anterior tibial artery was used, and with it the vena comitans between the anterior tibial and the extensor hallucis longus muscles. In the lower part of the leg, however, the vessels run superficially and have often been damaged by the original trauma or have been bound down in the overall wound reaction. Sometimes the dorsalis pedis artery is the preferable recipient vessel in the lower leg because this long, superficial artery can be easily turned proximally to join with the donor artery. A branch of the greater saphenous vein or a vena comitans is a convenient recipient vein (Fig. 27-6).

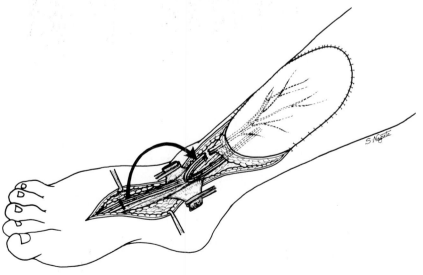

Fig. 27-6. Diagram showing the use of the dorsalis pedis vessels as recipient vessels for reconstruction of the lower leg.

SUMMARY

The data from our results with free flaps to the legs revealed a higher rate of success than seen in conventional flaps. In the lower leg a free flap transfer is often superior because of lack of sufficient local skin or muscles suitable for reconstruction.

REFERENCES

1. Godina, M.: Preferential use of end-to-side arterial anastomoses in free flap transfers, Plast. Reconstr. Surg. **64:**673, 1979.
2. Harii, K.: Microvascular free tissue transfers, World J. Surg. **3:**29, 1979.
3. Serafin, D., Georgiade, N., and Smith, D.: Comparison of free flaps with pedicled flaps for coverage of defects of the leg or foot, Plast. Reconstr. Surg. **59:** 492, 1977.
4. Taylor, G.I., and Watson, N.: One-stage repair of compound leg defects with free revascularized flaps of groin skin and iliac bone, Plast. Reconstr. Surg. **61:**494, 1978.
5. Taylor, G.I., Townsend, P., and Corlett, R.: Superiority of the deep circumflex iliac vessels as the supply for free groin flaps—clinical work, Plast. Reconstr. Surg. **64:**745, 1979.
6. Vasconez, L.O., Bostwick, J., and McCraw, J.: Coverage of exposed bone by muscle transposition and skin grafting, Plast. Reconstr. Surg. **53:**5, 1974.
7. White, W.L., et al.: Evaluation of 114 cross-leg flaps. In Skoog, T., and Ivy, R.H., editors: Transactions of the First Congress of the International Society of Plastic Surgeons, Baltimore, 1955, Williams & Wilkins Co.

Chapter 28

Microvascular flap transfer for coverage of exposed internal prosthesis

Marcus Castro Ferreira

The use of an internal prosthesis to replace long bones and joints has recently been developed in orthopedic surgery, and, despite a high success rate, some complications do occur.

One difficulty is a skin slough with exposure of the prosthesis. This frequently occurs when the prosthesis is placed under skin that is thin or poorly vascularized. The conventional method of treatment is removal of the prosthesis, closure of the skin by direct approximation or a skin flap, and delayed replacement of the prosthesis.

Attempts to provide skin cover for the exposed prosthesis are often complicated by persistent infection, fistulas, and sinuses. We were faced with one such case in which we used a free musculocutaneous flap to cover the prosthesis.

CASE REPORT

An 11-year-old male developed a Ewing's sarcoma on his right femur. An extensive resection was done that included two thirds of the femur, which was replaced with a metallic internal prosthesis (Fig. 28-1). The skin was sutured under tension. Postoperative treatment included radiotherapy and systemic chemotherapy.

The patient could walk well postoperatively, but 6 months later he sustained an injury to his right hip. Swelling and infection in the operated area developed, with resulting slough of the skin and exposure of the prosthesis (Fig. 28-2). Treatment by removal of the prosthesis and simple wound closure would probably have precluded any future chance of replacing the prosthesis and preserving the use of the limb.

Microvascular transfer of a musculocutaneous flap was then considered to provide a large segment of well-vascularized tissue to furnish coverage for the prosthesis.

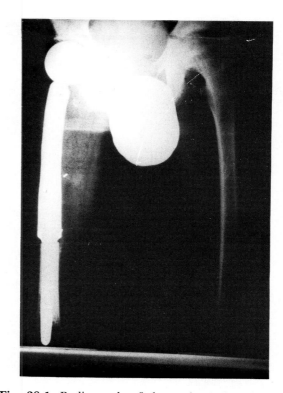

Fig. 28-1. Radiograph of the patient's lower limb. Two thirds of the femur was replaced with a metallic prosthesis.

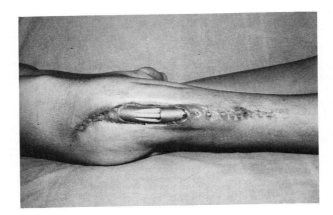

Fig. 28-2. Extent of exposure of the prosthesis on the lateral side of the thigh.

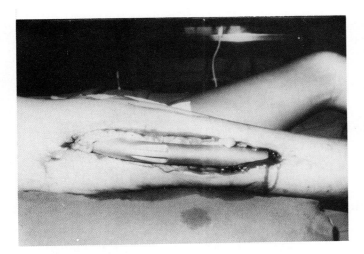

Fig. 28-3. After wound debridement.

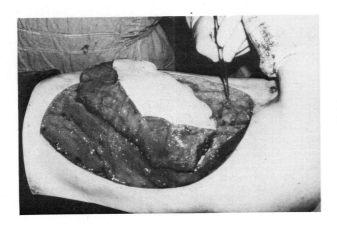

Fig. 28-4. Latissimus dorsi musculocutaneous flap elevated, the muscle in excess of the skin.

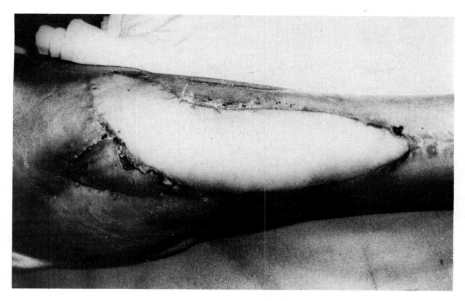

Fig. 28-5. One-month postoperative view of the flap showing good skin coverage and no infection.

The defect on the thigh was carefully debrided (Fig. 28-3); the lateral circumflex femoral artery and vein were dissected out on the medial aspect of the thigh.

A large latissimus dorsi musculocutaneous flap was designed with an island of skin large enough to close the defect on the thigh and an extended muscle segment to surround the prosthesis (Fig. 28-4). The thoracodorsal donor vessels were dissected and prepared for anastomosis. The flap was then transferred to the thigh, with the muscle completely encircling the prosthesis. The donor vascular pedicle was tunneled subcutaneously to the recipient vessels, and end-to-end microanastomoses were performed.

The vascular clamps were released, and good perfusion was immediately observed in the flap. The ischemic time was about 2 hours.

The skin island was sutured into the defect, and a small area of exposed muscle was covered with a skin graft.

The postoperative period was uneventful; the patient was given antibiotics, aspirin, dextran, and naftidrofuril (a vasodilator) for 1 week. The drains were taken out after 5 days. A small fistula draining a clear fluid persisted for 3 weeks and then closed. Major infection did not develop.

The patient was discharged after 10 days and resumed walking in 1 month. The quality of the transferred skin was excellent (Fig. 28-5). A patient follow-up of 1 year was uneventful.

Chapter 29

Augmented medial gastrocnemius myocutaneous island flap

Hsu Hsi Cheng

The medial gastrocnemius myocutaneous flap provides good covering for skin defects in the middle portion of the lower leg and for those overlying the upper portion of the tibia. However, for a skin defect in the distal portion of the lower leg, an ordinary medial gastrocnemius flap cannot be used.

For this purpose, two modifications are made. First, we increase the area of the flap by placing the posterior incision 2 cm farther posterior than usual and by placing the inferior incision just 2 cm above the medial malleolus. Thus we can gain 2 cm in width and 3 cm in length. (The distal portion of the unmodified flap is 5 cm above the medial malleolus.) Second, we detach the muscle origin, separating all structures except the neurovascular bundle so that it is converted into an island myocutaneous flap. This increases the distal arc of the flap by 5 to 6 cm. These basic steps bring heretofore inaccessible areas of the distal portion of the lower leg into range of the medial gastrocnemius flap.

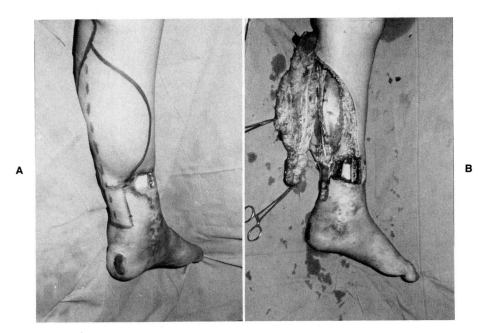

Fig. 29-1. **A,** The tibia and plate were exposed 3½ months after the injury. The incision was made 2 cm beyond the midline (dotted line) medially and 2 cm above the medial malleolus distally. **B,** The myocutaneous flap measured 22 by 10 cm.

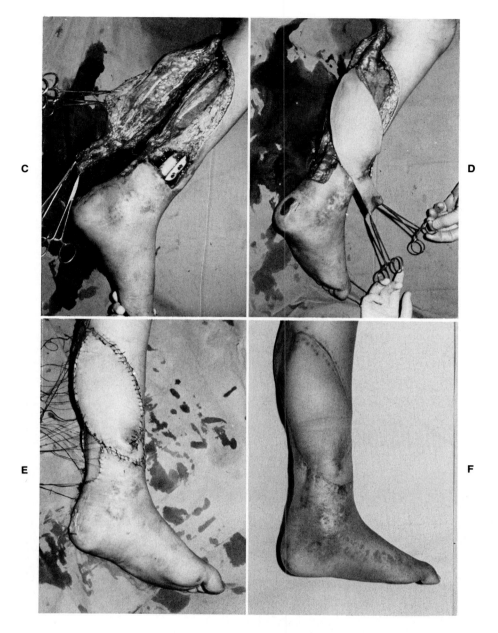

Fig. 29-1, cont'd. C and **D,** Following detachment of the origin of the gastrocnemius muscle, the flap can be advanced 5 cm distally. **E,** Immediate postoperative appearance after transfer of the flap. A free skin graft covers the donor area. **F,** Appearance 6 weeks after surgery.

CASE REPORT (Fig. 29-1)

The patient, a 27-year-old male, fell from a truck on December 25, 1980. The left lower leg was hit by a heavy object and sustained a compound fracture of the lower third of the tibia and fibula. Debridement was carried out immediately. A compression plate was applied after shortening the tibia. The skin was sutured directly. Ten

days later the skin over the lower third of the anteromedial part of the tibia necrosed, and the plate was exposed at the fracture site.

Transposition advancement of an augmented myocutaneous flap of the medial head of the gastrocnemius was performed on April 20, 1981 (3½ months after the injury). A flap measuring 10 by 22 cm was designed over

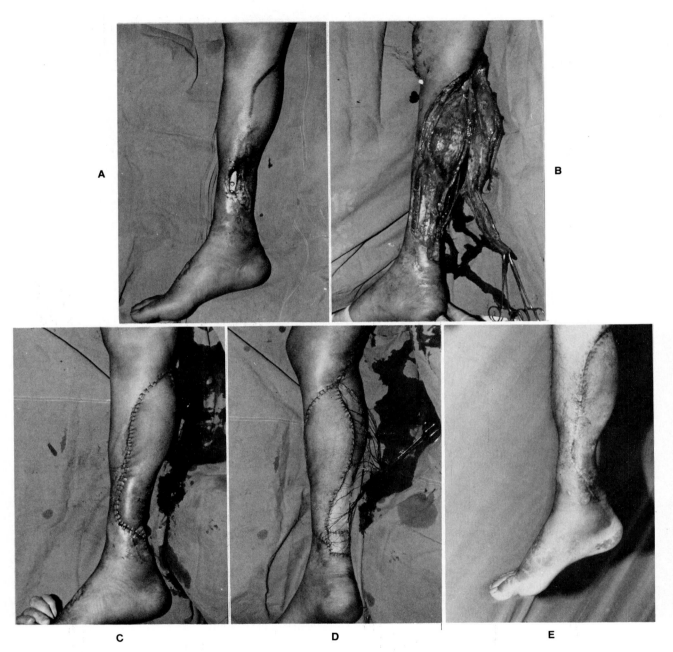

Fig. 29-2. A, Two months after injury the tibia and plate were exposed. **B,** Dissection of the gastrocnemius myocutaneous flap. **C** and **D,** Immediate postoperative appearance. **E,** Appearance 1½ months postoperatively.

the medial aspect of the lower leg. The anterior incision was parallel and adjacent to the anterior tibia. The flap extended to within 2 cm of the medial malleolus. In dissecting the flap, we preserved the Achilles tendon and paratenon. The greater saphenous vein was left intact at the base of the flap. The neurovascular bundle of the medial head was dissected and protected as the muscle origin was detached. Since the flap was completely freed except for the neurovascular bundle, it could be advanced distally along the longitudinal axis for a distance of 5 cm when the knee was flexed, as opposed to a maximum advancement of 2 cm before the muscle origin was detached.

A 7 by 5 cm skin defect remained after debridement of the wound. Transposition of the flap anteriorly and advancement inferiorly completely covered the wound. There was no tension on the vascular pedicle. However, the severed end of the muscle origin was advanced a short distance proximally and secured to the surrounding soft tissues to prevent inadvertent traction on the vascular pedicle. The donor defect at the posterior aspect of the lower leg was grafted with a thick split-thickness skin graft. The knee was immobilized in 30 degrees flexion with a long leg plaster splint.

The splint and sutures were removed 2 weeks postoperatively. The flap healed; however, there was partial necrosis at the margin of the skin graft. The graft on the Achilles tendon survived, and healing progressed without incident.

I have achieved a satisfactory result in another similar case, which was treated by the same technique (Fig. 29-2).

Part IX

Long bone transplantation in children

Chapter 30

Vascularized free transplants of the fibula in children

Alain L. Gilbert

The introduction of vascularized bone grafts has solved some difficulties associated with the loss of bone substance following surgery or trauma. Most recent publications deal with revascularized bone grafts for the replacement of long bone segments in adults. The fibula is the most frequent donor site, with iliac crest reserved for loss of both skin and bone.

In the child the problems are different in that conventional techniques are usually successful in dealing with bone loss after trauma or infection. Tumors, dystrophies, and formidable problems of congenital pseudarthrosis constitute the major indications for vascularized bone grafts in children. These indications are not rare, since in a personal series of 162 fibular bone grafts 41 were carried out in children.

ANATOMIC BASIS

Vascularization of the fibula has been studied by injections and dissections.[7]

The fibular diaphysis has a double vascular network—nutrient and periosteal. This double network arises from the peroneal artery, a branch of the tibioperoneal trunk. This artery invariably descends the length of the posteromedial border of the bone. It provides the musculoperiosteal and periosteal branches that ramify and anastomose at the periosteal surface. Two or three of these voluminous branches pass between the peroneus and soleus muscles to the skin of the leg. The existence of the direct periosteal branches allows preservation of the periosteal blood supply without the need for a muscular sleeve around the donor fibula.

The nutrient artery may arise directly from the peroneal artery or from a musculoperiosteal branch. The artery penetrates the middle third of the diaphysis, with a variation of 2.5 cm on either side. Inside the diaphysis the nutrient artery divides into a short ascending branch and a long descending branch. This anatomic pattern is a consistent one and the peroneal artery is reliable in its morphologic organization.

As with all epiphyses, the upper end of the fibula has a double vascularization—metaphyseal and epiphyseal. The metaphyseal vascularization arises from the peroneal artery; the epiphyseal vascularization arises from the descending branches of the inferior genicular artery and from ascending branches of the "artery of the neck" of the fibula, a branch of the anterior tibial artery. These two networks have rich anastomoses, and one alone would be sufficient to provide an epiphyseal blood supply.

OPERATING TECHNIQUE
Taking the fibular diaphysis

Several approaches to the fibular diaphysis have been described. Taylor[9] uses a posterior approach with the patient in a prone position; other surgeons place the patient on his back with the lower limbs internally rotated.[8] These approaches have in common an extensive, time-consuming dissection, taking the fibula with a substantial muscular sleeve to protect the periosteal vascular network.

The route of approach described here, which I have been using since 1976,[3] rests on two principles: (1) primary approach of the bone, and (2) taking the osteoperiosteum without a muscular sleeve, the vascular supply being essentially assured by the nutrient network.

Positioning. The graft can be taken with the patient in a prone, lateral, or supine position. We prefer a supine position, thigh and leg flexed, with the foot resting on the table. A slight internal rotation of the hip is helpful. A pneumatic tourniquet is used.

Approach. A midlateral approach is used, centered on the fibula. The positions of the two fibular epiphyses are marked on the skin. The midpoint of the diaphysis is also marked. The graft is then diagrammed on the skin, centered on the midpoint of the diaphysis, and the length measured. Accurate positioning helps avoid injury to the nutrient artery. The skin incision is made directly over the palpable fibular shaft, extending it 3 cm beyond each end of the diagram of the bone graft.

Once the aponeurosis is incised, the peroneal muscles appear. Dissection proceeds behind the peroneus longus muscle and in front of the soleus muscle. Separation of these two muscles brings the bone directly into view. The peroneal muscles are then retracted forward and detached from the bone, avoiding injury to the periosteum. The soleus is detached also, and care is taken to preserve the two or three pedicles that run on its surface. These pedicles arise from the peroneal artery and supply the lateral skin of the leg. If these vascular pedicles are preserved, it is possible to include a flap of skin with the fibula, since they are direct branches from the peroneal artery.

Anteriorly, dissection of the intermuscular septum exposes the anterior compartment of the leg. The extensor hallucis longus and extensor digitorum longus are detached, and dissection then proceeds to the interosseous membrane. The anterior tibial neurovascular bundle is carefully protected.

Posteriorly, the flexor hallucis longus is carefully detached from the bone and the peroneal vessels are seen for the first time. The interosseous membrane is incised close to the fibula along its entire length. The only remaining attachment is the tibialis posterior and its pedicle.

Taking the graft. Before proceeding the surgeon must know the exact length required for the graft. The length is marked out on the bone, and the periosteum is incised 2 cm beyond the upper and lower marks with a curved blade. In a child the periosteum has great osteogenic potential, and an extra sleeve is taken with the bone graft to potentiate healing. The periosteum is then incised cir-

cumferentially, and then the 2 cm sleeves are elevated above and below.

The bone is cut on the marks with a Gigli saw, and care is taken not to injure the vascular pedicle. Once the bone has been cut, it is grasped with a bone holder and retracted outward. At the level of the distal cut the peroneal pedicle is ligated and divided. The lower end of the graft is then lifted out of the wound. Under direct vision, the tibialis posterior muscle is detached from the bone, the intermuscular fascia is sectioned, the pedicle is dissected from below upward, and one comes promptly to the peroneotibial bifurcation. The graft is then totally free except for its peroneal pedicle. The tourniquet is released to obtain hemostasis and to verify the circulation of the graft. Abundant bright red bleeding must come from the medulla to confirm that the nutrient network is intact. The graft is left in situ while the recipient site is prepared. The pedicle is transected at the last moment.

Taking the proximal epiphysis

Positioning. The patient is supine, with flexion of the hip and knee and with internal rotation of the hip.

Incision. The incision follows the bony prominence of the fibula as far as the popliteal skin crease.

Dissection. The epiphysis is situated immediately under the skin. The difficult part of the dissection is freeing the head of the fibula from its muscular and ligamentous attachments (lateral collateral ligament of the knee and tibiofibular ligaments) without damaging the vascular supply. Dissection must be meticulous and orderly. It is essential to bear in mind the presence of the lateral popliteal nerve, which is in a vulnerable position.

Two pedicles must be identified and protected. Again, they will only be seen when the epiphysis is completely detached: (1) the peroneal pedicle with its ascending branch, and (2) the anterior tibial pedicle and the artery of the neck of the fibula.

It will not be necessary to sacrifice the anterior tibial pedicle; it will suffice to take only an 8 to 10 mm segment of the anterior tibial vessels that includes the epiphyseal arteries.

The anterior tibial artery is repaired, either by direct suturing or with a graft (Fig. 30-3). The vein can be divided at the tibioperoneal bifurcation; repair is unnecessary. The segment of the anterior tibial artery is then anastomosed to the proximal end of the peroneal artery; thus only one arterial anastomosis will be needed at the recipient site. Once the graft has been taken, the lateral collateral ligament must be reconstructed.

APPLICATIONS TO ORTHOPEDIC PEDIATRIC SURGERY

We have never had to use this method for post-traumatic loss of bone substance; classic methods have been satisfactory in children. Our major indications are for treatment of tumors, dystrophies, and, in particular, congenital pseudarthrosis.

CONGENITAL PSEUDARTHROSIS

Congenital pseudarthrosis is one of the most difficult problems facing the orthopedic surgeon. Its cause is unknown, and, though the majority of cases are associated with von Recklinghausen's neurofibromatosis, certain cases are distinct entities.

The problems of treatment are such that in the past the surgeon often had to resort to amputation. Even if healing is obtained by conventional techniques, it is at the price of multiple operations, prolonged hospitalizations, significant shortening of the limb, and major trophic problems.*

Since 1976 I have operated on thirty-one patients with congenital pseudarthrosis (Figs. 30-1 and 30-2). In one case the homolateral fibula was used; in all the other cases the contralateral fibula was used for the graft. In twenty-eight cases the leg was affected, and in three the forearm was the site of the pseudarthrosis.

The youngest of these patients was 7 months old; the oldest was 13 years old. At first this method was used only in older children who had undergone multiple operations and for whom amputation was being considered. The initial results were encouraging; we have progressively used the procedure in younger and younger children, until now it is the procedure of choice and is carried out as soon as the diagnosis is made.

A recently diagnosed pseudarthrosis without extensive bony destruction and without significant shortening presents a different problem from an old pseudarthrosis with a great deal of shortening. In the first situation the operation consists of complete resection of the affected area, including the periosteum, and its replacement with a graft from the contralateral fibula. In the second situation it is important to achieve equalization of the legs before healing takes place, because attempts at secondary lengthening of this area pose formidable

*References 1, 2, 4, 5, 6, 10.

problems. Lengthening is carried out with a Wagner apparatus, which is applied for 3 to 4 weeks. The fibular graft is done in a second stage.

The peroneal artery is sutured at each of its extremities to the recipient anterior tibial artery.

Bony fixation presents a major problem. Intramedullary fixation is contraindicated, since injury to the nutrient vessels would result. Fixation by oblique pins, metal wires, or simple plaster is inadequate and presents the risk of nonunion, of which I have seen five cases. The method of choice is as follows: (1) the two fragments of tibia are immobilized with a Wagner external fixation device, and (2) a 1 cm segment of posterior tibial cortex is preserved at each end of the defect. The graft is laid on these cortical ledges and is fixed at each end with a screw. Once the extremities begin to heal (toward the second month), the fixation device is replaced by plaster.

I feel it is important in children under 9 years of age to reconstruct the donor fibula to avoid a progressive valgus deformity of the ankle. A periosteocortical graft taken from the medial surface of the tibia is inserted into the defect, and it heals in about 2 months.

The results must be interpreted conservatively, since primary healing does not necessarily mean a satisfactory final result. Only twenty-six patients have had a follow-up of more than 1 year. All the patients healed in periods varying from 3 to 18 months. Fifteen patients showed primary healing with a delay of 4 to 6 months, the protective support having been removed an average of 1 month postoperatively. In eleven patients there was either a delay in healing or an angulation. This delay has been attributed to inadequate bony fixation or to premature removal of the external fixation device. This complication occasionally appeared early but was most often noted after the second month. In the leg we have reoperated seven times at the superior junction of the graft and twice at the inferior junction, with the addition of cancellous bone grafts and fixation by plate or pinning.

Thus when one compares these results with the more classic techniques[1,4,5,6,10] or with electrical stimulation,[2] the fibular grafts show more consistent healing; no case in this series required amputation. This technique is also applicable to younger children. Healing does not necessarily imply a good final result, because in certain children multiple operations have stiffened the foot and growth is diminished, with shortening of as much as 10 to 15 cm. This is too great a discrepancy to be cor-

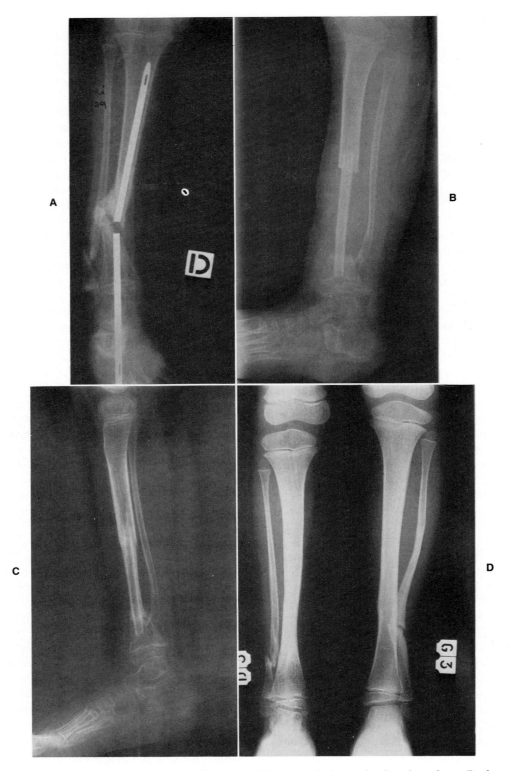

Fig. 30-1. Patient I. **A,** A 4-year-old female with congenital pseudarthrosis and von Recklinghausen's disease. Four previous operations failed. Preoperative view. **B,** The sclerotic bone has been resected and a 12 cm fibular graft transferred. **C,** Appearance at 2 months after surgery. The graft has healed on both sides. Note the thickening of the graft. **D,** One year later; the reconstructed tibia is on the left. There is still a slight length discrepancy to be corrected later. Note on the right the incomplete reconstruction of the fibula.

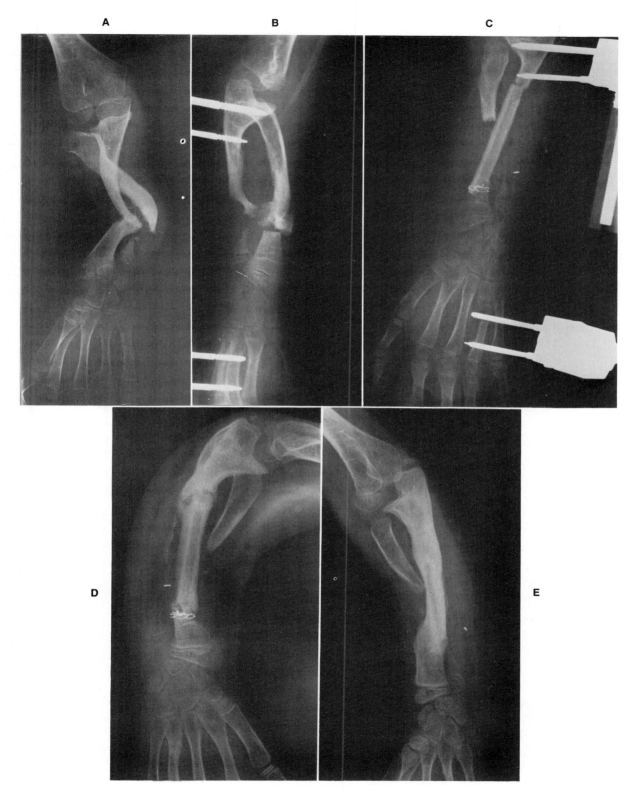

Fig. 30-2. Patient II. **A,** Congenital pseudarthrosis of the forearm in an 11-year-old female with neurofibromatosis, never treated. Preoperative appearance. **B,** Distraction is started with a Wagner lengthening device. **C,** Three weeks later a one-bone forearm is constructed by joining the proximal ulna to the distal radius with a fibular graft. **D,** After 4 months there is proximal union but distal nonunion. A cancellous bone graft is added. **E,** Result at 8 months.

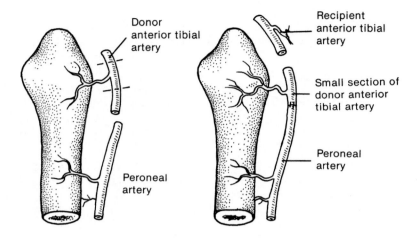

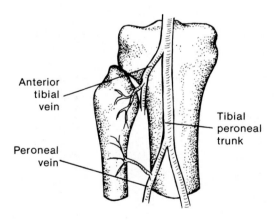

Posterior view
venous system

Fig. 30-3. Use of anterior tibial and peroneal vascular systems for the transfer of the epiphysis.

rected with certainty. It is thus desirable to operate on children at a very early age (before they begin walking) to avoid stiffening and shortening and above all, to allow the child to lead a normal life, free from long stays in the hospital with attendant interruptions of schooling and childhood activities.

TUMORS AND DYSTROPHIES

Defects resulting from the excision of various childhood tumors can be reconstructed with a vascularized fibular graft. These defects can be treated by conventional techniques, but healing is slow and precarious. Advantages of the vascularized fibular graft are the ample amount of bone available and the rapid healing that occurs. Again, fixation of the bones is a major problem.

I have reconstructed nine surgical defects secondary to tumor removal with vascularized fibular grafts, four times after multiple operations for the resection of fibrous dysplasia complicated by several fractures (superior third of femur, diaphysis, humeral), once following complete resection of the tibial diaphysis for a chondrosarcoma in a young child, and four times after excision of a giant cyst of the femur and humerus.

In these cases the loss of substance varied from 12 to 24 cm. In each case healing occurred within 4 months. Each of the two reconstructed femurs was supported by a large screw plate, and neither fibular graft showed appreciable thickening. One of them fractured a year after walking was resumed; it healed completely after the broken plate was replaced. It seems that special measures are necessary to encourage thickening of the fibular graft.

DISCUSSION

In general, reconstruction of major losses of bony substance in the child poses few problems. Often after osteomyelitis the periosteum persists and offers an excellent bed for a conventional graft. A vascularized graft may be indicated for extensive loss of substance (greater than 10 cm) following resection of a tumor, since it permits more rapid healing and a more physiologic reconstruction than a prosthetic diaphysis. The most interesting indication in the child is congenital pseudarthrosis, which as yet poses some unresolved therapeutic problems. A vascularized graft is doubly advantageous, because it allows rapid and early healing and negates the need for multiple operations, which are sources of stiffening and shortening. However, problems remain to be resolved that are either technical (bony fixation) or related to the unknown long-term outcome of these grafts and to the possibility of recurrence of the disease.

REFERENCES

1. Andersen, K.S.: Operative treatment of congenital pseudarthrosis of the tibia, Acta Orthop. Scand. **45:** 935, 1974.
2. Bassett, C.A., Caulo, N., and Kort, J.: Congenital pseudarthrosis of the tibia: treatment with pulsing electromagnetic fields, Clin. Orthop. **154:**136, 1981.
3. Gilbert, A.: Vascularized transfer of the fibular shaft, Int. J. Microsurg. **1:**100, 1979.
4. Morrissy, R.T., Roseborough, E.J., and Hall, J.E.: Congenital pseudarthrosis of the tibia, J. Bone Joint Surg. **63:**367, 1981.
5. Nove, J.: Pseudarthrose congenitale de jambe, Lyon Med. **3:**920, 1908.
6. Reichel, P.: Zur behandhing schwerer formen von pseudarthrosis, Arch. F. Klin. Chir. **71:**639, 1903.
7. Restrepo, J., Katz, D., and Gilbert, A.: Arterial vascularization of the proximal epiphysis and the diaphysis of the fibula, Int. J. Microsurg. **2:**48, 1980.
8. Tamai, S., et al.: Vascularized fibular transfer, Int. J. Microsurg. **2:**205, 1980.
9. Taylor, G., Miller, G., and Ham, F.: The free vascularized bone graft, Plast. Reconstr. Surg. **55:**533, 1975.
10. Van Nes, C.P.: Congenital pseudarthrosis of the leg, J. Bone Joint Surg. **48:**1467, 1966.

Chapter 31

Vascularized fibula transplantation: congenital pseudarthrosis and radial club hand

Susumu Tamai

In his orthopedic textbook Salter states: "Congenital pseudarthrosis of the tibia is the most difficult type of non-union confronting the orthopedic surgeon and requires special techniques of bone grafting for its correction."[3] In cases of congenital pseudarthrosis of the tibia, the defects or non-unions generally failed to unite after several conventional bone grafts or refractured postoperatively. The tibia itself often became sclerotic with an obstructed medullary canal and the surrounding soft tissues were often scarred as a result of several previous surgeries. In such conditions it is reasonable to use a living bone graft—in other words, a vascularized bone graft using the fibula as a final salvage operation.[1,2,4,5,6] Primary revascularized fibular grafts are now being used with increased frequency.

Congenital radial club hand is also a difficult condition to treat and to obtain anatomic restoration of both forearm bones. Growth of a grafted bone is problematic in the small child, and the vascularized fibula graft, with its proximal epiphysis, shows the greatest promise for anatomic reconstruction of the club hand. The major problem is that the smaller the child, the more difficult is isolation of the proximal fibula with its epiphyseal vessels.

From October 1976 to May 1981, we carried out seventeen vascularized fibula transplantations for the treatment of nonunion or massive bone defects in long bones. Among these patients were four children with congenital pseudarthrosis of the tibia. In two out of four the vascularized fibular graft was composed of bone that had regenerated after subperiosteal harvesting of a previous fibular

graft. Satisfactory bony union was obtained in all cases, with follow-up periods of 9 months to 3 years.

A child with radial club hand resulting from partial absence of the right radius received a free fibular transplantation in January 1980. Although the final outcome of the graft is still unknown because of the short time since the procedure, the operative technique and several problems encountered postoperatively will be described.

SURGICAL TECHNIQUES

As a rule a two-team approach is used to shorten the operating time.

Obtaining the fibular graft

An incision is made over the posterolateral margin of the fibula, and the superficial fascia is cut longitudinally between the soleus and the peroneus longus muscles. A plane is developed through the muscle tissue surrounding the fibula, leaving a 5 mm sleeve of muscle with the bone and carrying the dissection down to the interosseus membrane (Fig. 31-1, *arrow*). The peroneus brevis, extensor digitorum longus, and extensor hallucis longus muscles are thus freed from the anterolateral margin of the fibula extraperiosteally. Then the dissection is carried down to the flexor hallucis longus muscle, continuing until the peroneal vascular bundle comes into view medially. The 5 to 10 mm sleeve of muscle protects the nutrient and periosteal vessels from damage. At this point the fibula is sectioned according to measurement with an electric bone saw. The peroneal vascular bundle is ligated distally and cut (Fig. 31-2, *A*). Outward

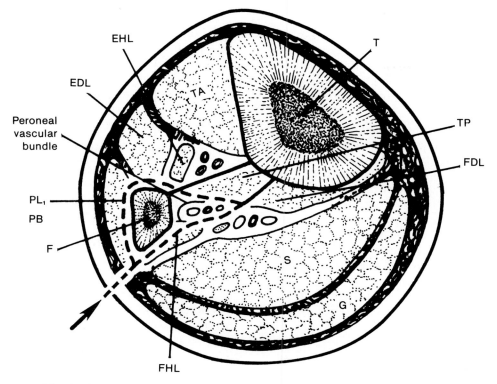

Fig. 31-1. Schematic drawing showing our surgical approach to the fibula.

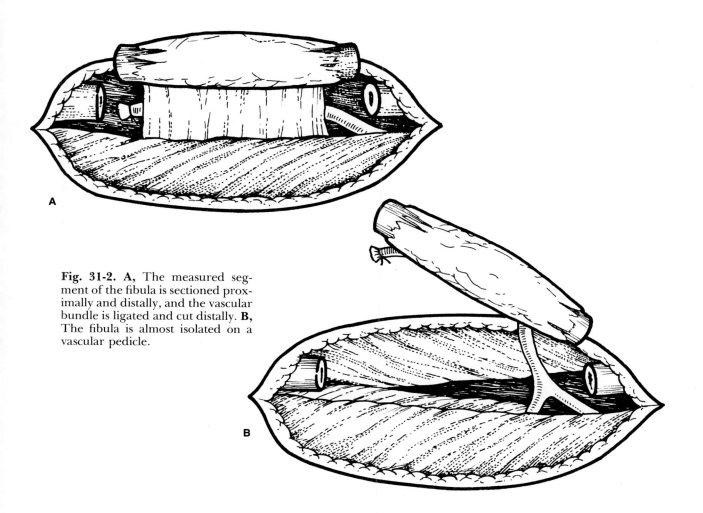

Fig. 31-2. A, The measured segment of the fibula is sectioned proximally and distally, and the vascular bundle is ligated and cut distally. **B,** The fibula is almost isolated on a vascular pedicle.

traction is placed on the distal end of the fibula, and it is detached from the interosseous membrane and the tibialis posterior muscle as the dissection is carried proximally. The origin of the peroneal vascular bundle is then identified further proximally; the fibular segment is now almost isolated on the vascular pedicle (Fig. 31-2, *B*). When the tourniquet is deflated, satisfactory bleeding from the cut end of the fibula or muscle sleeve must be seen. The graft is kept wet with warm saline-soaked gauze until the recipient site is ready for grafting.

When dissecting out the fibula with its proximal epiphysis, the skin incision is extended proximally up to the popliteal fossa, and the lateral head of the gastrocnemius muscle is elevated medially and laterally. The popliteal vessels, with the lateral inferior genicular artery and its concomitant vein, are known as the nutrient vessels to the proximal fibular epiphysis; they are exposed carefully. The origin of the soleus muscle on the fibula is transsected, leaving as large a sleeve of muscle as possible. The fibular collateral ligament is cut at its distal insertion from the fibula, and the tibiofibular articulation is separated, taking care not to damage the blood vessels that supply the head. The peroneal vascular system is left attached to the fibular shaft, as noted previously.

Preparation of the recipient site

In congenital pseudarthrosis of the tibia, the involved tibia is exposed extraperiosteally by making a longitudinal incision on the anterior aspect of the leg. Depending on the preoperative angiogram, the anterior tibial artery or the posterior tibial artery and its concomitant veins are carefully exposed and isolated as the recipient vessels. The tibia is cut above and below the area of the pseudarthrosis with an electric bone saw, and the pseudarthrosis is removed with the surrounding scar tissue.

In radial club hand a zigzag incision is made on the radial aspect of the forearm, and any fibrous bands or remnants are carefully removed from the distal forearm. The radial artery may be absent; in such an event, either the anterior or the posterior interosseus artery can be isolated as the recipient artery. Recipient veins are easily found.

Complete isolation of the donor fibula

The peroneal vascular bundle is ligated at its origin, freeing the fibular segment for transplantation. In grafts of the proximal fibula the lateral inferior genicular artery and the concomitant vein are also ligated and cut.

Transplantation

Fixation of the bone is performed first. The surgeon may choose among several fixation methods. In tibial defects we prefer to insert the ends of the fibula into the medullary canal (Fig. 31-3, *B* and *C*). However, if there is a discrepancy in size, one end of the fibula may be fixed to the tibia in a side-to-side fashion. The application of an extraskeletal fixation device is also useful in some cases.

Under an operating microscope the peroneal artery of the donor fibula is anastomosed to the recipient artery end to end and then two concomitant veins are anastomosed in the same fashion, using 9-0 monofilament nylon sutures. After the completion of the vascular anastomoses, the air tourniquet is deflated and the circulation is restored. It is essential to see satisfactory bleeding from the tissues surrounding the grafted fibula.

In transplanting the proximal epiphysis of the fibula in a small child with a radial club hand, one encounters problems resulting from congenital abnormalities of the radial artery and from the small size of the lateral inferior genicular artery and its concomitant vein. It may be difficult to obtain an accurate anatomic position of the grafted fibular head in the wrist joint because of the size and shape of the head of the fibula. The details of the operation will be described in the case report.

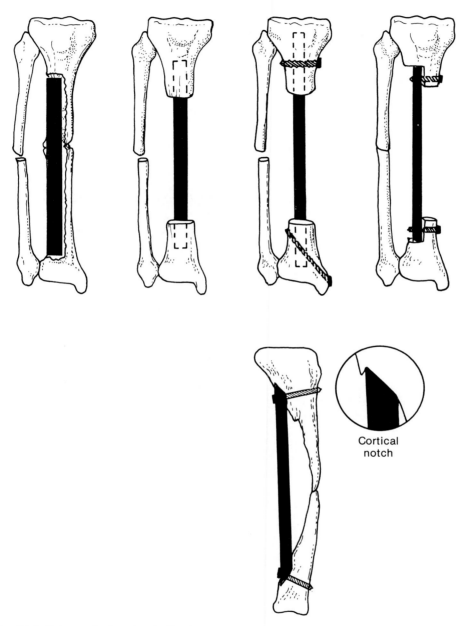

Cortical
notch

Fig. 31-3. Schematic drawing indicating several modes of bone fixation when the vascularized fibula is grafted to the tibia.

CASE REPORT
Patient I

An 8-year-old female had been treated in our hospital since the age of 1 year for congenital pseudarthrosis of her left tibia (caused by von Recklinghausen's disease). Despite seven conventional bone grafting procedures in 8 years, pseudarthrosis remained with resultant shortening and anterior bowing of the leg. A vascularized fibular graft taken from the right leg was performed, using a type of bypass bone grafting. Bony union was noted on the radiograph at 1 month and union was completed at 5 months postoperatively. The grafted bone became more hypertrophic month by month, and after 20 months the space between the original tibia shaft and the grafted fibula was almost fully occupied with new bone. A corrective osteotomy at the supramalleolar level was done at 2 years, and perfect union was obtained. Three years postoperatively she can walk without a non-weight-bearing brace and crutch (Fig. 31-4, *A* and *B*).

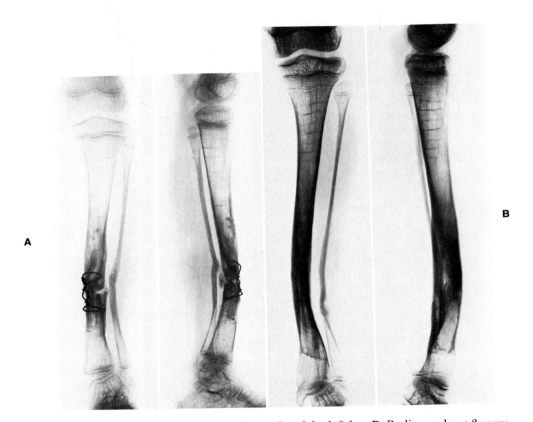

Fig. 31-4. Patient I. **A,** Preoperative radiographs of the left leg. **B,** Radiographs at 3 years demonstrate perfect union of the grafted fibula, with significant hypertrophy. The deformity was corrected with a supramalleolar osteotomy at 2 years, and it united well.

Patient II

A 14-year-old male with congenital pseudarthrosis of his left tibia had undergone five previous operations, all of which were unsuccessful, including an autogenous fibular shaft graft several years before. The fibula had been resected subperiosteally, and regenerated bone subsequently filled the remaining periosteal sheath. As a final procedure we used the regenerated fibula as a vascularized bone graft. The preoperative angiogram revealed an intact peroneal artery. The regenerated fibula seemed to receive its periosteal blood supply only from the peroneal artery, but during the operation, when the fibula was revascularized following vascular anastomoses, sufficient bleeding from the periosteal sleeve and the medullary canal was noted. We used the same technique as for patient I (bypass bone grafting). Bony union, however, was delayed, taking approximately 1 year. Even at 2 years 6 months postoperatively, the space between the graft and the recipient tibia is still open, without hypertrophy of the graft (Fig. 31-5).

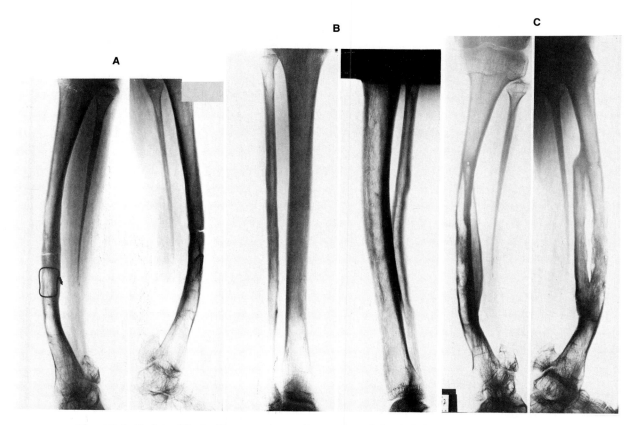

Fig. 31-5. Patient II. **A,** Preoperative radiographs of the left leg. **B,** The right fibula regenerated subperiosteally after being previously resected for a graft. **C,** Radiographs at 2 years, 6 months reveal perfect union at both ends of the bypassed graft, but no hypertrophy is seen.

Patient III

A 14-year-old female was treated in our hospital for congenital pseudarthrosis of her right tibia. She had also undergone four bone grafting procedures since the age of 3, but bony union had not been achieved. In this case, as with patient II, the contralateral fibula had been used as a donor bone several years before. The radiograph of her right leg showed the typical findings of a congenital pseudarthrosis of the tibia. On the left leg the shape of the regenerated fibula was not entirely normal in appearance. At surgery the distal end of the graft was fitted into the medullary cavity of the distal tibia. The cortex of the proximal end of the tibia was partially resected, and the proximal end of the fibula was fixed with a screw in a side-to-side fashion. Nine months after grafting, bony union at the proximal end and enlargement of the graft had still not been obtained. An additional iliac bone graft fixed at the proximal end with Kirschner wires led to successful union at 1 year (Fig. 31-6).

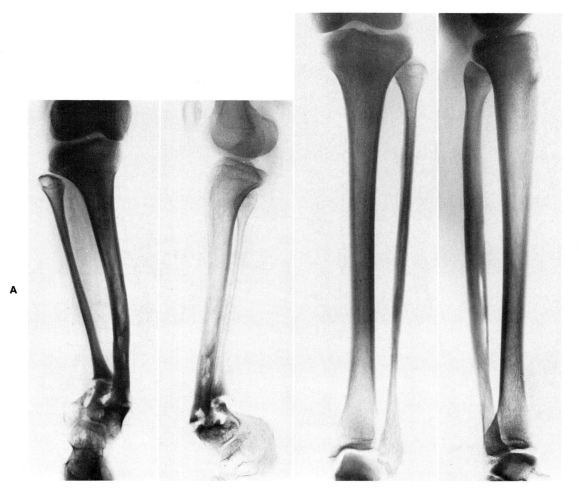

Fig. 31-6. Patient III. **A,** Preoperative radiograph of the right leg. **B,** Regenerated left fibula.

C

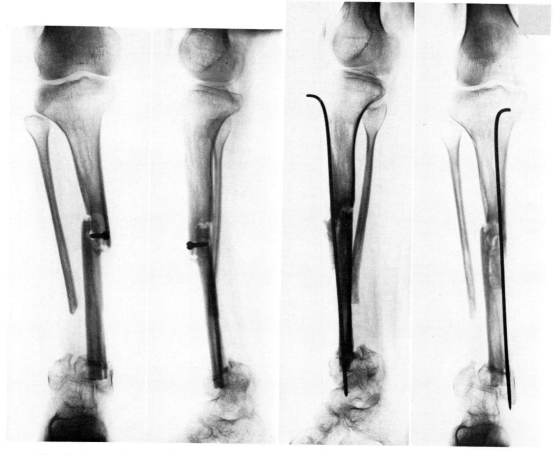

D

Fig. 31-6, cont'd. C, Radiograph at 9 months demonstrates nonunion at the proximal end, with loosening around the screw. **D,** After an additional iliac bone graft and Kirschner wire fixation, union was obtained at 1 year postoperatively.

Patient IV

A 5-year-old female had been treated in a city hospital for congenital pseudarthrosis of the left tibia (caused by von Recklinghausen's disease); four unsuccessful operations had been performed. When she came to our hospital, a typical pseudarthrosis was noted just proximal to the ankle joint. At surgery the diseased segment of the tibia, including the nonunion site, was resected and the contralateral fibula was grafted. At 1 month significant enlargement of the graft was seen. Although the distal end of the graft was well united, bony union at the proximal end was still not present at 7 months. An additional iliac bone graft with Kirschner wire fixation was carried out, and union was almost complete at 9 months. At 1 year perfect bony union and enlargement of the graft had been obtained (Fig. 31-7, *A* and *B*).

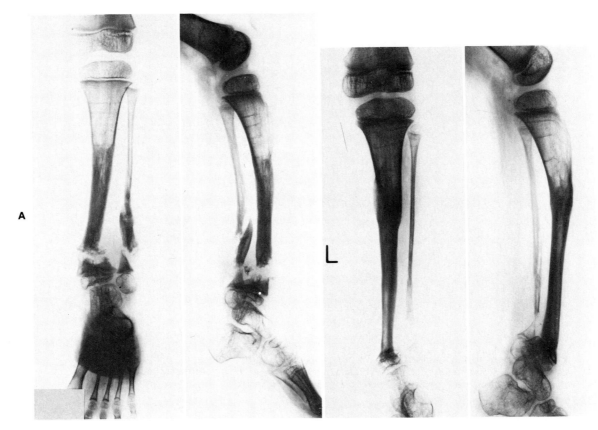

Fig. 31-7. Patient IV. **A,** Preoperative radiograph of the left leg. **B,** Radiograph at 1 year postoperatively demonstrates complete union at both ends, with significant thickening of the graft.

Patient V

A 3-year, 4-month-old male had a congenital radial club hand caused by a partial defect of the right distal radius. There were several associated anomalies in both hands, and the preoperative radiograph revealed an absence of the distal two thirds of the radius in the right forearm (Fig. 31-8, *A* and *B*). On January 24, 1980, the right fibula, including its proximal epiphysis, was transplanted to the right forearm to reconstruct the radial defect. During surgery the right proximal fibula, 7 cm in length, was isolated with the peroneal vascular system and the lateral inferior genicular artery and vein. Fig. 31-8, *C,* shows the fibular head almost isolated on its vascular pedicle. Since the radial artery was absent in the right forearm, the anterior interosseous artery and a subcutaneous vein were used as the recipient vessels. We affixed the proximal fibula to the proximal radius, using a bone peg with its head placed in the wrist joint. Because the fibular head was somewhat larger than a normal distal radius, it was necessary to use a Kirschner wire for fixation between the ulna and the graft. Using a T-shaped vein graft to the anterior interosseous artery (Fig. 31-8, *D*) the peroneal artery and vein anastomoses were performed first. When we released the arterial clamps after completing the anastomosis of the inferior lateral genicular artery, no bleeding was seen from the concomitant vein, but the epiphysis showed a satisfactory ooze of blood from the periosteum. The end of the geniculate artery was then sutured to a subcutaneous vein, making an arteriovenous fistula. After some time the graft gained its normal color along with sufficient oozing, and the wound was closed, followed by placement of a long arm cast for immobilization. One month postoperatively the Kirschner wire was removed and a miniosteotaxis was applied to obtain further correction of the anatomic relationships of the grafted bone and wrist joint. Three months after bony union was completed, the osteotaxis was removed. At 9 months, to obtain further correction of the deformity, shortening and a correction osteotomy of the ulna were carried out. A ligamentous reconstruction of the distal radioulnar joint was performed at the same time. At 1 year and 4 months alignment of the forearm bones looked much better than preoperatively, with an 80 degree range of motion. However, epiphyseal growth cannot be detected as yet, and further follow-up evaluation will be necessary (Fig. 31-8, *E*).

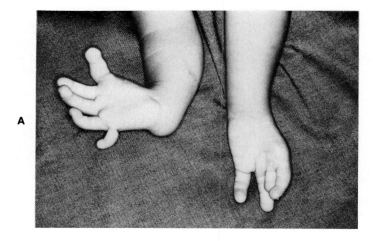

Fig. 31-8. Patient V. **A,** Preoperative appearance of both hands, with multiple anomalies of the digits.

Continued.

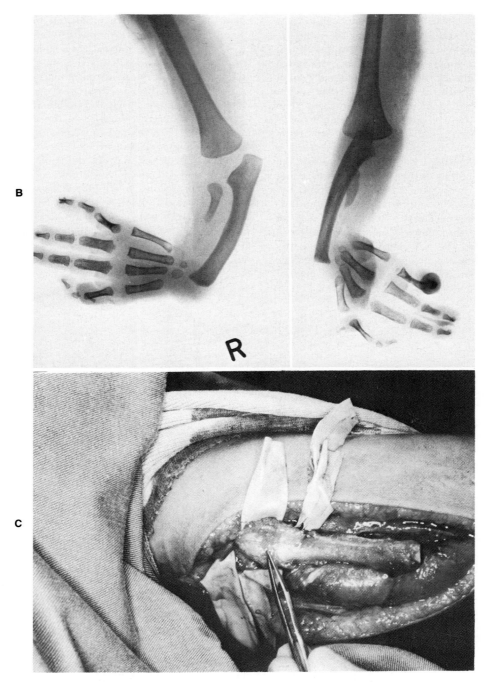

Fig. 31-8, cont'd. B, Preoperative radiographs of the right forearm and hand. **C,** At surgery the fibular head is almost isolated on a vascular pedicle.

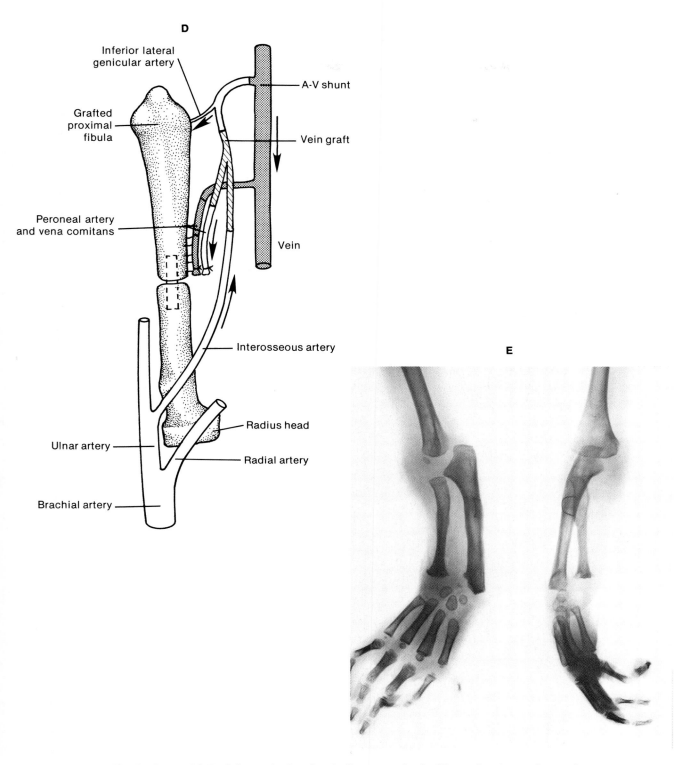

D

Inferior lateral genicular artery

A-V shunt

Grafted proximal fibula

Vein graft

Peroneal artery and vena comitans

Vein

Interosseous artery

Ulnar artery

Radius head

Radial artery

Brachial artery

E

Fig. 31-8, cont'd. D, Schematic drawing indicates method of bone fixation and vascular anastomoses between recipient and donor. **E,** Radiographs at 1 year, 4 months postoperatively. A malalignment at the wrist joint remains, and growth of the grafted proximal fibula is in question.

REFERENCES

1. Chen, Z.W., and Bao, Y.S.: Microsurgery in China, Clin. Plast. Surg. **7:**437, 1980.
2. Gilbert, A.: Vascularized transfer of the fibular shaft, Intern. J. Microsurg. **1:**100, 1979.
3. Salter, R.B.: Textbook of disorders and injuries of the musculoskeletal system, Baltimore, 1970, The Williams & Wilkins Co., p. 95.
4. Tamai, S., et al.: Vascularized fibula transplantation: a report of 8 cases in the treatment of traumatic bony defect or pseudarthrosis of long bones, Intern. J. Microsurg. **2:**205, 1980.
5. Taylor, G., et al.: The free vascularized bone graft, Plast. Reconstr. Surg. **55:**533, 1975.
6. Weiland, A.J., et al.: Free vascularized bone grafts in surgery of the upper extremity, J. Hand Surg. **4:**129, 1979.

Chapter 32

Experimental vascularized growth plate transfers

Kenneth L.B. Brown

Richard L. Cruess

Rollin K. Daniel

Pierre J. Marie

Tadeusz Lyczakowski

The possibility of restoring or providing increased length of a bone through the transplantation of a growing epiphysis has challenged surgeons for over 70 years. The first successful clinical epiphyseal transplant was reported by Straub.[23] He transferred a strip of bone and epiphysis from the normal tibia to the opposite tibia, which had been destroyed by osteomyelitis. Apparently some growth continued, but this was later disputed by Haas,[10] who reviewed the radiographs and found no evidence of growth. Haas attempted an experimental series himself, with little success.

Over the years several other case reports have followed, some successful,[1,25,26] others failures.[7,21] Freeman[8] reviewed epiphyseal transfers and reported a case he had operated on. In eleven cases of epiphyseal transfer reported by Wilson[27] only one patient showed radiographic evidence of longitudinal growth. Rank[17] reviewed six cases of epiphyseal transfer to correct congenital bone deformities. The epiphyses were transplanted as free grafts or in staged composite flaps. Less than half showed continued growth of the transplanted segment on follow-up radiographic examination. Radiographic measurement of growth following epiphyseal transplantation is unreliable, since it is difficult to assess the contribution of the epiphysis at the other end of the bone. In addition, Spira et al.[21,22] have shown that the growth plate may appear open radiologically, even though on histologic examination it is nonfunctional.

There have been several experimental studies of conventional epiphyseal transfers.* One of the best studies using conventional nonvascularized transfers was completed by Harris et al.[11] Only half of the autogenous transfers were successful by their criteria. Of those that survived, up to two thirds of normal growth occurred. It was concluded that the transplant must survive an avascular period before successful incorporation can occur or true longitudinal growth can resume. This avascular period lasts for 7 to 10 days, and during this time the graft is nourished only by tissue fluid. This is insufficient for survival of most cartilage cells, because they must be in close proximity to blood vessels to survive and function properly. This experiment demonstrated the exquisite sensitivity of the growth plate to ischemia and indicates why success in epiphyseal transplantation has been so elusive. From a review of the literature it is evident that nonvascularized epiphyseal transfers generally give variable and usually unsatisfactory results. Even in those cases in which growth reportedly continues, the segment rarely grows normally,

The work discussed in this chapter was sponsored by a grant from the Medical Research Council of Canada.

*References 2, 4, 11, 12, 13, 18, 19.

and at maturity the transplanted segment is usually smaller than the contralateral side.

With the recent use of microsurgery in free tissue transfers, it was only natural that the problem of epiphyseal transplantation would be readdressed. Isolated experimental studies and clinical reports of toe-to-thumb transfer in children have indicated that successful growth can occur following transplantation and microvascular anastomoses of the essential vasculature.*

BLOOD SUPPLY OF THE GROWTH PLATE

A knowledge of the basic anatomy and vasculature of the epiphyseal cartilage plate is necessary to understand why growth plate transplantation has been so difficult. The growth plate is a cartilaginous structure containing four distinct zones: (1) the reserve zone, (2) the zone of proliferation, (3) the zone of hypertrophy, and (4) the zone of calcification. There are three main sources of blood supply to the cartilage growth plate (Fig. 32-1). The epiphyseal vessels (E vessels) provide nourishment for cells in the reserve and proliferative zones. Four fifths of the metaphyseal supply is provided by the nutrient artery and one fifth from the periosteal vessels. The metaphyseal vessels end in closed vascular loops just beneath the growth plate and are crucial to the process of cartilage calcification. This is a key step in the conversion of cartilage to primary bony spongiosa, a process called "enchondral ossification." At the periphery of the plate the perichondral vessels provide the blood supply for the pericondral ossification groove. This area is essential for growth in width of the bone and for metaphyseal remodeling.

EXPERIMENTAL MODEL

Experimental studies have shown that occlusion of the epiphyseal vessels leads to rapid death of the whole physis and early closure.[3,21,24] Capillaries from the metaphyseal side invade the devitalized area, leading to bony bridging within 10 days of the vascular interruption. Destruction of the metaphyseal vessels causes a rapid cellular proliferation, leading to a greatly increased width of the growth plate. After a week the number of cells in the hypertrophic zone increases from the normal 10 to 16 cells to 60 to 90 cells. Eventually a fatigue fracture occurs, leading to vascular invasion and calcification.

*References 5, 6, 7, 9, 14, 15, 16, 20, 28, 29.

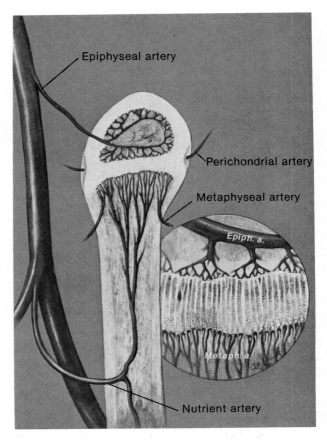

Fig. 32-1. Anatomy and blood supply of the proximal fibula. The nutrient artery is derived from the peroneal artery, which is a branch of the posterior tibial artery. The main epiphyseal supply is from the lateral inferior geniculate artery. Both blood supplies are preserved with the popliteal vascular pedicle.

We recently completed an experimental study of free vascularized growth plate transfers in dogs. Detailed anatomic studies, using plastic and latex injections, and barium microangiography showed that the dog's fibula is a suitable model, since its vascular anatomy is similar to humans. Other advantages are that its nutrient vessels are of sufficient size to ensure a high patency rate, and it bears relatively little weight. In the dog the main nutrient artery supply to the fibula is a branch of the peroneal artery that comes off the posterior tibial artery. The nutrient artery enters the fibula in its middle third. The main epiphyseal supply is from the lateral inferior genicular artery. To preserve all of the blood supplies while requiring only one arterial and venous anastomosis, the fibula and its proximal epiphysis were transferred using the popliteal vessels as the vascular pedicle. The size of these vessels ranged from 1.0 to 2.3 mm, the aver-

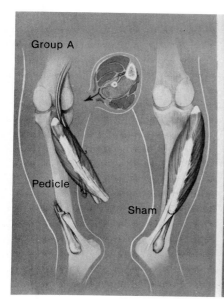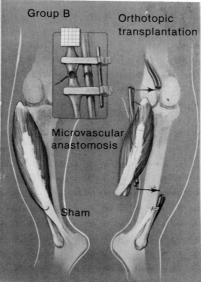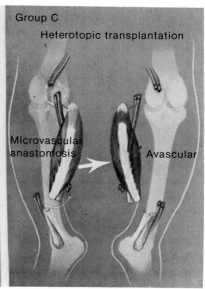

Fig. 32-2. In group A the proximal fibula and surrounding muscles are isolated on the popliteal artery as a pedicle. Insert shows the plane of dissection. In group B the vessels are transected, the transplant is replaced in its bed, and microvascular anastomoses performed. In both these groups a sham operation is performed on the opposite limb. In group C two complete dissections are done, the fibulas are switched to the opposite legs, and microvascular anastomoses are performed on one side only. The other transplant remains avascular.

age being 1.8 mm in diameter. The entire trifurcation was removed distally with the fibula, its surrounding muscle cuff, and a periosteal strip from the tibia.

Our study population of forty-eight dogs of different ages and breeds was divided into three groups. In each dog one limb was used as an internal control. In group A (Fig. 32-2, *A*) the fibula and its surrounding muscular envelope was completely removed from its bed as described, but the transplant remained attached by its popliteal vessels. A sham operation was performed on the opposite limb. We felt this would be a more valid control, since cutting the bone would stimulate growth, thus making histologic comparisons more accurate. With both legs injured the dog would either avoid weight-bearing entirely or else use both legs for ambulation. The purpose of this group was to show that the essential blood supply for survival and function of the growth plate was preserved by our chosen pedicle.

In group B (Fig. 32-2, *B*) the same operating procedure was carried out, except that the popliteal artery and vein were transected and the transplant was removed. It was then replaced in its bed, and microvascular anastomoses were performed. The average ischemic time was 48 minutes. By

comparing the monthly growth to the sham control fibula, we were able to determine how closely the growth approximated normal.

In group C (Fig. 32-2, *C*) both fibulas were removed in an identical manner. They were then transferred to the opposite limbs, but only one side had anastomoses performed. The other transplant was left avascular. The anterior tibial artery was reanastomosed distally, as well as the popliteal vessels. The ischemic time in this group averaged 1 hour and 20 minutes. In all limbs the fibula was fused to the distal tibia with a plate or screws. By doing this any possible contribution to longitudinal growth from the distal fibular epiphysis was eliminated, and the radiopaque screws served as useful markers for measurement of growth radiographically.

The forty-eight dogs were sacrificed at 1, 2, 4, 8, 12, 16, and 26 weeks postoperatively. Multiple methods of assessment were used to be certain that the growth plate was alive and functioning. Radiographs were used to measure monthly growth of the transplants. A standard technique was used, and the monthly increase in growth was measured from the physis proximally to the internal fixation device distally. The two sides were then compared. We tried to use bone scans to monitor vascularity

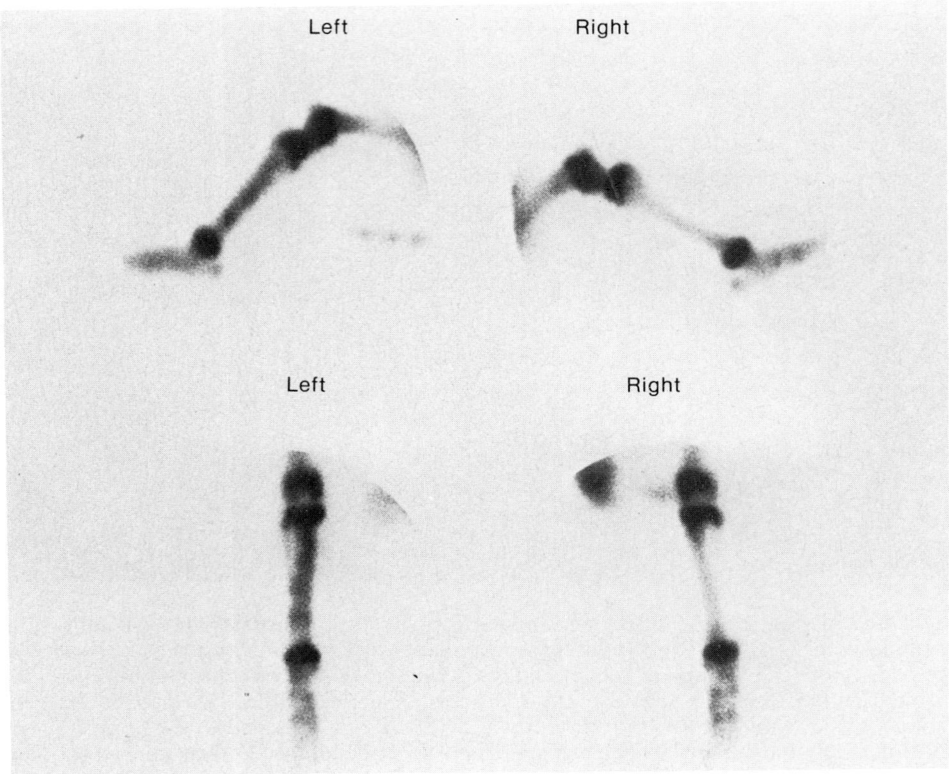

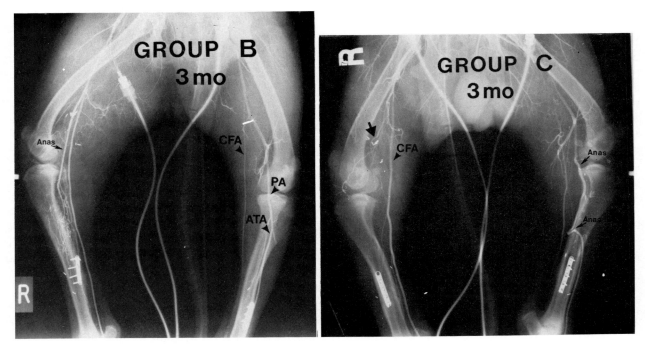

Fig. 32-3. The bone scans are difficult to interpret because the adjacent physes are so hot and the fibula is much smaller than the adjacent tibia. On the left is the vascularized graft; on the right is the sham operated control.

Fig. 32-4. A and **B,** Angiograms showing patent anastomoses at 3 months. In group C the anterior tibial vessels have been reanastomosed as well as the popliteal vessels. (*Anas* = anastomoses; *CFA* = caudal femoral artery; *PA* = popliteal artery; *ATA* = anterior tibial artery.)

postoperatively but found them to be impossible to interpret (Fig. 32-3). The much larger tibia blocked out the uptake in the fibula. This occurred even when a pinhole collumator was used. Angiograms were used to study the effects of surgery on vascularity in the dogs' hindlimbs. Fig. 32-4, *A*, shows a group B dog in which the left leg is the control limb with a normal canine vascular tree. The right leg has an abundant collateral circulation that has developed because the popliteal vessels were transected. In the group C dog (Fig. 32-4, *B*) the left leg contains the vascular anastomoses and is identical to the vascularized right leg in the group B dog. The right limb contains a nonvascularized free fibula transplant, and the caudal femoral vessels have hypertrophied to preserve viability of the limb following ligation of the popliteal vessels.

Before the dogs were sacrificed, two doses of tetracycline were given several days apart to label new bone formation. Only living bone is capable of becoming dual labeled. At sacrifice the limbs were explored to find the anastomoses and check for patency. To determine viability of the growth plates more precisely, autoradiographs were prepared. This is the most accurate method of demonstrating cartilage viability, since the cells must be alive to take up the radioactive material. H^3 proline is utilized by the cartilage cells for protein synthesis and matrix production. The tritiated thymidine is incorporated into DNA just before mitotic division so that only actively dividing cells are labeled.

RESULTS

We found no differences between the pedicled (group A) and the orthotopically transplanted fibulas (group B). One week after transplantation the gross appearance of the sham and orthotopically transplanted fibulas were similar except for changes in the muscle cuff. During the first week, safranin O and proline stains are a little less dense on the side with the vascular anastomoses, but by 2 weeks both sides become indistinguishable (Figs. 32-5 and 32-6). The identical morphologic appearance is preserved throughout all of the study intervals. During the 6 months of growth, the fibulas with the vascular anastomoses grew an average of 37 mm, while the sham operated control fibulas grew an average of 40 mm (Fig. 32-7). Grossly, there is little to distinguish the two sides other than the remodeling that has occurred in the epiphysis on the transplanted side (Fig. 32-8). Histologically the two sides are very similar (Fig. 32-9). For group B dogs as a whole the average monthly

growth measured on the orthotopically transplanted side was 6 ± 3 mm. This growth rate was significantly different (P<0.01) from the average monthly growth on the control sham operated limb which was 7 ± 3 mm. This difference was not surprising, considering the magnitude of the surgical operation. The wide range in monthly growth resulted from variable growth potentials in dogs of different ages and breeds.

In group C animals there was never any growth measured in the avascular control fibula. Although there was no difference in growth rate of the free vascularized epiphyseal transplants in groups B and C, the surgical procedures were a little different. In group C the anterior tibial vessels were reanastomosed distally as well as the popliteal vessels, while in group B the transplanted fibula received all of the blood flow from the popliteal artery without any distal runoff into the anterior tibial system. Radiologic study showed evidence of some resorp-

Text continued on p. 301.

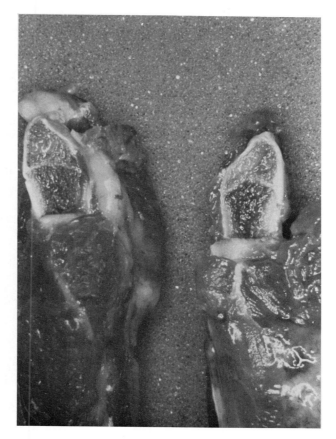

Fig. 32-5. Gross appearance 2 weeks postoperatively shows the vascularized transplant on the right and the sham operated control graft on the left.

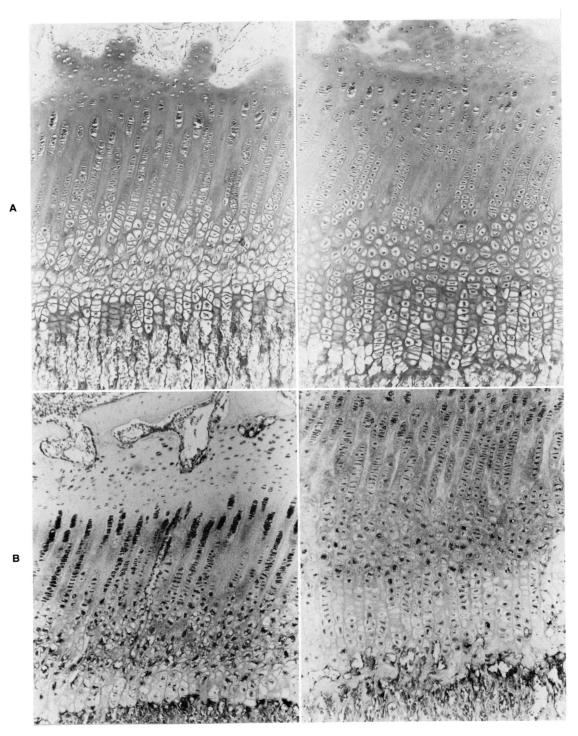

Fig. 32-6. Histologic appearance of the epiphyses shown in Fig. 32-5. The photographs on the right are from the free vascularized transplant. **A,** Safranin O stain showing normal morphologic appearance. **B,** Proline autoradiograph demonstrating normal protein synthesis on both sides.

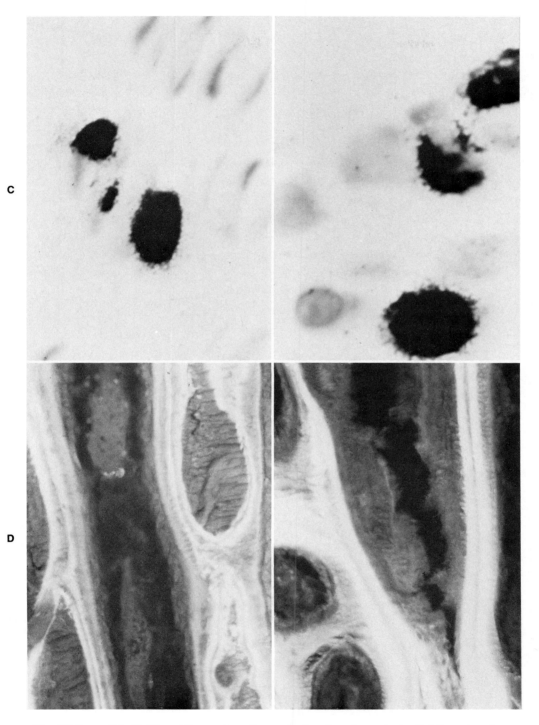

Fig. 32-6, cont'd. C, Thymidine autoradiograph showing the actively dividing chondro-cytes. **D,** Tetracycline labeling of new bone formation in both specimens.

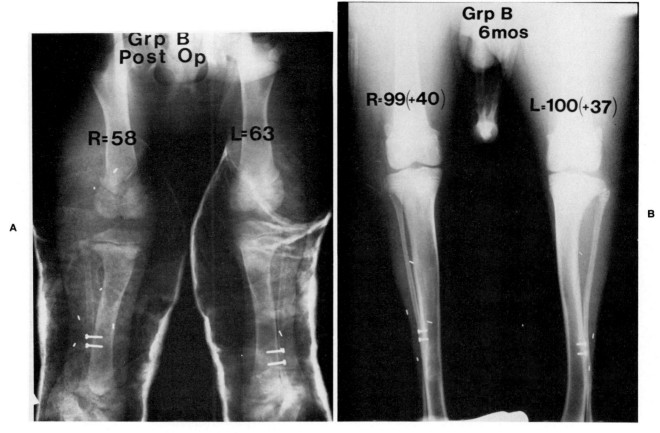

Fig. 32-7. Radiographs from a group B dog. The fibula in the right leg has been transplanted orthotopically. The left leg is the sham operated control. **A,** Immediately after surgery. **B,** After 6 months of growth.

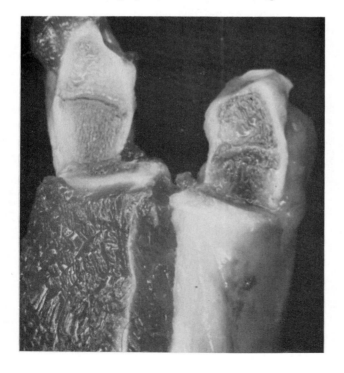

Fig. 32-8. Gross appearance 6 months after transplantation is seen on the right. The growth plate and marrow are similar to the sham operated left side, but there is evidence of remodeling in the vascularized epiphysis.

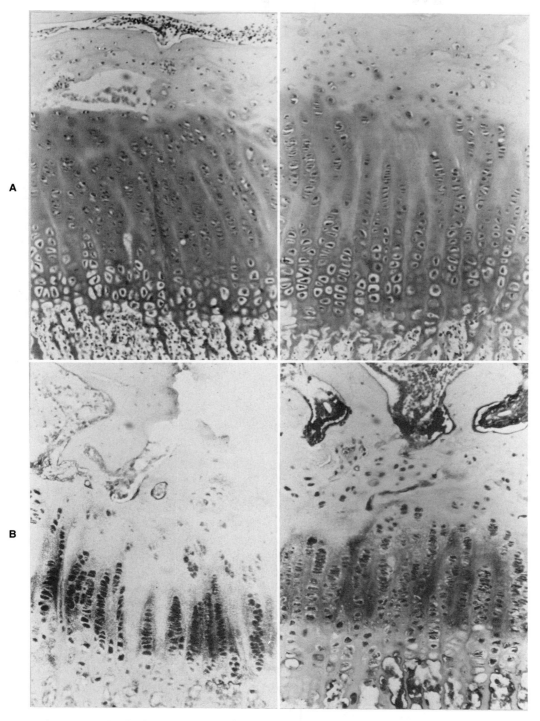

Fig. 32-9. Histologic appearance of specimens seen in Fig. 32-8. The right side is the revascularized fibula, the left is the sham operated control leg. **A,** Safranin O stain. **B,** Proline stain.

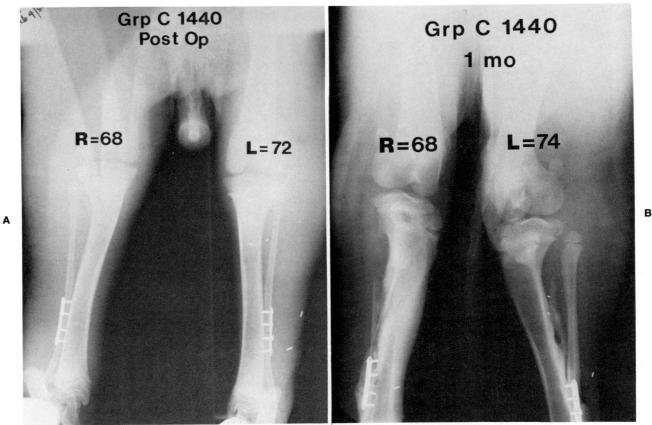

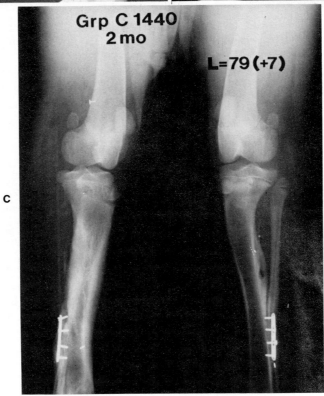

Fig. 32-10. Radiographs showing the resorption that occurs in avascular transplants. **A,** Radiograph immediately after surgery; **B,** one month after surgery; **C,** two months after surgery.

tion in every avascular transplant. In many cases the bone disappeared completely or remained as a small ossicle (Fig. 32-10). The resorption occurred because the thick cuff of avascular muscle prevented early revascularization and the non-weight-bearing function of the transplanted fibula encouraged bony resorption. During the first month the differences between the two sides in group C were most notable on the autoradiographs, since significant resorption had not always occurred on x-ray examination and the differences in standard histologic stains were not always striking (Figs. 32-11 and 32-12). At no interval was there ever any uptake of tritiated proline or thymidine in the avascular physis. By 6 months after transplantation the vascularized growth plates grew an average of 41 mm and appeared normal, whereas the avascular transplants were only represented by a spicule of bone and fibrocartilage (Figs. 32-13 to 32-15).

Only one dog died postoperatively; this occurred 1 month after transplantation and resulted from distemper. He was replaced in our study. We had one anastomosis failure because of venous thrombosis. This occurred in a group B animal who was sacrificed at 1 week. Histologically the findings were identical to group C animals. There were six postoperative infections. All but one occurred in group C animals, and all on the avascular side. Most were low-grade infections that resolved without treatment. The one other infection occurred in the sham-operated control limb of a group B dog. No limbs with microvascular anastomoses became infected. This study shows that long-term survival and useful growth can occur following free vascularized growth plate transplantation.

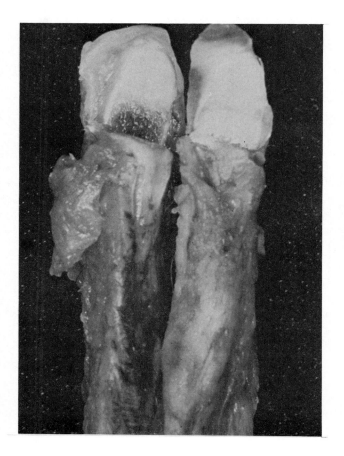

Fig. 32-11. Gross appearance of group C dog at 2 weeks. The marrow in the avascular transplant (right) is dead, while that on the anastomosed side (left) looks viable.

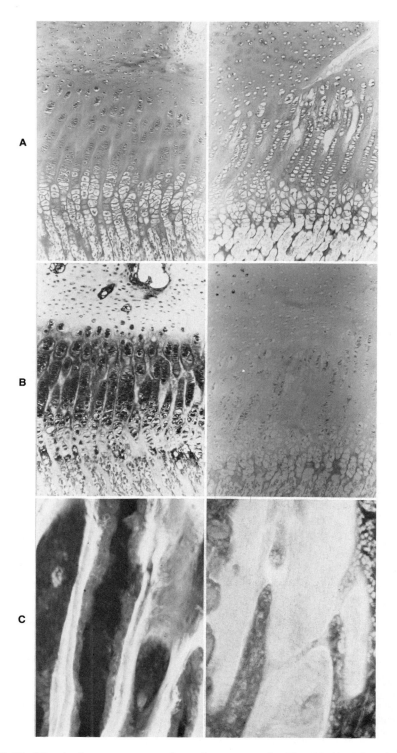

Fig. 32-12. Histologic appearance of specimens seen in Fig. 32-11. The right side is avascular, the left side is from the vascularized fibula. **A,** Safranin O—very pale staining on the right. Most of the lacunae are devoid of cells. **B,** There is no proline uptake on the nonvascularized side. **C,** There has been no tetracycline uptake on the right side.

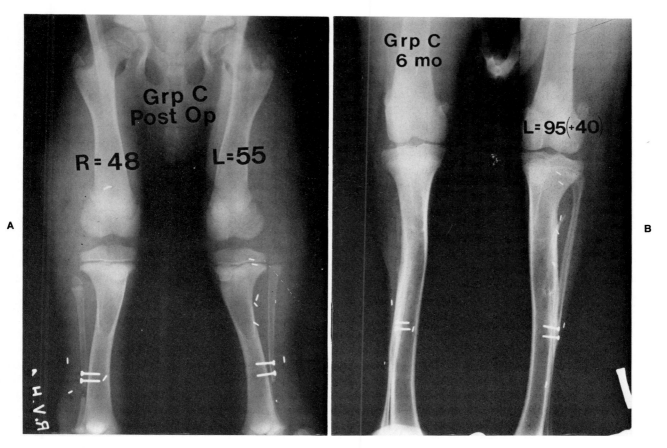

Fig. 32-13. Group C dog at 6 months. **A,** Appearance immediately after surgery. **B,** Amount of growth that has occurred by 6 months. In the right leg with the avascular fibula there has been no growth, and only a thin spicule of bone and fibrocartilage remains.

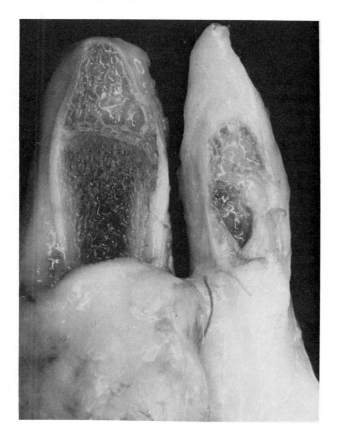

Fig. 32-14. Gross appearance of the fibulas seen in Fig. 32-13. The right specimen is avascular.

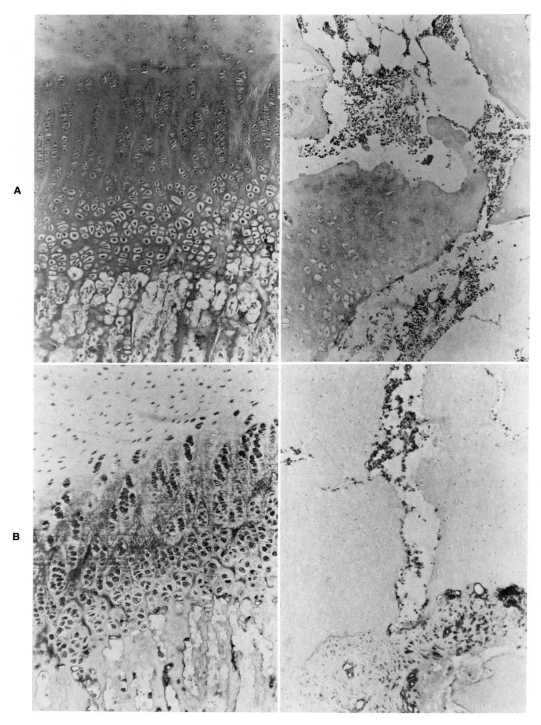

Fig. 32-15. Histologic appearance of transplant seen in Figs. 32-13 and 32-14. **A,** The right side has become revascularized, but there is no evidence of the growth plate structure. **B,** The cartilage seen on the right side is not metabolically active, since there is no proline uptake. Some marrow cells have taken up the proline, indicating their viability.

DISCUSSION

These results cannot be exactly extrapolated for application in children, since there are other problems to be considered. Our model maintained every possible blood supply to the growth plate to obtain near normal growth. This would not be possible in children since the use of such a thick muscle cuff would lead to significant donor site morbidity. We don't know how the transplant would function with a thinner muscle cuff, but theoretically it should not be as successful, since some of the periosteal supply would surely be disrupted. The sacrifice of the popliteal artery and vein in a child and the insertion of vein grafts would expose the child's normal limb to a significant risk of ischemia. Since the lateral inferior genicular artery in children is very tiny, anastomosis of this vessel to preserve epiphyseal blood supply would be very difficult and the failure rate high, resulting in growth arrest. Perhaps with more experience some of these technical problems can be overcome.

Another unanswered question concerning free vascularized epiphyseal grafts is the pattern of growth and time of closure following transplantation. For example, if the transplanted fibula were used as a replacement for a congenitally absent radius, would it grow at the same rate and fuse at the same time as the opposite fibula or would it adopt the growth pattern of the radius? The growth potential of the proximal fibular epiphysis might be further compromised when it is subjected to compressive forces caused by weight-bearing or the correction of a deformity.

Our experimental work supports clinical experience that suggests that after failure of anastomoses, a free vascularized bone graft with a thick muscle cuff does not behave as a conventional bone autograft. Our data show that the dead muscle cuff acts as a barrier to revascularization of the bone graft and the bundle of necrotic muscle acts as a nidus for infection. These findings support the current recommendation for taking vascularized bone grafts: a cuff of muscle is left around the vascular pedicle only to protect the vessels during dissection, not to preserve periosteal blood supply. Only the nonvascularized grafts became infected in our study, which suggests that vascularized free bone transplants may be more resistant to infection. In addition to possible enhanced resistance to infection, vascularized bone grafts have a greater potential for antibiotic penetration. Further work in this area may help refine the indications for free vascularized bone transfers.

SUMMARY

Free vascularized epiphyseal transplantation shows promise for aiding in the solution of many difficult pediatric surgical problems. We strongly believe that continued experimental work is necessary before widespread use in children can be recommended.

REFERENCES

1. Barr, J.S.: Autogenous epiphyseal transplant, J. Bone Joint Surg. **36A:**688, 1954.
2. Bisgard, J.D.: Transplanted epiphyseal cartilage, Arch. Surg. **39:**1028, 1939.
3. Brashear, H.R.: Epiphyseal avascular necrosis and its relation to longitudinal bone growth, J. Bone Joint Surg. **45A:**1423, 1963.
4. Calderwood, J.W.: The effect of hyperbaric oxygen on the transplantation of epiphyseal growth cartilage in the rabbit, J. Bone Joint Surg. **56B:**753, 1974.
5. Donski, P.K., Carwell, G.R., and Sharzer, L.A.: Growth in revascularized bone grafts in young puppies, Plast. Reconstr. Surg. **64:**239, 1979.
6. Donski, P.K., and O'Brien, B.: Free microvascular epiphyseal transplantation: an experimental study in dogs, Br. J. Plast. Surg. **33:**169, 1980.
7. Eades, J.W., and Peacock, E.E.: Autogenous transplantation of an interphalangeal joint and proximal phalangeal epiphyses: case report and ten year follow-up, J. Bone Joint Surg. **48A:**775, 1966.
8. Freeman, B.S.: The results of epiphyseal transplant by flap and by free graft: a brief survey, Plast. Reconstr. Surg. **36:**227, 1965.
9. Furnas, D.W.: Growth and development in replanted forelimbs, Plast. Reconstr. Surg. **46:**445, 1970.
10. Haas, S.L.: Further observation on the transplantation of the epiphyseal cartilage plate, Surg. Gynecol. Obstet. **52:**958, 1931.
11. Harris, W.R., Martin, R., and Tile, M.: Transplantation of epiphyseal plates, J. Bone Joint Surg. **47A:**897, 1965.
12. Heikel, H.V.A.: Experimental epiphyseal transplantation, Part I, Acta Orthop. Scand. **29:**257, 1960; Part II, Acta Orthop. Scand. **30:**1, 1960; Part III, Acta Orthop. Scand. **36:**371, 1965.
13. Hoffman, S., Siffert, R.S., and Simon, B.E.: Experimental and clinical experiences in epiphyseal transplantation, Plast. Reconstr. Surg. **50:**58, 1972.
14. Hurwitz, P.J.: Experimental transplantation of small joints by microvascular anastomoses, Plast. Reconstr. Surg. **64:**221, 1979.
15. Mathes, S.J., Buchannan, R., and Weeks, P.M.: Microvascular joint transplantation with epiphyseal growth, J. Hand Surg. **5:**586, 1980.
16. O'Brien, B.M.: Microvascular free bone and joint transfer. In O'Brien, B.M., editor: Microvascular reconstructive surgery, New York, 1977, Churchill-Livingstone, p. 267.
17. Rank, B.K.: Long-term results of epiphyseal transplants in congenital deformities of the hand, Plast. Reconstr. Surg. **61:**321, 1978.

18. Ring, P.A.: Excision and reimplantation of the epiphyseal cartilage of the rabbit, J. Anat. **89:**231, 1955.
19. Ring, P.A.: Transplantation of epiphyseal cartilage, J. Bone Joint Surg. **37B:**642, 1955.
20. Snowdy, H.A., Omer, G.E., and Sherman, F.C.: Longitudinal growth of a free toe phalanx transplant to a finger, J. Hand Surg. **5:**71, 1980.
21. Spira, E., and Farin, I.: The vascular supply to the epiphyseal plate under normal and pathological conditions, Acta Orthop. Scand. **38:**1, 1967.
22. Spira, E., Farin, I., and Hashomer, T.: Epiphyseal transplantation, J. Bone Joint Surg. **46A:**1278, 1964.
23. Straub, G.F.: Anatomical survival, growth and physiological function of an epiphyseal bone transplant, Surg. Gynecol. Obstet. **48:**687, 1929.

24. Trueta, J., Amato, V.P.: The vascular contribution to osteogenesis, J. Bone Joint Surg. **42B:**571, 1960.
25. Wenger, H.L.: Transplantation of epiphyseal cartilage, Arch. Surg. **50:**148, 1945.
26. Whitesides, E.S.: Normal growth in a transplanted epiphysis, J. Bone Joint Surg. **59A:**546, 1977.
27. Wilson, J.N.: Epiphyseal transplantation, J. Bone Joint Surg. **48A:**245, 1966.
28. Wray, R.C., Jr., Mathes, S.M., Young, V.L., and Weeks, P.M.: Free vascularized whole-joint transplants with ununited epiphyses, Plast. Reconstr. Surg. **67:**519, 1981.
29. Zaleske, D.J., et al.: Growth plate behavior in whole joint replantation in the rabbit, J. Bone Joint Surg. **64A:**249, 1982.

Part X

Muscle transplantation

Chapter 33

Muscle transplantation: making it function

Ralph T. Manktelow

Muscle transplantation with the use of microvascular anastomoses is a clinical reality. The muscle, with or without its overlying skin, is frequently transplanted to provide a well-vascularized soft tissue cover. The addition of a motor nerve repair should provide a contractile capability to the transplanted muscle. The possibility of transplanting functioning muscle presents many tempting reconstructive possibilities to the reconstructive surgeon. Two areas of application are reconstruction in facial paralysis and the replacement of missing skeletal muscle. This chapter will concentrate on the restoration of skeletal movement with functioning free muscle transplantation.

Tamai[6] established the applicability of this procedure in an experimental model in 1970. He demonstrated the functional capability in the rectus femoris of the dog. In 1973 a surgical team at the Sixth People's Hospital in Shanghai successfully transplanted the lateral portion of the pectoralis major muscle to the forearm to replace finger flexor musculature in a patient who had sustained a Volkmann's contracture. This patient obtained a good range of motion and muscle strength.[5] I reported my initial experience with two cases in 1978; since that time, I have used the procedure on sixteen occasions to replace skeletal musculature. The technique that evolved from this experience is described in this chapter.

INDICATIONS FOR MUSCLE TRANSPLANTATION

Muscle transplantation is indicated for a patient who has sustained a major loss of skeletal musculature that has produced a significant functional deficit that cannot be reconstructed by simpler means. This usually means that local tendons are not available for transfer. The causes have been direct trauma to the forearm, producing loss of musculature (either directly or secondary to Volkmann's ischemic paralysis), electrical burns, or aftereffects of gas gangrene. The operation has also been used in paralysis following brachial plexus injury; however, its status in this condition is not yet clear.

A number of conditions must be satisfied before muscle transplantation is feasible. The surgeon must adhere to all of the principles applied to any tendon transfer. The arm and hand must have mobile joints, good skin cover, and a bed suitable for the receipt of the transplanted tendon and muscle. The proximal joints should be stable with suitable balancing muscles. A high level of patient motivation is also a prerequisite.

PREOPERATIVE PLANNING

Although the surgical technique for replacement of forearm flexor musculature will be described here, the principles are the same for any anatomic area.

Angiograms are required for assessing the arterial vasculature in the damaged recipient limb. This allows suitable vessel selection for the arterial anastomosis. Superficial veins or venae comitantes are suitable for venous return. The selection of a suitable motor nerve is critical to the success of the procedure. The nerve must be an undamaged motor nerve without a sensory component. In the flexor aspect of the forearm, the motor nerve branches to the superficialis or the anterior interosseous nerve are suitable. From the clinical examination it is usually possible to determine which motor nerve is likely to be present. If there is uncertainty, however, the surgeon should do a preliminary procedure to explore for a motor nerve and ascertain its axonal integrity through a biopsy at the expected site of nerve repair.

The incision must be planned to allow good

exposure of the neurovascular structures and to provide flap coverage at the site of tendon repair and over the distal muscle. The proximal portion of the muscle may be covered with a split-thickness skin graft.

OPERATING TECHNIQUE

A two-team approach is preferred, with one team preparing the forearm, the other preparing the muscle. The muscle is completely separated from its site of origin, except for the vascular pedicle. This allows an assessment of the adequacy of the pedicle to supply the entire muscle to be transplanted. Dissection of the forearm requires the development of suitable flaps, identification and preparation of the flexor tendons that are to be attached to the muscle, preparation of the neurovascular structures, and exposure of the medial epicondyle to which the muscle will be attached.

When the muscle has been separated from its origin, it should be promptly transferred to the arm and positioned for the repair of all structures. Arterial and venous anastomoses should be done first to minimize the ischemic time. The muscle should be positioned in such a way that the nerve repair can be placed as close to the muscle as possible to minimize the duration of muscle denervation and atrophy. A meticulous fascicular repair is done with interrupted 11-0 nylon sutures. The muscle is then attached firmly to the medial epicondyle and surrounding fascia and inserted into the flexor tendons.

The selection of the correct tension is critical to the development of good muscle function. In their normal state, muscles are under tension. There are two methods of judging the adequacy of muscle tension. If extensor and intrinsic musculature is intact, the posture of the fingers on completion of the tendon repairs will indicate the adequacy of the tension. The fingers should sit in a position of function or in slightly more flexion on completion of the repair. However, the patient may not have normal antagonistic musculature, and an alternate technique of determining tension will be required. This alternate technique begins while the muscle is still in its site of origin. The muscle is stretched to its normal maximum extension by manipulation of the extremity. It is then tattooed with marks on the belly at fixed intervals, such as every 5 cm. It can then be assumed that the muscle can be safely stretched to this length when it is transferred. Following revascularization and attachment of the muscle's origin, it is then stretched out in the forearm until the markers are spaced at 5 cm intervals. This will require considerable tension to be placed on the muscle. The wrist and fingers are then extended, and adjacent points on the transplanted muscle's tendon and the flexor tendons to the fingers can be noted and suitably marked. This is the point at which the muscle tendon should be sutured to the flexor tendons. Using this technique, the surgeon can be assured that the muscle will allow full finger and wrist extension. If a muscle has been chosen whose normal excursion is greater than the 7 cm necessary to provide full finger flexion in any position of the wrist, on reinnervation the muscle will have the potential to provide full finger movement. Flap coverage must be provided over the muscle tendon junction and the distal portion of the muscle to allow it to glide. This may be a local flap from the forearm or a flap that is carried with the muscle as a musculocutaneous flap.

POSTOPERATIVE MANAGEMENT

Immediate postoperative management is the same as for any free vascularized flap to the extremity. The patient must be kept warm and well perfused to maintain a good peripheral circulation. The wrists and fingers are positioned in flexion to relax the junction between the muscle transplant and the finger flexor tendons.

At 3 weeks after surgery, passive wrist and finger extension is begun until a full range is obtained. When reinnervation occurs, usually at 2 to 4 months after transplantation, the patient is encouraged to do active finger flexion. Between 6 months and a year, the patient will develop a full range of finger flexion and can be started on a program of active resisted exercises. These exercises should be done daily and the amount of resistance applied increased as muscle strength improves. This may involve the use of springs, pulleys, weights, and various other devices that will create a resistance to finger flexion. It is our experience that muscle strength will plateau between 2 and 3 years after transplantation.

CASE REPORT
Patient I

In 1974 a 22-year-old male injured his right forearm in an industrial accident. Initial treatment consisted of debridement of nonvascular muscle, internal fixation of fractures of the radius and ulna, and skin grafts. When the patient was referred to us 2 years later, his arm had an hourglass deformity (Fig. 33-1, *A*). There was no long flexor or extensor musculature to the fingers or thumb. Extensor carpi radialis longus and brachioradialis muscles were present, with one half of their normal strength. The median and ulnar nerve supply to the hand was virtually normal, with good intrinsic function and sensation present. The passive range of motion at the finger and wrist joints was normal. Relaxing the wrist extensor produced finger extension by the tenodesis effect of the adherent extensor digitorum communis over the distal forearm.

The inferior four fifths of the ipsilateral sternal head of the pectoralis major muscle was transplanted to his forearm. Six individual branches of the anterior inter-osseous nerve were sutured to six nerves of the pectoralis major. The anterior interosseous artery was sutured to the pectoral artery, and two venous anastomoses were done. The flexor digitorum profundus and flexor pollicis longus tendons were attached to the muscle. A split-thickness skin graft was applied directly to the muscle belly, since direct closure was not possible because of the bulk of muscle transferred.

Gentle passive extension was begun at 2 weeks after transplantation, and nearly full finger extension was obtained at 6 weeks. Active muscle contraction began at 3 months, and a program of resisted finger exercises was begun 6 months after surgery. The patient developed a full range of finger flexion, and with relaxation the muscle allowed full finger and wrist extension (Fig. 33-1, *A* to *E*).

Muscle strength and bulk increased rapidly for 2 years, after which there was a gradual increase in strength to the present (Fig. 33-1, *F*). The patient is now employed in heavy construction work.

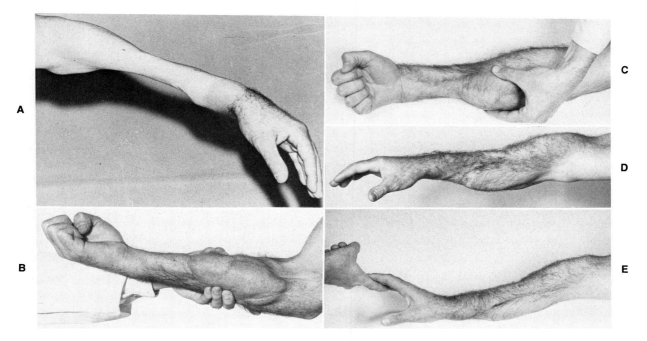

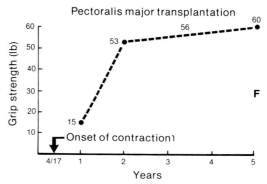

Fig. 33-1. A, Twenty-four-year-old male with hourglass deformity of the forearm secondary to a loss of flexor and extensor musculature. (From Manktelow, R.T., and McKee, N.H.: Free muscle transplantation to provide active finger flexion, J. Hand Surg. **3:**416, 1978.) **B,** Fourteen months after transplantation of four fifths of the sternal head of the pectoralis major muscle and reinnervation, the patient developed a full range of finger flexion and return of muscle bulk. **C,** Four years after surgery the muscle has increased in bulk, as seen between the examiner's fingers and thumb. A flexor pollicis longus tendon-lengthening procedure has been done to balance the finger and thumb movements. **D,** Active finger and thumb extension was developed with a brachioradialis transfer. **E,** With muscle relaxation, good passive wrist and finger extension is possible. **F,** Chart demonstrates progress in grip strength over time.

Patient II

An 11-year-old male lost the musculature of the anterior compartment of his right leg when the blades of a power lawn mower struck it repeatedly. We saw him 2 years after his injury, at which time he had a complete foot drop (Fig. 33-2, *A* and *B*). A Tinel's sign was present over the scar just anterior to the head of the fibula.

On May 31, 1978, a contralateral gracilis muscle transplantation was done (Fig. 33-2, *C* and *D*). Vascularization was accomplished with an end-to-side anastomosis between the artery to the gracilis and the anterior tibial artery and end-to-end anastomoses between the venae comitantes. The motor nerve to the gracilis was sutured to a branch of the deep peroneal nerve. The muscle was fixed to the lateral aspect of the proximal tibia, and the tendon was inserted through a drill hole in the cuboid. The muscle healed well; a portion of the distal skin flap necrosed and required a split-thickness skin graft. Three months postoperatively reinnervation began; strength increased until approximately 1½ years after surgery. The patient developed good contraction in the muscle (Fig. 33-2, *E* to *G*). This extended his foot to 80 degrees against gravity and gave him sufficient support to eliminate his drop-foot brace. He now functions well, running and playing most sports.

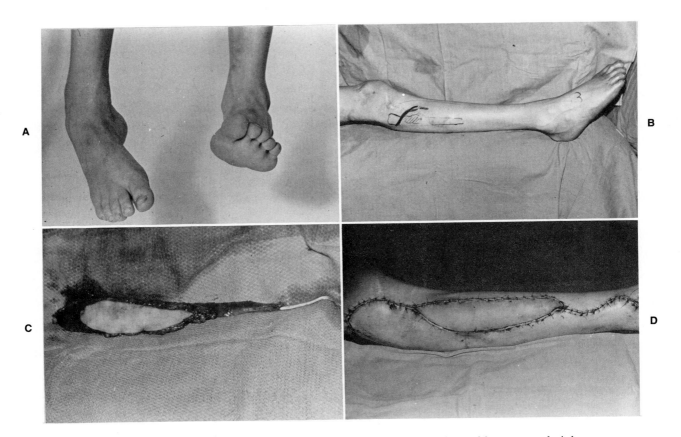

Fig. 33-2. A, Following anterior compartment injury, patient is unable to extend right ankle. **B,** Expected location of peroneal nerve and anterior tibial artery shown on injured leg. **C,** Myocutaneous gracilis is prepared for transplantation. Long tendon suitable for distal fixation is seen to right. **D,** Immediately following transplantation of muscle and insetting of cutaneous flap.

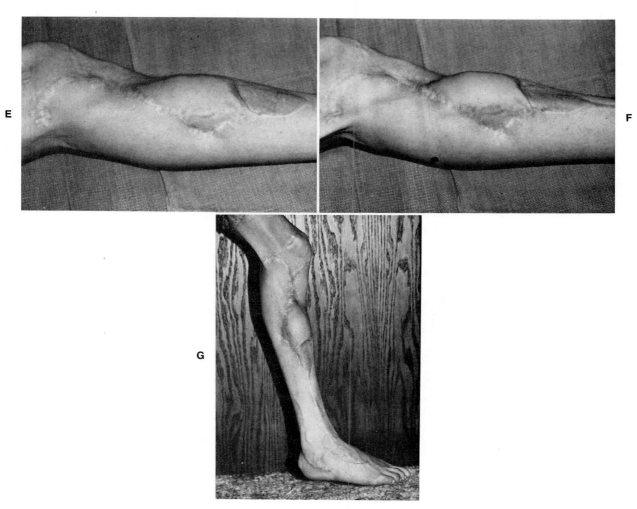

Fig. 33-2, cont'd. E, Muscle in relaxation. Skin graft was applied on distal portion of muscle following necrosis of overlying skin. **F,** Muscle contraction. **G,** Contracting muscle supports foot against gravity, dorsiflexing foot to 80 degrees.

MUSCLE SELECTION

Many muscles have been used for functioning muscle transplantation, including the gracilis, pectoralis major, pectoralis minor, latissimus dorsi, rectus femoris, brachioradialis, and extensor digitorum brevis. Most of our experience has been with the gracilis muscle. It has a number of significant advantages. The neurovascular bundle is of adequate size for microvascular anastomosis and is 5 to 6 cm long, which allows some latitude in placement of the muscle.

The dynamic requirements for finger flexion are a range of contraction of at least 7 cm and adequate strength and stamina. The gracilis supplies these requirements without difficulty. Using a single gracilis to power all four flexor tendons, one can expect a maximum of 50% of the grip strength normally present in the hand. Other muscles such as the pectoralis major and latissimus dorsi have the advantage of carrying a good cutaneous flap with them that is more reliable than the gracilis over its distal portion. Frequently the arm will be so damaged that existing skin coverage over the tendons at the wrist will not be suitable for covering repairs; in such a case skin is readily furnished by including it with the donor muscle as a myocutaneous flap. If the latissimus dorsi is used, it should be placed so that its insertion is attached to the flexor tendons and its origin to the medial epicondyle; this provides a suitable structure for suturing to the flexor tendons. The pectoralis major is a more complicated muscle, with four to ten separate motor nerve branches, all of which have independently functioning muscular territories.[3] In addition, this muscle does not have a good tendon insertion and it is necessary to suture the flexor tendons into the muscle bellies themselves. The technique of removing these muscles has been described previously.[1]

SUMMARY

The primary advantage of this procedure is that it provides a functioning muscle in situations in which standard tendon transfers are not possible. All of the principles that apply to tendon transfers are relevant to this procedure, and a good motor nerve that can be sutured to the muscle must be present in the recipient area. It is possible to obtain a range of motion and strength of contraction that are greater than those obtained by standard tendon transfers such as the extensor carpi radialis longus to the flexor digitorum profundus.

The major disadvantages of this procedure are the time it takes before the forearm becomes functional and the complexity of the procedure. Because of the interval between denervation and reinnervation, a functioning range of finger flexion cannot be expected for 6 to 12 months. At this time the hand will be useful only for light activities; it will take another 6 months to a year before a powerful grip function is obtained. This is in contrast to the standard tendon transfers, which provide a good grip strength at 3 to 4 months. Another disadvantage is the time that is lost if the procedure fails. One may wait for 6 months to a year hoping for reinnervation, while the patient's unimproved life-style goes on. Our experience with sixteen muscle transplantations to the skeleton includes one total failure and one partial failure—all others survived. Twelve caes of forearm muscle transplantation have been followed for 3 years, and the results have been described in detail. Nine of these patients obtained a full range of finger motion with the wrist stationary, and five patients had nearly a full range of finger motion with the wrist both flexed and extended. The maximum grip strength obtained was 42 pounds for a gracilis and 60 pounds for a pectoralis major transplant. The grip strength depends on the level of nerve regeneration, proper muscle tension, and motivation of the patient.

ACKNOWLEDGMENT

I have the pleasure of working with Drs. R.M. Zuker and N.H. McKee; I acknowledge their contributions and assistance in the development of muscle transplantation techniques.

REFERENCES

1. Manktelow, R.T.: Free muscle flaps. In Green, D.P., editor: Operative hand surgery, Vol. 1, New York, 1982, Churchill Livingstone, p. 861.
2. Manktelow, R.T., and McKee, N.H.: Free muscle transplantation to provide active finger flexion, J. Hand Surg. **3:**416, 1978.
3. Manktelow, R.T., McKee, N.H., and Vettese, T.: An anatomical study of the pectoralis major muscle as related to functioning free muscle transplantation, Plast. Reconstr. Surg. **65:**610, 1980.
4. Manktelow, R.T., Zuker, R.M., and McKee, N.H.: Functioning free muscle transplantation, J. Hand Surg. (In Press.)
5. Shanghai Sixth People's Hospital: Free muscle transplantation by microsurgical neurovascular anastomoses, Chin. Med. J. **2:**47, 1976.
6. Tamai, S., et al.: Free muscle transplants in dogs with microsurgical neurovascular anastomoses, Plast. Reconstr. Surg. **46:**219, 1970.

Chapter 34

Free muscle graft: clinical and experimental studies

Yoshikazu Ikuta

Eiji Hatano

Kaoru Yoshioka

The attempt to graft muscles has a long history, beginning with Zielonko (1874) and others.[12] The first graft using a neurovascular anastomosis was performed by Tamai in 1970[10] and was applied clinically by Harii,[2] Ikuta,[3] and others.[6,7,8,9] In preparation for clinical application we performed experiments on dogs and found that a muscle graft incorporating a vascular anastomosis and nerve suture was superior to any other method.[5] However, some still claim that adequate functional recovery can be achieved by the procedure described by Thompson, which does not employ any form of anastomosis or suture.[13] Therefore we decided to undertake a full review of the problems and performed the following series of experiments.

EXPERIMENTAL STUDIES
Viability of muscle fibers in free muscle graft

The anterior tibial muscle of rats weighing 250 g was used. The neurovascular bundle entering the muscle belly was isolated. The proximal and distal ends of the muscle were then reattached in their original sites. Next the muscle was transected at the middle and then repaired with 8-0 monofilament nylon suture.

Fig. 34-1 shows Mallory's stained specimens obtained at 10 days and at 4 weeks after surgery. As shown in Fig. 34-1, *A*, the distal portion (the free graft portion in which both the nerves and vessels had been severed) showed coagulation necrosis in the central portion, surrounded by a proliferation of granulation tissue; generalized swelling was

seen. Under high magnification several layers of viable muscle fibers were seen in the periphery of the distal portion. The details of this experimental study were reported,[4] and the following conclusions were drawn:

1. In the so-called free muscle graft in which the neurovascular bundle is not retained, muscle cells of the superficial layer will survive, but the central portion, which constitutes practically all of the muscle belly, will become fibrotic.
2. Muscle fibers in which there is good circulation will return to show an almost normal histologic pattern by the third week after surgery.
3. Even when a portion of the muscle is severed in areas where the neurovascular bundle is intact, the muscle cells will survive along almost the full length of the muscle.

Muscular changes resulting from denervation and reinnervation

The circulation in the anterior tibial muscle of rats was left intact, whereas the nerve was excised to prevent reinnervation, and comparisons were made with the healthy side (Fig. 34-2, *A*). The difference in the wet weight ratio is shown in Fig. 34-3. The wet weight dropped below 40% in comparison with the healthy side at 3 weeks following surgery and steadily decreased to 20% at 10 weeks. A separate group was used to study the nerve, which, after transection, was repaired with a single suture of 10-0 monofilament nylon. Five weeks af-

315

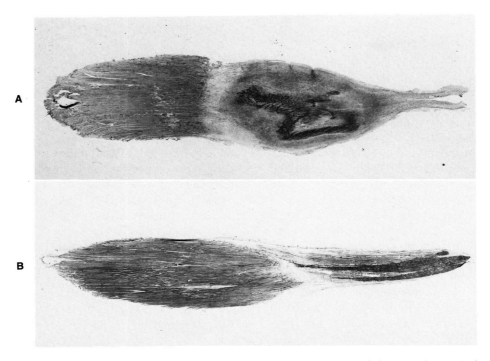

Fig. 34-1. Microscopic findings. **A,** Proximal vascular portion of the muscle at 10 days after surgery. **B,** Distal avascular portion (Mallory's stain). Proximal portion is almost normal muscle but distal is fibrotic at 4 weeks after surgery (×5).

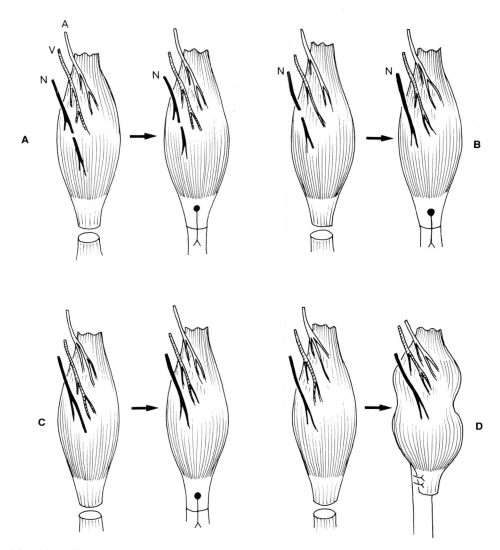

Fig. 34-2. The anterior tibial muscle of rats was used and divided into four groups: **A,** Denervation; **B,** reinnervation; **C,** normal tension; and **D,** reduced tension.

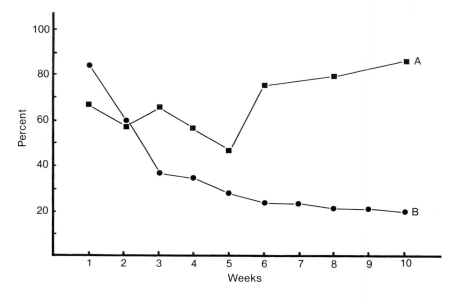

Fig. 34-3. The changes of muscle wet weight caused by **(A)** denervation and **(B)** reinnervation.

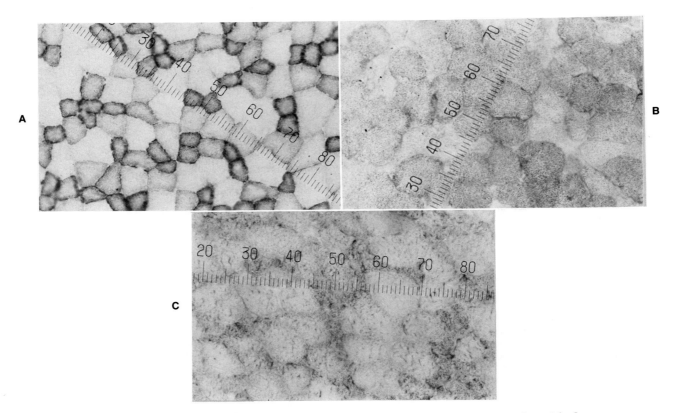

Fig. 34-4. Microscopic findings with succinic dehydrogenase stain. **A,** Normal muscle fibers (×100). **B,** Denervated muscle at 4 weeks after surgery (×200). **C,** Denervated muscle at 7 weeks after surgery (×200).

ter surgery the wet weight dropped to its lowest point, 40% of the healthy side, but gradually increased thereafter, reaching 80% at 10 weeks (Fig. 34-3).

The interval changes in the muscle fibers were observed by succinic dehydrogenase stain. Fig. 34-4 shows the normal and denervated muscle at 4 and 7 weeks after surgery. The deeply stained fibers are Type I, and those lightly stained are Type II; the moderately stained are intermediate fibers.[1] The denervated group stained poorly; distinction between Types I and II cannot be made, and the outline of the muscle fibers is not clear. These findings are more noticeable at 7 weeks than at 4 weeks after surgery.

However, in a muscle in which a neurorrhaphy has been done (Fig. 34-2, *B*), type grouping can be seen at 4 weeks after surgery (Fig. 34-5, *A*), and at 10 weeks a clear outline of the muscle fibers can be seen with distinct representations of both Types I and II, as shown in the lower part of Fig. 34-5, *B*. Groupings of Type I and II fibers can also be seen.

Fig. 34-6 shows a histogram of the muscle fibers grouped by diameter. The solid line is the affected side and the dotted line shows the healthy side. At 1 week after surgery both Types I and II are reduced in size, and at 3 weeks Type II becomes half its original size.

On the other hand, although there is muscle fiber atrophy at 5 weeks after surgery, at 10 weeks both Types I and II are restored to normal, and at 23 weeks the Type I fibers are even larger than the control side (Fig. 34-7).

These experimental results indicate that the most important point for restoring function in the grafted muscle is reinnervation. To achieve this it is important to choose a recipient nerve with many motor fibers and to make the junction with the donor nerve as close to the muscle belly as possible to induce early reinnervation.

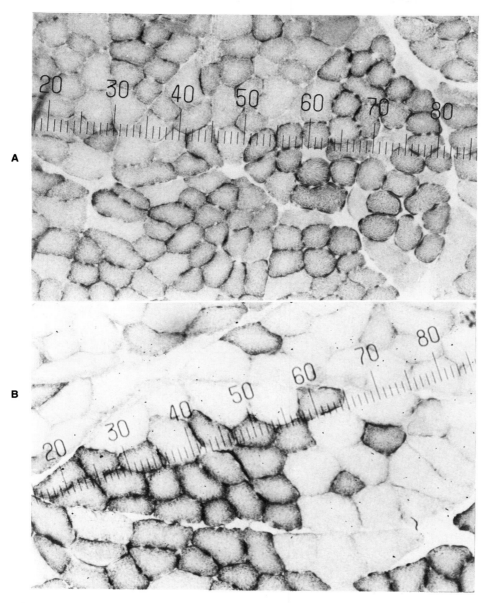

Fig. 34-5. Microscopic findings with succinic dehydrogenase stain. **A,** Reinnervated muscle at 4 weeks after surgery. **B,** Reinnervated muscle at 10 weeks after surgery. A clear outline of the muscle fibers and distinction by stain of types I and II can be made as shown in the lower portion (×100).

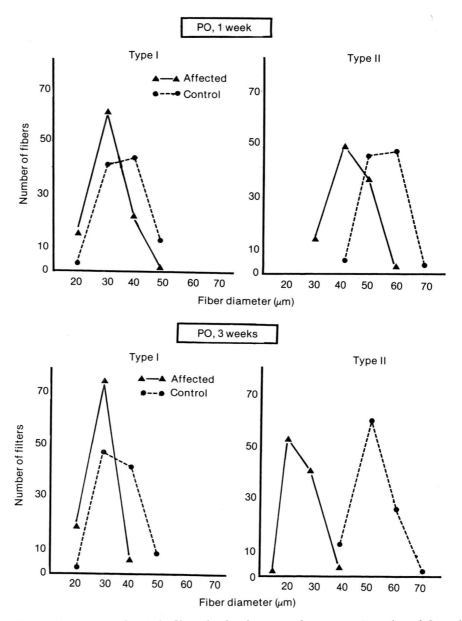

Fig. 34-6. Histograms of muscle fibers in the denervated group at 1 week and 3 weeks after surgery.

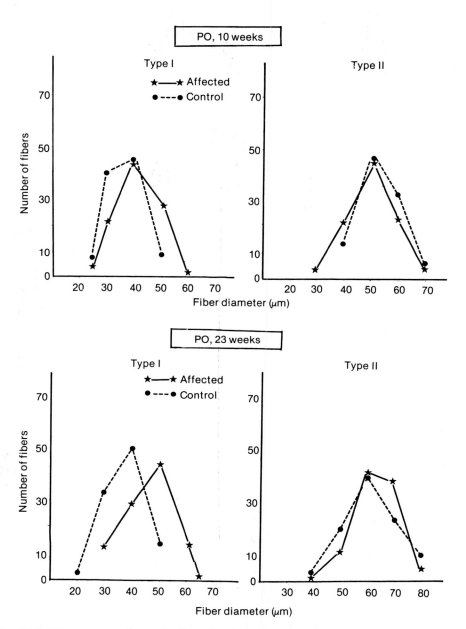

Fig. 34-7. Histograms of muscle fibers in the reinnervated group at 10 weeks and 23 weeks after surgery.

Grafted muscle tension and muscular changes

When the muscle belly is too long to graft to a particular recipient site, a portion of the distal end must be resected. Our experiments indicate that such a resection does not have too deleterious an effect on the proximal portion. Generally one would think that the length of the muscle belly should be about the same length as the muscle defect; but then how should the degree of joint flexion be determined? Or, how should we judge the tension for the grafted muscle? To resolve this problem, the following experiment was performed.

The anterior tibial muscle of rats was used, as in the other experiments. After freeing the muscle, sparing the neurovascular bundle, the distal portion was not resutured to the original tendon but rather was shortened by 5 mm and sutured side to side to the neighboring extensor hallucis longus tendon as shown in Fig. 34-2, *D*. A control procedure was done on the opposite side, simply transecting and repairing the contralateral tendon (Fig. 34-2, *C*).

After tenotomy the group sutured at normal tension showed hardly any change in wet weight, whereas the group that received 5 mm shortening of the tendon showed a decrease to 60% of normal at 6 weeks but recovered to almost the same level as the normal tension group at 10 weeks (Fig. 34-8).

The histogram in Fig. 34-9 shows the muscle fibers by type as distinguished by succinic dehydrogenase stain. By the tenth week the diameters of both Type I and II fibers are slightly increased, but at 20 weeks no clear distinction between the two can be made. No change can be observed at 3 and 7 weeks after surgery in the normal tension group. Thus we concluded that it is best to graft the muscle at normal tension. Clinically this is accomplished by grafting a muscle of suitable length and adjusting the angle of the joints so that normal tension can be attained.

Neurorrhaphy was performed to determine the correlation between reinnervation and muscle tension, but the results of this series were about the same as the former series. In other words, at about 1 month after surgery the grafted muscle decreased to 60% of the size of the control but at 6 months was restored to 95% of the control in the normal tension group and 90% in the weak tension group.

Atrophy of denervated muscle and effect of low frequency stimulation

Atrophy of the grafted muscle is unavoidable; therefore keeping the degree of atrophy to the minimum is very important, since it will make possible early functional training and rapid muscle recovery. Since it is evident that atrophy is caused by loss of stimulation from the peripheral nerves to

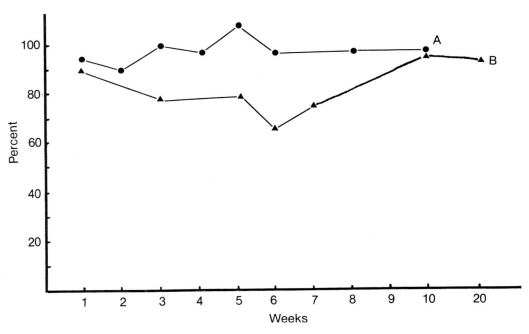

Fig. 34-8. The changes of muscle wet weight **(A)** in the tenotomy group (normal tension) and **(B)** in the reduced tension group.

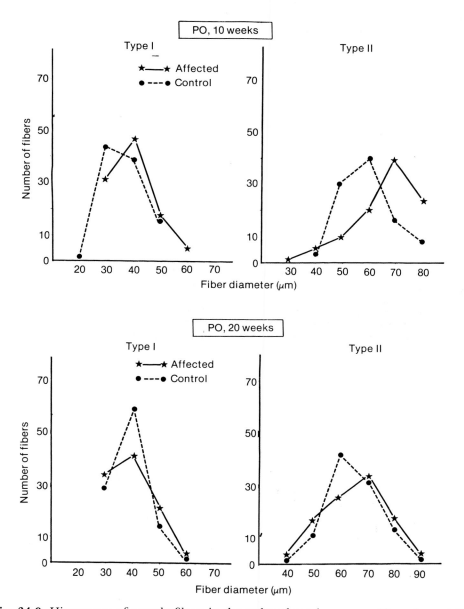

Fig. 34-9. Histograms of muscle fibers in the reduced tension group 10 weeks and 20 weeks after surgery.

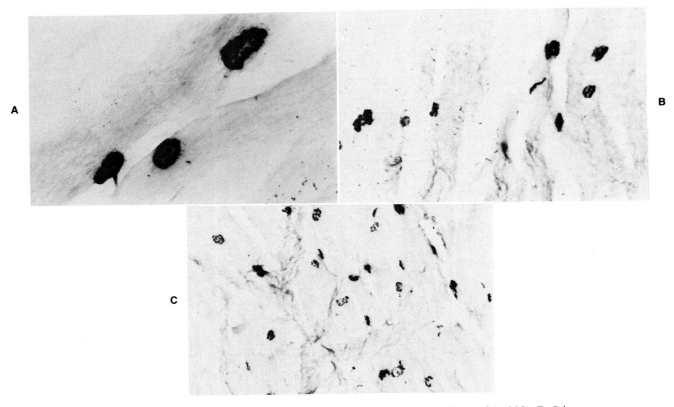

Fig. 34-10. Motor end-plates stained by Wachstein's method. **A,** Normal (×200). **B,** Stimulation to the denervated muscle 3 weeks after surgery (×100). **C,** Without stimulation 3 weeks after surgery (×100).

the end-plate of the myocytes, would it not be possible to reduce the degree of atrophy by finding something to substitute for this stimulation pathway? To answer this we applied low frequency stimulation to the muscle.

The experiment was performed by denervating the right anterior tibial muscle of rats. The muscle was then stimulated from the skin surface at a frequency of 5 Hz, a duration of 0.1 msec, 30 volts for 1 hour each day from the first to the fourth week. Fig. 34-10, *A,* shows findings of the normal motor end-plate, Fig. 34-10, *B,* shows the state in which stimulation was performed after denervation, and Fig. 34-10, *C,* shows those without stimulation.

In both groups that underwent surgery, deformation of the end-plate can be seen. Staining is poor and the synaptic folds show fragmentation, indistinctness, and diminished numbers. However, the shape and stain characteristics are better preserved in the group that received stimulation. Even after 4 weeks the same degenerative pattern seen at the third week was noted in the end-plate

in both the stimulated and nonstimulated groups (Fig. 34-11).

From these experiments we concluded that degeneration occurs at the motor end-plate as a result of denervation. When low frequency stimulation is administered, the degree of degeneration is slightly less.

Fig. 34-12 shows the difference in wet weight of the anterior tibial muscle of stimulated and nonstimulated rats. Those with stimulated muscle had a slightly smaller degree of atrophy.

Restoration of muscular power in muscle graft

The rectus femoris muscle of rabbits weighing 3 kg was used as a typical free muscle graft. The arterial anastomosis was a typical 0.6 mm anastomosis. The venous anastomosis was modified, with the vein followed to a larger proximal trunk 1.2 mm in diameter, which was chosen as the site of anastomosis. The length of the muscle belly was about 7 cm (Fig. 34-13). In group I the muscle was resutured in its original length, whereas in group

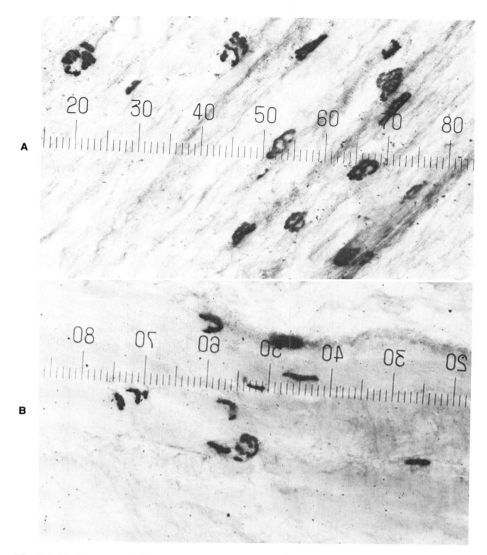

Fig. 34-11. Motor end-plates at 4 weeks after surgery. **A,** Stimulated (×200); **B,** nonstimulated (×200).

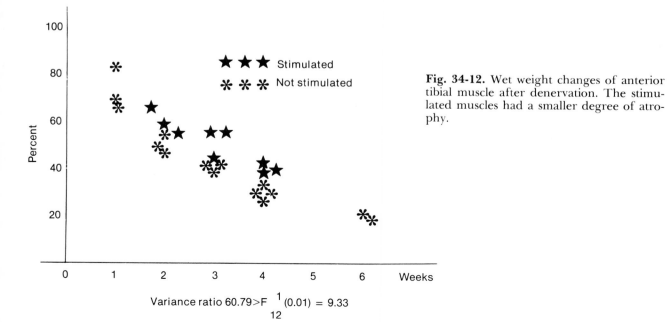

Fig. 34-12. Wet weight changes of anterior tibial muscle after denervation. The stimulated muscles had a smaller degree of atrophy.

Variance ratio $60.79 > F^{1}(0.01) = 9.33$

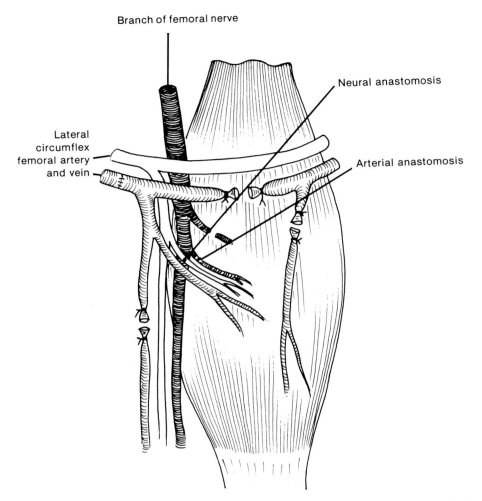

Branch of femoral nerve

Neural anastomosis

Lateral
circumflex
femoral artery
and vein

Arterial anastomosis

Fig. 34-13. Muscle graft of the rectus femoris muscle of rabbits. Arrows indicate the sites of vascular and neural anastomoses. The artery entering the muscle was 0.6 mm in diameter. Anastomosis was possible, but the veins were too small; thus anastomosis of the vein was performed at a more proximal site. The length of the muscle belly was about 7 cm.

II it was reduced in length by 2 cm before resuturing.

Fig. 34-14 shows the changes in wet weight of the grafted muscle. The solid circles represent the group with normal tension and the asterisks indicate the group with weak tension. The wet weight in both groups dropped to about 60% of that of the healthy side but gradually improved thereafter. At 6 months the group with normal tension reached 95%, whereas the group with weak tension reached about 90% of normal.

An effective means of measuring functional restoration of a grafted muscle is to check its contractile power.[11] Fig. 34-15 shows the method we used. The exposed nerve was stimulated and the contractile power of the muscle was measured by a force transducer, evaluating both twitch tension and tetanic tension.

The muscular power measured by twitch tension recovered to about 20% in both groups at 1 month after surgery and gradually increased thereafter, the group with normal tension reaching about 90% of the healthy side, and the group with weak tension reaching about 60% at 6 months. The muscular power measured by tetanic tension reached approximately 60% at about 2 months and 70% and 60%, respectively, at about 6 months in both groups.

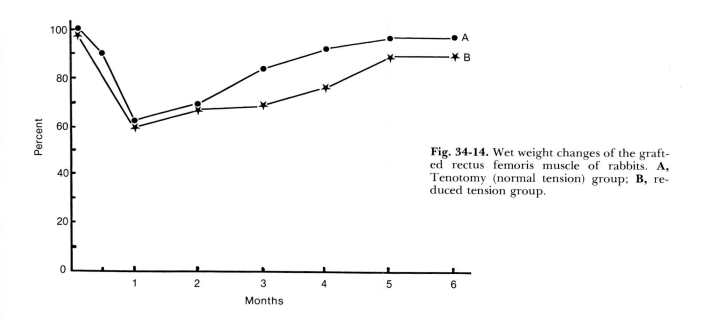

Fig. 34-14. Wet weight changes of the grafted rectus femoris muscle of rabbits. **A,** Tenotomy (normal tension) group; **B,** reduced tension group.

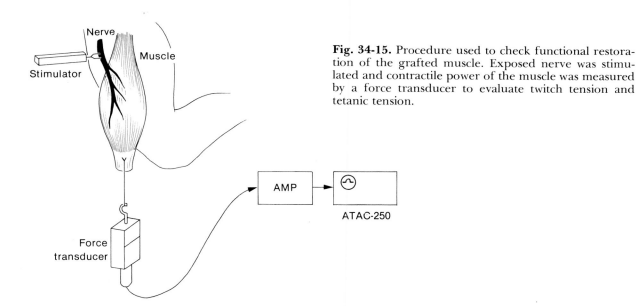

Fig. 34-15. Procedure used to check functional restoration of the grafted muscle. Exposed nerve was stimulated and contractile power of the muscle was measured by a force transducer to evaluate twitch tension and tetanic tension.

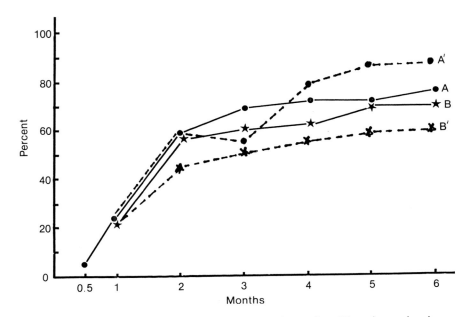

Fig. 34-16. Muscle force in twitch tension and tetanic tension. Tetanic tension in muscle under normal tension *(A)*; twitch tension in muscle under normal tension *(A')*; tetanic tension in muscle under reduced tension *(B)*; and twitch tension in muscle under reduced tension *(B')*.

Table 34-1. Clinical cases of free muscle graft (1975-1980)

Sex	Age	Diagnosis	Recipient site	Donor site	Result
M	6	Volkmann's contracture	Right forearm	Pectoralis major	Success
M	12	Volkmann's contracture	Left forearm	Gracilis	Success
M	11	Brachial plexus paralysis	Right upper arm	Gracilis	Success
F	20	Poliomyelitis	Right upper arm	Gracilis	Failure
M	21	Poliomyelitis	Left upper arm	Gracilis	Failure
M	6	Volkmann's contracture	Right forearm	Semitendinosus and skin	Success
F	5	Volkmann's contracture	Right forearm	Gracilis	Success
M	21	Volkmann's contracture	Left forearm	Gracilis and skin	Success
M	8	Volkmann's contracture	Left forearm	Gracilis and skin	Success

This series of experiments indicates that muscular power recovers to at least a measurable degree at 1 month after surgery and to 60% at 6 months (Fig. 34-16).

SUMMARY OF EXPERIMENTAL STUDIES

Three important factors influence the functional recovery of the grafted muscle—circulation, reinnervation of the motor nerve, and muscle training. Circulation in the muscle is influenced by the type of vascular anastomosis and the size of vessels. If another good source of vascularity is available in the affected area, the artery should be anastomosed not end to side but end to end.

Tension of the grafted muscle is not as impor-tant for functional recovery as previously thought, but ideally, normal tension should be sought.

For the transferred muscle to function well, the donor motor nerve of the muscle must recover and provide reinnervation of the muscle fibers as soon as possible. Ideally a pure motor branch with a matching funicular pattern is selected as a recipient. When identification of a pure motor branch is not possible, a mixed branch is selected. The anterior interosseous nerve in a case of Volkmann's contracture is an example. The site of the nerve anastomosis should be near the muscle entry to induce early reinnervation.

Finally, we emphasize the importance of post-operative stimulation and training of the grafted muscle.

CLINICAL CASES

Nine patients underwent free muscle graft procedures involving the upper extremity from 1975 to 1980. Their ages ranged from 5 to 21 years; seven were males and two were females. The causes of paralysis or damage to the muscle were ischemic contracture following supracondylar fracture in six cases, poliomyelitis in two cases, and a brachial plexus injury in one case.

In seven patients the gracilis muscle was selected as the muscle to be transferred, while the pectoralis major muscle and semitendinosus muscle were used in the other two. In three cases the gracilis muscle and semitendinosus muscle were removed together with the overlying—a so-called musculocutaneous flap technique. Functional recovery was confirmed in seven patients (Table 34-1).

REFERENCES

1. Dubowitz, V., and Pearse, A.G.E.: A comparative histochemical study of oxidative enzyme and phosphorylase activity in skeletal muscle, Histochemie **2:** 105, 1960.
2. Harii, K., Ohmori, K., and Torii, S.: Free gracilis muscle transplantation with microneurovascular anastomoses for the treatment of facial paralysis: a preliminary report, Plast. Reconstr. Surg. **57:**133, 1976.
3. Ikuta, Y., Kubo, T., and Tsuge, K.: Free muscle transplantation by microsurgical technique to treat severe Volkmann's contracture, Plast. Reconstr. Surg. **58:**407, 1976.
4. Ikuta, Y., Yoshioka, K., and Tsuge, K.: Free muscle grafts as applied to brachial plexus injury—case report and experimental study, Ann. Acad. Med. **8:** 454, 1979.
5. Kubo, T., Ikuta, Y., and Tsuge, K.: Free muscle transplantation in dogs by microneurovascular anastomoses, Plast. Reconstr. Surg. **57:**495, 1976.
6. Manktelow, R.T., and McKee, N.H.: Free muscle transplantation to provide active finger flexion, J. Hand Surg. **3:**416, 1978.
7. Maxwell, G.P., Stueber, K., and Hoopes, J.E.: A free latissimus dorsi myocutaneous flap: case report, Plast. Reconstr. Surg. **62:**462, 1978.
8. Shenk, R.: Free muscle transplantation and composite skin transplantation by microvascular anastomoses, Orthop. Clin. North Am. **8:**367, 1977.
9. Six Peoples Hospital, Microvascular Service, Shanghai: Free muscle transplantation by microsurgical neurovascular anastomoses, Chin. Med. J. **2:**47, 1976.
10. Tamai, S., et al.: Free muscle transplants in dogs with microsurgical neurovascular anastomoses, Plast. Reconstr. Surg. **46:**219, 1970.
11. Terzis, J.K., Sweet, R.C., Dykes, R.W., and Williams, H.B.: Recovery of function in free muscle transplants using microneurovascular anastomoses, J. Hand Surg. **3:**37, 1978.
12. Thompson, N.: Investigation of autogenous skeletal muscle free grafts in the dog—with a report on a successful free graft of skeletal muscle in man, Transplantation **12:**373, 1971.
13. Thompson, N.: On free muscle transplantation by microsurgical technique for Volkmann's contracture, (letter to the editor), Plast. Reconstr. Surg. **60:** 104, 1977.

Chapter 35

Gracilis muscle transplantation in the management of lower extremity osteomyelitis

Stephen J. Mathes

Muscle transposition flaps are now frequently used in the management of difficult lower extremity wounds. During the acute phase of management of an open fracture, a muscle flap can provide vascularized tissue to cover the exposed bone, preventing further wound desiccation and bacterial invasion. With stable wound coverage provided by the transposed muscle flap, fracture healing may proceed in an environment of healthy soft tissue.

When infection occurs at the site of prior bone injury, conservative methods of bone debridement and antibiotic therapy are often ineffective, even when soft tissue coverage appears adequate. Osteomyelitis from contiguous foci[9] is commonly observed in the tibia because of injury-related loss of periosteal and endosteal circulation.[1] Sequestrectomy and antibiotic therapy, combined with transposition of a muscle flap into the bone defect, has been demonstrated to be an effective method to provide stable coverage and obtain resolution of osteomyelitis.[3,6,7,8]

The distal leg, ankle, and foot are not readily covered by vascularized tissue because safe local muscle or axial flaps are not available. With the development of microvascular techniques, it is now possible to transplant muscle from a distant site into areas where local muscle flaps are either unavailable or inadequate in size for coverage of the defect.

During the last 6 years the gracilis muscle has been transplanted by microvascular techniques to the distal lower extremity for the management of chronic osteomyelitis. The addition of this operative procedure to the regimen of culture-specific antibiotic therapy and sequestrectomy has resulted in uniform success in management of osteomyelitis in sixteen consecutive patients. Experimental and clinical evidence suggests that the positive effect of the muscle flap in treating chronic osteomyelitis is related to the increased blood supply it provides; thus the components of the host defense mechanism (immunoglobulins, complements, and phagocytic leukocytes), oxygen, and antibiotics are more effectively delivered to the wound.[2,4]

The three specific components of treatment (culture-specific antibiotics, sequestrectomy, and muscle transplantation) are presented in this chapter, with an emphasis on the rationale for their use and specific details of technique and results.

ANTIBIOTICS

Preliminary cultures of the sinus tract and specific cultures of the involved bone are obtained at the time of sequestrectomy. Most often, specific therapy is directed toward both *Staphylococcus* (present in 60% of wound cultures) and gram negative organisms (mixture of *Pseudomonas*, *Bacteroides* and *Enterococcus*, present in 81% of cultures). Most patients have had previous intense antibiotic therapy, but wound drainage has persisted. Failure of antibiotic therapy alone appears to be related to poor circulation at the wound site. An osteomyelitic wound is characterized by a predominance of scar tissue with minimal vascular ingrowth and osteoblast function. After sequestrectomy and muscle transplantation into the defect, culture-specific antibiotic therapy is continued for 10 days to 6 weeks. Future studies will define the exact antibiotic requirements in the postoperative period.

SEQUESTRECTOMY

Aggressive debridement is required to remove infected devascularized bone and adjacent fibrotic soft tissue. Failure of the standard methods of treatment of osteomyelitis with sequestrectomy and antibiotic therapy may in part reflect a reluctance to aggressively debride involved bone. Since immediate coverage of the defect is provided by muscle transplantation, the reconstructive surgeon may remove all infected bone, cartilage, and soft tissue at the site of chronic osteomyelitis. Although we have not seen loss of bone stability resulting from this extensive bone debridement, nonetheless, subsequent bone grafts may be carried out after the infection has resolved. We have successfully used such delayed bone grafting procedures for nonunion of long bones and for fusion of an unstable ankle.

MUSCLE TRANSPLANTATION

The muscle selected should have the following characteristics:

1. Single dominant, or major vascular pedicle[6]
2. Adequate muscle size to fill the bony defect
3. Minimal donor site functional and contour defect

The gracilis is the muscle of choice for coverage of a bony defect following sequestrectomy for distal lower extremity osteomyelitis. This muscle has a type II circulation[5]: single dominant pedicle (medial femoral circumflex artery and paired venae comitantes) and a minor pedicle, which is routinely divided without adverse effect on muscle circulation. Loss of function at the donor site is minimal, since the adductors longus and magnus muscles preserve function. The donor scar is located in the medial superior thigh. The muscle is transplanted without its overlying skin. This minimizes bulk at the recipient site and any deformity at the donor site from skin excision in the thigh.

The soft tissue defect in chronic osteomyelitis of the distal lower extremity is usually small. The purpose of the muscle flap is to fill the sequestrectomy site; thus a large muscle flap is rarely required. Usually the gracilis muscle is trimmed until just large enough to fill only the bony defect, avoiding excessive bulk at the recipient site.

The latissimus dorsi muscle is the preferred flap in (1) osteomyelitis of a large segment of the tibia (greater than 15 cm) or (2) a large soft tissue defect associated with an infected acute fracture site.

The latissimus dorsi has a type V circulation[5]: a single major vascular pedicle, the thoracodorsal artery, and veins entering adjacent to the muscle insertion. This pedicle will support the muscle when circulation is restored by microvascular techniques at the recipient site.

Like the gracilis, the latissimus muscle is used primarily to fill the bony defect and then tailored to avoid excessive bulk. For both gracilis and latissimus dorsi muscle transplants, skin grafts are placed over exposed muscle to complete coverage of the defect.

OPERATING TECHNIQUE

A two-team approach is used. The gracilis muscle is obtained from the opposite leg. The adductor longus is retracted and the medial femoral circumflex artery and paired venae comitantes are dissected to their junction with the profunda femoris artery and vein. At this level a pedicle length of 6 centimeters is obtained. The pedicle is not divided until the second team has completely prepared the recipient site.

The sequestrectomy is then performed under tourniquet control with a separate set of instruments to avoid contamination of the donor site. After bone debridement the recipient vessels are isolated in proximity to the wound.

An arteriogram is routinely obtained before surgery to locate a suitable recipient vessel. If either the anterior tibial or posterior tibial artery has been interrupted from prior leg trauma, the remaining normal vessel is used as the recipient. End-to-side arterial and venous anastomoses are used so that the distal circulation is not impaired. If a normal-appearing arterial stump is found near the defect, this artery may be used as the recipient. If both of the major distal vessels of the leg are damaged, vein grafts should be used to extend the pedicle far enough for anastomosis at a healthy site.

Our single failure resulted from an attempt to use abnormal recipient vessels near the site of sequestrectomy. When normal arterial and venous recipient vessels are identified, the tourniquet is deflated and hemostasis obtained. The vascular pedicle to the gracilis muscle is divided and then revascularized by anastomosis to the isolated recipient vessels. After circulation is restored to the muscle flap, the muscle is tailored to fit the sequestrectomy defect precisely. A closed suction system is placed beneath the muscle to ensure muscle adherence to the bone and to avoid seroma formation. Skin grafts are meshed and placed over the exposed muscle belly. The leg is immobilized with a plaster splint.

POSTOPERATIVE CARE

The patient is given dextran and aspirin for 5 days. The muscle is frequently examined for adequate color and capillary bleeding during the first 24 hours. If the circulation appears impaired, anesthetic is administered, an examination is performed, and if needed, revascularization is attempted.

Antibiotic therapy is maintained for 10 days (or longer if needed). Ambulation without weight-bearing on the involved extremity is started in 3 to 4 weeks. A compressive stocking, used to avoid flap edema, is continued for 3 months.

If bone stability is not in question, ambulation is allowed after 6 weeks. If further procedures are required, such as bone grafts for nonunion or ankle fusion, they are delayed until approximately 3 months.

CASE REPORT

Three patients with osteomyelitis following lower extremity trauma demonstrate the technique of gracilis muscle transplantation (Figs. 35-1 to 35-3). Although infection had persisted 5 (Fig. 35-1) to 35 (Fig. 35-2) years, bone union had remained stable. Symptoms of pain, chronic purulent drainage, and repeated episodes of cellulitis were noted by these patients, despite numerous surgical efforts at treatment.

Preoperative evaluation includes standard radiographs (Fig. 35-2, *B*) and arteriograms of the involved lower extremity (Fig. 35-2, *C*). Since the infection involves primarily bone, the skin defect is usually small (Figs. 35-1, *A* and *B*; 35-2, *A*; and 35-3, *A* and *B*). The gracilis muscle is correspondingly tailored to avoid excess muscle bulk (Figs. 35-1, *C*; 35-2, *D*; and 35-3, *C*). The pedicle of the muscle is anastomosed end to side to the recipient vessels (Fig. 35-2, *E*), and thus circulation to the distal leg and foot is not altered. Suction drains and careful suturing technique ensure that the muscle has close contact with the walls of the bony debridement site (Figs. 35-1, *D* and *E*, and 35-3, *D*). Skin grafts placed over the exposed muscle are meshed. The meshed skin adheres to the irregular surface of the muscle (Fig. 35-3, *E*).

In these patients, follow-up views taken at 2 years (Figs. 35-1, *F* and *G*, and 35-2, *F*) and 8 months (Figs. 35-3, *F* and *G*) demonstrate stable wound coverage. These patients are fully ambulatory and show no recurrence of infection. Moderate muscle atrophy ensures normal leg contour (Figs. 35-1, *F* and *G*; 35-2, *F*; and 35-3, *F* and *G*). Since the mesh graft is unexpanded, there is minimal skin irregularity. Postoperative radiographs (Fig. 35-1, *H*) show persistence of the bony defect, which is now filled with muscle. The bone does not regenerate in this area. The bone has remained stable in these patients despite aggressive debridement.

Text continued on p. 338.

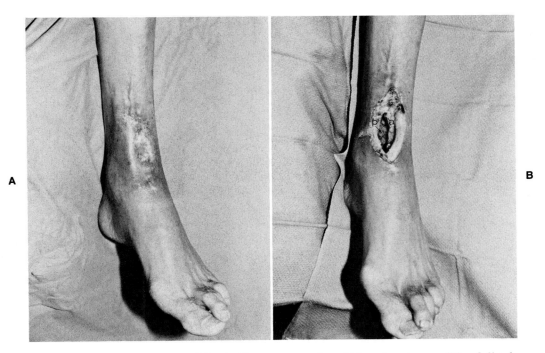

Fig. 35-1. Distal leg osteomyelitis. **A,** Sinus tract to site of chronic osteomyelitis of distal tibia. Twelve prior procedures over 24 years have failed to cure chronic infection. **B,** Defect following debridement of distal tibia. (*a* = anterior cortex, *p* = posterior cortex.) (**A** to **H** from Mathes, S.J., Alpert, B.S., and Chang, N.: Use of muscle flap in chronic osteomyelitis: experimental and clinical correlation. Plast. Reconstr. Surg. **69:**815, 1982.)

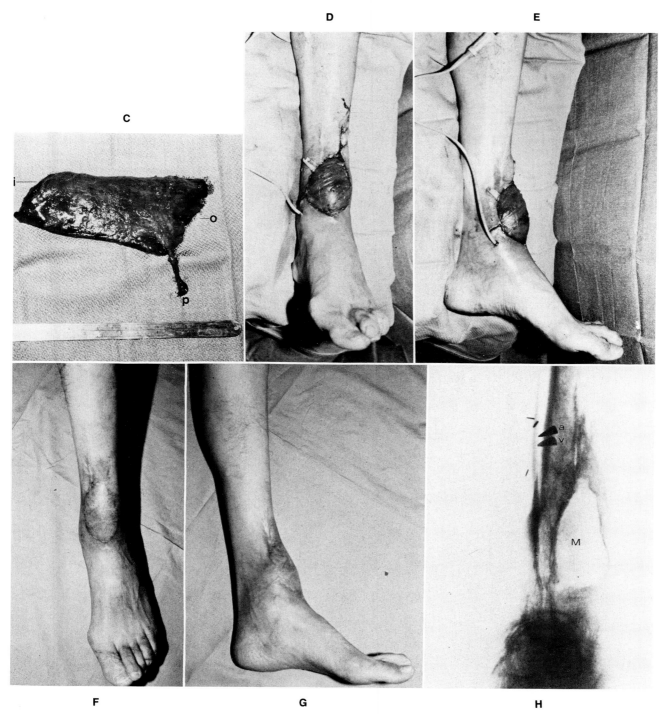

Fig. 35-1, cont'd. C, Gracilis muscle from opposite leg ready for transplantation to distal tibia bone defect. Note: muscle is tailored to fill defect with excision of muscle from origin (*o*) and insertion (*i*). (*p* = muscle vascular pedicle.) **D,** Muscle inset into bone defect. Exposed muscle covered with skin graft. **E,** Lateral view demonstrates muscle inset with minimal excess muscle bulk. **F,** Anterior postoperative view 2 years after muscle transplantation with no recurrence of infection. **G,** Lateral view. Stable wound coverage with adequate contour provided by muscle flap with skin grafts. **H,** Anterior radiograph 2 years after gracilis (*M*) transplantation. Bone does not replace muscle within bone cavity. Intact fibula and posterior tibia cortex provides bone stability.

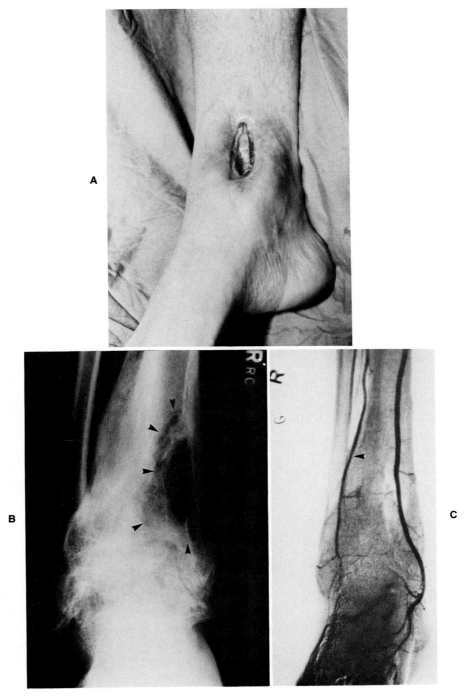

Fig. 35-2. Chronic osteomyelitis—distal tibia. **A,** Chronic osteomyelitis at site of prior open tibia fracture. Nine prior procedures over the last 35 years have failed to cure chronic infection. **B,** Radiograph of distal tibia demonstrates radiolucency *(arrows)* typical of bone defect associated with chronic osteomyelitis. **C,** Arteriogram demonstrates patency of both anterior and posterior tibial arteries at site of osteomyelitis. Anterior tibial artery and vein *(arrow)* are selected as recipient vessels for muscle flap transplantation. (**A** to **F** from Mathes, S., and Nahai, F.: Clinical applications for muscle and musculocutaneous flaps, St. Louis, 1982, The C.V. Mosby Co.)

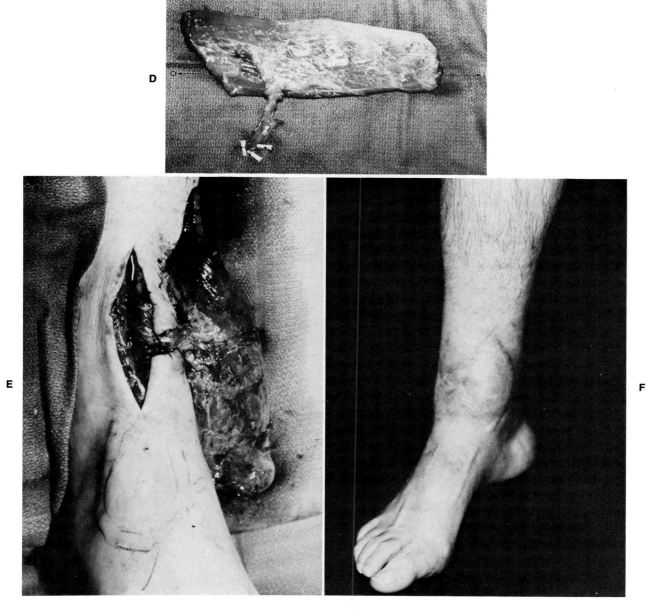

Fig. 35-2, cont'd. D, Gracilis muscle ready for transplantation. Muscle tailored to fill defect with excision of muscle from origin *(o)* and insertion *(i)*. (*a* = medial femoral circumflex artery, *v* = venae comitantes.) **E,** Gracilis vascularized by end-to-side anastomosis of medial femoral circumflex artery and venae comitantes with anterior tibial artery and vein. **F,** Lateral view of leg demonstrates stable wound coverage without recurrent infection 2 years after reconstructive surgery.

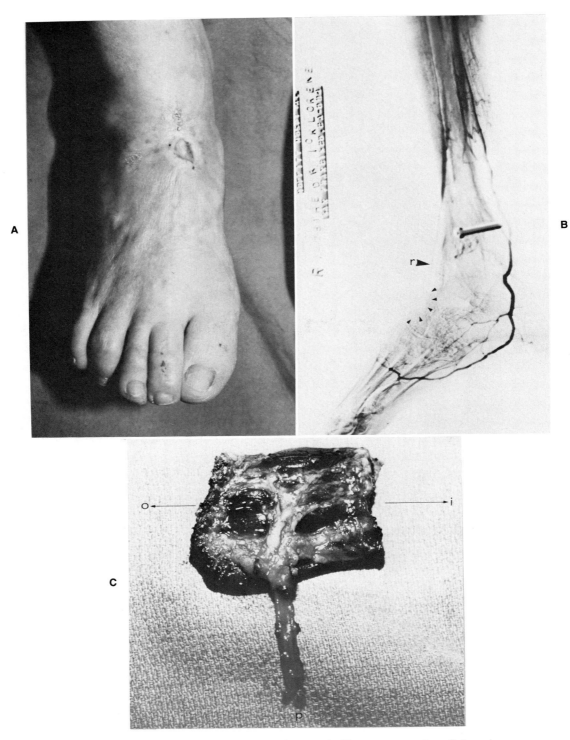

Fig. 35-3. Chronic osteomyelitis of tarsal bones. **A,** Sinus tract to site of chronic osteo-myelitis. Three prior procedures over 5 years have failed to cure this chronic infection. **B,** Arteriogram demonstrates interruption of anterior tibia artery at site of injury. Arrow *(r)* indicates proximal vessel normal and this site selected for recipient site. Small arrows denote site of bone infection. **C,** Gracilis muscle ready for transplantation. Majority of muscle excised from both origin *(o)* and insertion *(i)*, since bone defect is small. (*p* = muscle vascular pedicle.)

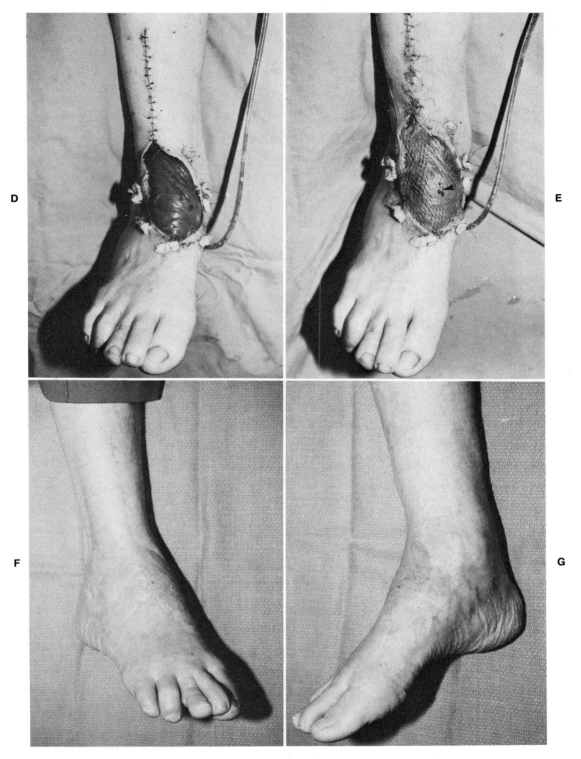

Fig. 35-3, cont'd. D, Muscle inset into site of bone debridement. **E,** Meshed skin grafts placed over exposed muscle. Note capillary bleeding at site of small incision with an 11 blade confirms intact muscle circulation. **F,** Eight months after muscle transplantation, with no recurrence of infection. **G,** Lateral view. Stable wound coverage with adequate contour provided by muscle flap with skin grafts.

RESULTS

In sixteen consecutive patients, the gracilis muscle has been successfully used for treatment of chronic osteomyelitis of the tibia and tarsal bone. In a recent review,[4] our initial eleven patients showed resolution of chronic bone infection with no relapse after follow-ups averaging 1.8 years. The patients were reevaluated 6 months after completion of this report. One patient required amputation of the involved extremity following vascular complications associated with an orthopedic reconstructive procedure to correct nonunion. Negative bone cultures were noted at the time of the amputation. The remaining patients are all ambulatory and have stable wound coverage. None have shown evidence of recurrent infection.

SUMMARY

Repeated sequestrectomy with muscle flap coverage of the defect should be considered for cases of chronic osteomyelitis in the lower extremity that have failed to respond to culture-specific antibiotic therapy and aggressive bone debridement. In the distal leg, ankle, or foot, local muscle flap transposition techniques are generally not possible. When local muscle flaps are either unavailable or inadequate in size to fill the sequestrectomy site, muscle transplantation is used in conjunciton with culture-specific antibiotic therapy.

REFERENCES

1. Byrd, H.S., Cierny, G. III, and Tebetts, J.B.: The management of open tibial fractures with associated soft tissue loss: external pin fixation with early flap coverage, Plast. Reconstr. Surg. **68**:73, 1981.
2. Chang, N., and Mathes, S.J.: Comparison of the effect of bacterial inoculation in musculocutaneous and random pattern flaps, Plast. Reconstr. Surg. **70**:1, 1982.
3. Ger, R.: Muscle transposition for treatment and prevention of chronic post-traumatic osteomyelitis of the tibia, J. Bone Joint Surg. **59A**:784, 1977.
4. Mathes, S.J., Alpert, B.S., and Chang, N.: Use of the muscle flap in chronic osteomyelitis: experimental and clinical correlations, Plast. Reconstr. Surg. **69**: 815, 1982.
5. Mathes, S.J., and Nahai, F.: Classification of the vascular anatomy of muscles: experimental and clinical correlation, Plast. Reconstr. Surg. **67**:177, 1981.
6. Mathes, S.J., Vasconez, L.O., and Jurkiewicz, M.J.: Extension and further application of muscle transposition, Plast. Reconstr. Surg. **60**:6, 1977.
7. Stark, W.J.: The use of pedicled muscle flaps in the surgical treatment of chronic osteomyelitis resulting from compound fractures, J. Bone Joint Surg. **28**: 343, 1946.
8. Vasconez, L.O., Bostwick, J. III, and McCraw, J.: Coverage of exposed bone by muscle transplantation and skin grafting, Plast. Reconstr. Surg. **53**:526, 1974.
9. Waldvogel, F.A., Medoff, G., and Swartz, M.N.: Osteomyelitis: a review of clinical features, therapeutic considerations and unusual aspects, Part II. N. Engl. J. Med. **282**:260, 1970.

Part XI

Peripheral nerves

Chapter 36

Microsurgery of peripheral nerves: selection for and timing of the operation

David G. Kline

Two critical factors in the management of peripheral nerve injuries are the selection of patients and the timing of surgery. Injury of a nerve sets cycles of degeneration and regeneration into motion. Wallerian degeneration occurs not only at the site of injury but also along a retrograde segment of the proximal stump. In addition, the entire distal nerve stump, the motor end plates ("distal inputs") and the muscle itself undergo degenerative changes over a period of days to months.[2] Restoration of function can only be brought about by successful initiation of nerve regeneration. Any nerve that is injured "incontinuity" will regenerate, and its axons will reach the distal stump; however, critical to success is the quality of this regeneration.[3,8] Frequent branching and/or endoneurial scar may diminish the caliber of the new axons and the quality of the myelin coating; in such cases function will not return even if the axons reach distal inputs. To encourage the regenerative process the surgeon must select the correct operation at the correct time and must know when to withhold surgery.[15]

SELECTION FOR OPERATION

First we must ask: is an operation necessary? Some nerve injuries improve spontaneously with skillful nonoperative management. The need for surgery will depend in part on whether or not the neurologic deficit is complete or incomplete and whether the deficit is serious.[6] Incomplete injuries with partial sensory loss tend to improve spontaneously, whereas complete injuries usually do not. Incomplete loss may take any of several forms.

Mild injury to the entire cross section of the nerve is a common form. Although the entire nerve is affected, the signs are limited to muscle weakness rather than paralysis and mild sensory loss, even in autonomous zones of the nerve. Function always improves with time unless there is compression or entrapment from formation of traumatic aneurysms, arteriovenous fistulae, excessive callus, or wound fibrosis.

Another form of incomplete loss is *injury to only part of the cross section of the nerve*. The neurologic loss may or may not be complete for the limited sector of injury. If the nerve deficit of this limited sector of nerve is severe and if recovery does not occur with time, a partial or "split" repair may be fruitful. If an incomplete injury of the median nerve involves the sensory fascicles, repair may be needed, even though the motor fascicles are intact. Incomplete lesions of either type may be associated with pain that does not respond to medical treatment yet that is not causalgic. Internal neurolysis or partial nerve repair may diminish the pain in such cases.

If there is complete loss of function distal to the injury, surgical exploration is usually indicated. If a nerve transection is discovered at exploration, nerve repair is mandatory. (The possibility that a transected human nerve will reunite or regenerate is remote.)

The possible gains from operation must be carefully weighed. Repair of a lower C8 or D1 root, a lower trunk, or a medial cord in the presence of neurologic signs suggesting a complete lesion is unlikely to yield improvement in an adult; however, it may be worthwhile in a child. Proximal, complete lesions of the peroneal nerve seldom recover, even in children. Repairs of the radial nerve, musculocutaneous nerve, or the tibial nerve have a better prognosis and should be given serious consideration. Also, the components of the brachial plexus or lumbosacral plexus that give rise to these three nerves may respond well to repairs. Even if prognosis for return of function is in doubt, exploration may still be warranted, since in experienced hands the risk of harm is small. The decision to operate for relief of pain requires complex judgment, since the results of this surgery are unpredictable.

TIMING OF OPERATION

The severity of the lesion and presence of continuity of the nerve are important factors in the selection and timing of an operation. Sharp injuries from knives, razors, and glass or metallic objects are likely to cause transection of the nerve; if the neurologic deficit is complete, early exploration and primary repair may be important. Unfortunately few prospective studies offer evidence to help with this decision.[5] We have used Seddon's[10] and Sunderland's[12] guidelines for primary repair in selected lesions. If a complete nerve deficit is associated with a sharp laceration, we promptly explore the wound. If the nerve is not completely divided (15% to 20% of cases), it will sometimes be contused, even after a sharp cut. If the bruising and hematoma with complete division are minimal and the epineurium has been divided in a sharp "neat" fashion, primary end-to-end epineurial suture repair is carried out. If the stumps are bruised or if the epineurium is ragged, the stumps are "tacked" to adjacent fascial planes at different levels to minimize retraction. At the time of delayed repair, 2 to 4 weeks later, the surgeon determines the extent of nerve resection that will yield healthy axons proximally and tubular structure with minimal scar distally. He resects and repairs accordingly. Our results with this approach are equal to our results with secondary repair.

Primary repair is particularly important in sharp, transecting injuries of the brachial plexus, the sciatic nerve, or the femoral nerve. When exploration is carried out promptly, the structures are easier to identify and appose accurately. The need for nerve grafts is diminished because the stumps have not yet retracted. However, primary repair must be reserved for the "neatly" divided nerve; efforts at suturing contused stumps will lead to failure.

Prompt exploration must also be considered for a nerve that is compressed by a traumatic aneurysm, an arteriovenous fistula, or a case in which progressive deficit is noted. Expeditious resection of the vascular mass can prevent a permanent deficit. Sometimes a hematoma can cause nerve compression in the shoulder, the popliteal area, or the subgluteal space, and immediate drainage is in order. Brachial artery spasm can cause ischemia and infarction of volar forearm musculature with compression and palsies of the median, ulnar, and even the radial nerve; in the leg, anterior compartment swelling can lead to a peroneal nerve palsy. Fasciotomy in such cases will decrease intratissue pressure, and neurolysis will sometimes minimize secondary nerve compression and prevent a Volkmann's contracture or anterior compartment syndrome.

Since most serious injuries leave the nerves in-continuity with a mixture of types of injury, exploration is usually delayed for several months. Typical situations would be gunshot wounds, fractures, contusions, or even surgical mishaps. Delay for several months will permit spontaneous recovery of the neuropraxic elements; elements of axonotmesis will have time to regenerate, and areas of neurotmesis will have time to become evident. Assessment of these elements is facilitated by intraoperative stimulation and recording.[3,5,8] If loss is complete or severe and if signs of clinical or electrical recovery are not seen in 2 to 3 months, then exploration is in order. With severe contusive, stretching injuries, the nerve lesion may be lengthy, and further delay (4 months) from the time of injury may be needed for spontaneous regeneration. Both stimulation and stimulation-recording techniques are necessary for intraoperative assessment of the lesion in-continuity, whether it is focal or lengthy (as a result of stretch).

OPERATING TECHNIQUE

Good surgical exposure permits accurate anatomic identification of the injured areas.[4] Proper positioning of the patient facilitates the surgical approach and affords relaxation of the nerves if necessary. Limbs must be draped out in full view to allow for observation of any limb movements; $2.5\times$ to $3.5\times$ surgical loupes are used for surgery on most peripheral nerves. The operating microscope is used for digital nerve repairs, for some cranial nerve repairs, and for internal neurolysis and split nerve repairs (where a portion of the fascicular structure is spared and a portion is repaired by suture or grafts. Dissection progresses from areas of normal tissues toward the area of injury. Adjacent major vessels such as the axillary or brachial artery and vein are freed up and retracted to gain exposure.

Lesions not in-continuity

After a period of delay, stumps of nerves *not* in-continuity will form a proximal neuroma and a distal glioma. These nerves are the last to be freed from the surrounding soft tissue. The stumps are then gently pulled together to determine the need for further mobilization, for sacrifice of unimportant branches, or for nerve transposition (Fig. 36-1).

The stumps are then sectioned back to healthy neural tissue proximally and to healthy fascicular structure distally (Fig. 36-2). A pair of lateral epineurial sutures are then preplaced, tied simultaneously, and used as stay sutures. The ends of the stumps are gently placed in accurate apposition. Then epineurial interrupted sutures are placed at close intervals on the upper surface of the nerve. Major bundles and fascicular groups are oriented

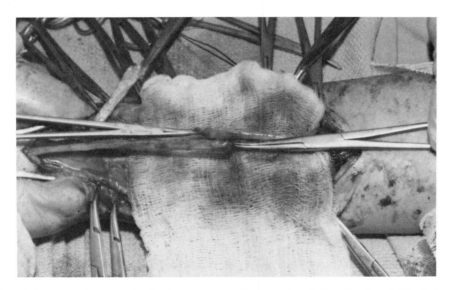

Fig. 36-1. Secondary repair of ulnar nerve at forearm level. Proximal and distal stumps have been mobilized and are placed on gentle traction by hemostats grasping stumps before they are trimmed back to healthy neural tissue. This provides an estimate of whether or not end-to-end repair without the use of grafts is possible.

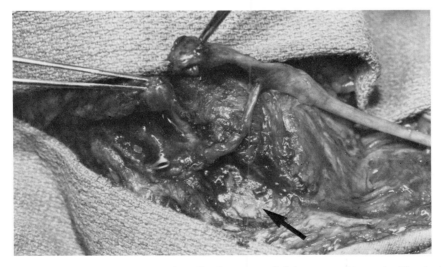

Fig. 36-2. Peroneal nerve transection distal to superficial peroneal branch. Head of the fibula has been rongeured down *(arrow)*, preliminary to an end-to-end repair. Stumps are ready to be sectioned back to healthy tissue.

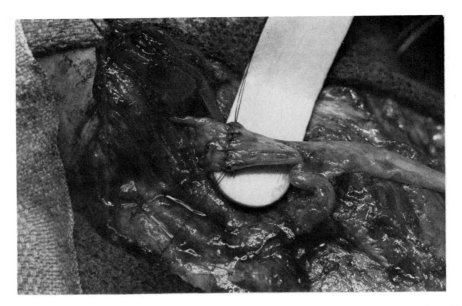

Fig. 36-3. End-to-end repair of transected peroneal nerve. Some attempt was made to line up the major bundles of fascicles as the epineurial sutures were placed, almost giving the appearance of a fascicular repair.

and aligned, and with the help of the stay sutures, the posterior wall is rotated for repair.

The repair site is then gently rolled and palpated between thumb and forefinger and the suture line is given a final inspection to confirm its integrity. The repair site is placed in an area as free of scar as possible. We do not use wrappers or cuffs around the repair, nor have we had experience with cuffs of epineurium, pull-out sutures, and so forth.[1,11]

In primary repair of a transected nerve, less mobilization is needed to gain length. Sharp transection of the stumps is carried out, cleanly trimming any ragged edges of epineurium. Some resection of contused and hemorrhagic tissue from both stumps is usually necessary. Bundles and fascicular groups are carefully aligned and repaired with epineural sutures (Fig. 36-3).

Lesions in-continuity

The neuroma in-continuity is exposed with meticulous, sharp dissection and then is inspected and gently palpated.[16] The nerve is stimulated above and below the lesion to see if musculature distal to it will contract.[8] Such contraction suggests that functional regeneration is progressing through the lesion, and it may antedate voluntary contraction return by as much as 6 weeks. Care must be taken not to misinterpret muscle contraction from stimulation of nerve branches proximal to the lesion.

Stimulus is conducted through the tips of bipolar electrodes made of No. 18 stainless steel or platinum alloy. The electrodes are bent in the shape of a shepherd's crook to cradle the nerve. They are placed 1 to 2 cm apart. Stimulus output is provided by a Grass stimulator, which can be adjusted to vary the voltage, duration, and frequency of the stimuli. A stimulus isolation unit is used to reduce the chance of producing a ground loop between patient and equipment.

The nerve action potential (NAP) is then recorded. Similar bipolar electrodes are used for stimulation and recording; the recording is accomplished by a preamplifier and oscilloscope. It is best to elevate the portions of the nerve to be stimulated from the field.[5,13] The stimulus device and the recording apparatus are first tested on intact proximal nerve branches. Then the nerve to be tested is elevated from the field and the electrodes are applied. A short duration (0.02 to 0.08 msec) stimulus is used with a relatively high voltage. Stimuli of longer duration tend to cause artifacts that can interfere with evoked NAPs. Amplification is usually between 50 μv and 0.5 mv per division with filters set within the range of 3.0 and 0.1. Once a proximal potential is obtained, recording electrodes are moved through the lesion in-continuity. Then amplification is increased and the distal stump is searched for a NAP (Fig. 36-4). If a NAP is present, it indicates that adequate nerve regeneration is underway; thus total resection is not needed and

Ulnar nerve—upper arm 3 months after injection injury

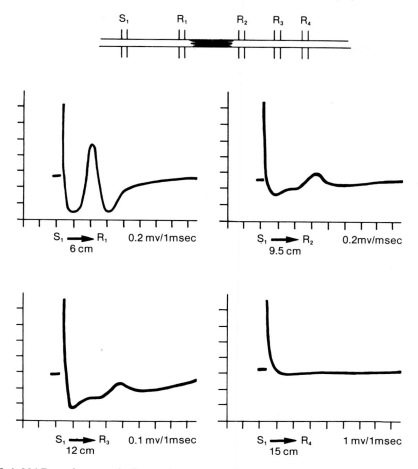

Fig. 36-4. NAP tracings made from ulnar nerve of a patient who received an injection in the right ulnar nerve at upper arm level 3 months before. Despite complete ulnar deficit clinically and electrically, the nerve was regenerating, and as can be seen by these tracings, a NAP could be traced to 12 cm but not 15 cm distal to the stimulation site. As a result only an external neurolysis was done, and the patient has made an acceptable recovery over the last 2 years.

neurolysis will suffice. An external neurolysis is usually chosen, removing scar from the epineurium but *not* splitting the region of injury into individual fascicles or bundles (Fig. 36-5). Over 90% of cases having a NAP 2 or more months after injury will regain significant function with only a neurolysis. If after 2 months or more a NAP is not recorded, then resection of the lesion in-continuity is planned. We preplace two lateral orientation sutures proximally and two distally. These are looped around on either side of the lesion, and as resection is carried out, realignment is retained. The site of suture placement is judged by inspection and gentle palpation of the neuroma. If the extent of damage has been misjudged and resec-

tion is inadequate, the sutures are simply replaced and further resection is carried out. After verifying that healthy fascicular structures have been gained proximally and distally, we tie the preplaced lateral sutures so that the stumps gently oppose one another. Then interrupted epineurial sutures are closely placed both anteriorly and posteriorly.

If repair without tension is not possible after efforts at mobilization, limb flexion, and nerve transposition, grafts will be necessary. End-to-end repair is superior *if* it can be done without tension.[4] Interfascicular sural grafts are effective if they are properly placed and relatively short in length. For the last 8 years we have been using

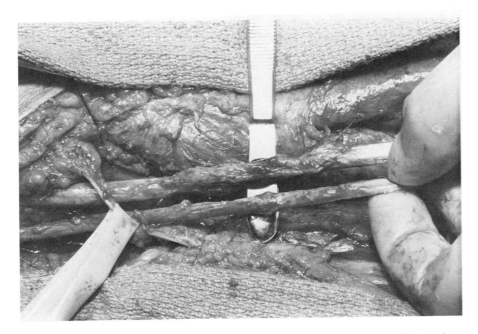

Fig. 36-5. Gunshot injury to midthigh sciatic nerve. Nerve has been split into its two divisions and each individually evaluated by stimulation and stimulation-and-recording studies. A NAP could be recorded across the peroneal injury but not through the tibial injury.

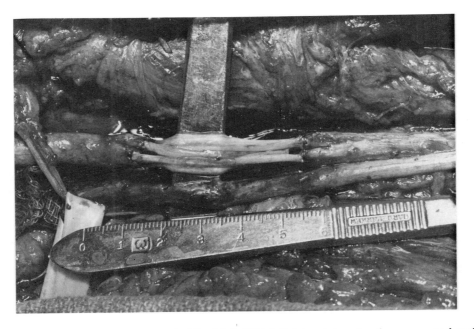

Fig. 36-6. Sciatic complex shown in Fig. 36-5. Tibial division injury has been resected and sural interfascicular grafts have been used to span the gap created since end-to-end repair was not feasible. Only an external neurolysis was done to the peroneal division.

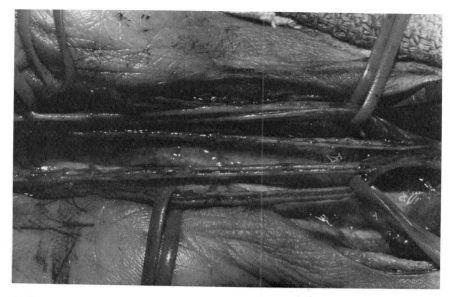

Fig. 36-7. Internal neurolysis on median nerve at palmar level. Nerve had been previously injured during carpal tunnel release, and the patient, although having acceptable function, had severe pain with hyperesthesia and hyperpathia in the median distribution. Some, but not complete, relief of the pain was gained by the internal neurolysis.

grafts whenever there is any question about maintaining an end-to-end repair.[7] Major fascicles or fascicular groupings are exposed on both the proximal and distal stumps, and the ends of the sural grafts are placed in opposition by one or two sutures,[7,9] aligning grafts and fasciculi groups with accuracy. Grafts should be longer than the gap so that they are under no tension at all (Fig. 36-6). To harvest the sural nerve graft we usually use a mildly curvilinear vertical incision. The incision begins just superior and lateral to the lateral malleolus and extends up along the lateral part of the Achilles tendon; it then curves medially to reach the midposterior calf region. If there is any question about distinguishing the sural nerve from its neighboring vessels, a NAP recording will settle the issue.

Occasionally a NAP will be recorded, even though on inspection and palpation it is obvious that at least a portion of the cross section of the nerve is severely damaged. Any functioning fasciculi can be identified by separating the nerve into its components and recording each group individually.[13,14] If some fascicular groups conduct evoked NAPs and some do not, a split repair is done. Fasciculi that do not conduct are resected and are replaced with sural or antebrachial cutaneous nerve grafts; fasciculi that do conduct receive only external neurolysis. Internal neurolysis is usually reserved for the lesion that causes severe noncausal-

gic pain and that does not respond to sympathetic blocks or analgesics (Fig. 36-7). Careful, internal neurolysis under magnification is then sometimes of value. It is best to first separate the major fascicles or bundles of small fascicles in normal tissue proximal and distal to the injury site. Then they are dissected and traced through the injury site itself.

SUMMARY OF OPERATIONS
Sharp soft tissue lacerations with severe distal deficit

1. The mechanism of the injury usually results from a knife, razor blade, or occasionally glass.
2. If the nerve has been transected in a neat fashion with "tidy" epineurium, a primary repair may be of value.
3. If the stumps are contused and the epineurium is ragged, a secondary repair at 2 to 4 weeks is best. The stumps should be tacked down to adjacent but separate fascial levels to maintain length.
4. In 15% to 20% of cases, neural elements will still have gross continuity as a result of either partial transection or contusion. Such an injury is best evaluated at 8 weeks, when the presence or absence of regeneration can be documented by intraoperative electrical studies and either split repair or neurolysis can be done.
5. Primary repair is especially indicated for prox-

imal injuries to brachial plexus elements and sciatic and femoral nerves.

Blunt soft tissue lacerations with severe distal deficit

1. The mechanism of the injury usually results from metal, animal bite, chainsaw, or occasionally glass.
2. The stumps are usually contused, and transection of the epineurium is ragged. Delayed repair (2 to 4 weeks) is best so that resection to healthy tissue is ensured. If visualized acutely, the stumps should be tacked to separate fascial levels to maintain length.
3. Such injuries are more likely to have lesions incontinuity than sharp lesions (20% to 30% of cases) and here delayed exploration (8 weeks) is best so that electrical studies as well as inspection can determine the need for resection.
4. Partially divided elements may need split graft repair providing the portion in-continuity has electrical evidence of function and/or regeneration.

Gunshot wounds and focal contusions caused by fractures with severe distal deficit

1. A baseline clinical evaluation of the entire limb is carried out.
2. An acute operation is indicated for vascular injury, including an aneurysm or arteriovenous fistula complicating neural injury, some bone injuries, and an occasional patient with severe pain and a shell fragment or other foreign body embedded in nerve.
3. A baseline electromyogram is done at about 3 weeks.
4. Clinical and electrical follow-up including physical therapy is carried out over the next 2 to 3 months. If function does not improve clinically or electrically, exploration is done.
5. The surgeon should be prepared to evaluate the lesion in-continuity by both stimulation and stimulation and recording (NAP) studies.
6. If there is no electrical evidence of regeneration, resection and either end-to-end suture or graft repair is indicated.

Initial management of stretch injuries with severe distal deficit

1. A baseline clinical evaluation is done. With brachial plexus injuries, Horner's syndrome, winging of the scapula or other proximal paralysis, and vertebral column or even spinal cord injury should be checked for. Vascular injury is less likely than with gunshot wounds, but can occur.
2. Myelography is indicated for brachial and pelvic stretch injuries once blood is cleared from the cerebrospinal fluid.
3. A baseline electromyogram is done at about 3 weeks. Brachial plexus injuries should also have sensory NAP studies done.
4. Clinical and electrical follow-up including physical therapy is carried out over the next 4 months. If function does not improve clinically or electrically, then exploration *may* be indicated for some cases (see below).
5. Some distal stretch palsies or those partial to each element may improve with time. Those complete to one or more elements are less likely to improve.

Operative management of stretch injuries

1. Effective repair may not be possible and thus exploration is not indicated in these instances:
   A. In the presence of signs of proximal paralysis such as paraspinal and/or rhomboid denervation, and in brachial plexus injuries, winging of the scapula, paralysis of diaphragm, or total pectoralis palsy.
   B. In the presence of meningoceles at multiple levels. This is a relative contraindication, since a meningocele or failure to fill a root sleeve does not absolutely preclude repair at other levels without such change, even though their presence stands against it. In a few instances, even roots with such myelographic changes can regenerate spontaneously or be successfully repaired.
   C. Horner's syndrome stands against successful repair of lower plexus roots.
   D. Sensory NAPs recorded from multiple peripheral nerves indicates preganglionic lesions, but the absence of sensory NAPs does not preclude it.
2. Most repairable plexus elements will still be in-continuity, whereas distal stretches to nerves such as peroneal may not have continuity.
3. Electrical evaluation of in-continuity but stretch-injured elements is important, since 20% to 25% will be regenerating despite total distal deficit and can be proven by 4 months.
4. Despite proper screening and selection of brachial plexus stretch injuries for operation, some elements will still not be reparable because of the proximal extent of damage to roots or excessive length of injury.

REFERENCES

1. Braun, R.M.: Epineurial nerve repair. In Omer, G., and Spinner, M., editors: Management of peripheral nerve problems, Philadelphia, 1980, W.B. Saunders Co., p. 366.
2. Guttmann, E., and Young, J.Z.: Reinnervation of muscle after various periods of atrophy, J. Anat. **78:** 15, 1944.
3. Hudson, A., and Hunter, D.: Timing of peripheral nerve repairs: important local neuropathological factors, Clin. Neurosurg. 24:391, 1977.
4. Kline, D.G.: Macroscopic and microscopic concomitants of nerve repair, Clin. Neurosurg. 26:582, 1979.
5. Kline, D.G.: Timing for exploration of nerve lesions and evaluation of the neuroma in continuity, Clin. Orthop. **163:**42, 1982.
6. Kline, D.G., and Judice, D.: Operative management of selected brachial plexus lesions, J. Neurosurg. **58:** 631, 1983.
7. Millesi, H., Meissl, G., and Berger, A.: Further experience with interfascicular grafting of median, ulnar and radial nerves, J. Bone Joint Surg. **58B:**209, 1976.
8. Nulsen, F.E., and Kline, D.G.: Acute injuries of peripheral nerves. In Youmans, J.R., editor: Neurological surgery, Vol. 2, Philadelphia, 1973, W.B. Saunders Co., p. 1089.
9. Samii, M.: Modern aspects of peripheral and cranial nerve surgery. In Advances and technical standards, New York, 1975, Springer-Verlag.
10. Seddon, H.: Surgical disorders of peripheral nerves, Baltimore, 1972, The Williams & Wilkins Co.
11. Snyder, C.C., et al.: Intraneural neurorrhaphy: a preliminary clinical and histological evaluation, Ann. Surg. **167:**691, 1968.
12. Sunderland, S.: Nerves and nerve injuries, Edinburgh, 1972, Churchill-Livingstone.
13. Terzis, J.K., Dykes, R.W., and Hakstian, R.W.: Electrophysiologic recordings in peripheral nerve surgery: a review, J. Hand Surg. **1:**52, 1976.
14. Williams, H.G., and Terzis, J.: Single fascicular recording: an intraoperative diagnostic tool for the management of peripheral nerve lesions, Plast. Reconstr. Surg. **57:**562, 1976.
15. Woodhall, B., and Beebe, G.: Peripheral nerve regeneration, V.A. Medical Monograph, Washington, D.C., 1957, U.S. Government Printing Office.
16. Zachary, R.B., and Roaf, R.: Lesions in continuity. In Seddon, H.J., editor: Peripheral nerve injuries, London, 1954, Her Majesty's Stationery Office, Medical Research Council Special Report Series #282.

Part XII

Lymphatics

Chapter 37

Microsurgery of peripheral nerves: neurolyses, nerve grafts, brachial plexus injuries

Hanno Millesi

In March 1971 I had the opportunity to present my personal thoughts on the management of peripheral nerve lesions and my experience with nerve grafts, performed by microsurgical techniques, at the annual meeting of the American Society for Surgery of the Hand in San Francisco.

Microsurgery of peripheral nerves was introduced by Smith[76] and Kurze[39] and further developed by Millesi et al.[48,55] Other authors regarded this technique as unrewarding.[5,20] At the same meeting in San Francisco, Ashworth[1] still favored mobilization of the nerves and acceptance of some tension to achieve an end-to-end repair in large defects. Though success with nerve grafts had been reported previously,[6,7,72] this procedure seemed to elicit little confidence at that time.[62,78,80]

Thirteen years have passed. What has developed during these years? What is our position now?

MICROSURGICAL TECHNIQUE

Microsurgery has now been well accepted, and today advanced peripheral nerve surgery without a microscope and microsurgical technique can scarcely be imagined. Current debate centers on the use of only a few sutures to approximate fascicles or fascicle groups, relying on natural fibrin clotting for coaptation, versus the use of several sutures per fascicle.[28] Foucher et al.[24] concluded that the result is inversely proportional to the number of stitches. It is evident that if some tension is accepted, more sutures have to be used. It is also evident that we should reduce surgical trauma to a minimum. Since these goals conflict, the surgeon must accept a compromise.

TENSION AT THE SITE OF COAPTATION

It is now well established that tension beyond a certain limit affects nerve regeneration unfavorably.[50,54,57,60,61] If one plots tension on the repair against size of the defect, the correlation between an increase in tension with an increase in the gap in the nerve is striking (Fig. 37-1). Rushworth et al.[64] are the only ones who feel that tension has a favorable effect on nerve regeneration. Their data do not support their conclusion. The level at which tension is detrimental might vary in different species and even in different individuals. Some tension can be accepted if the surgeon uses a proper technique. This means that the surgeon accepts some tension at the expense of increased surgical trauma (more sutures). Beyond a certain level the adverse effect of tension becomes more and more evident. This relationship is particularly important when nerve grafts are used.

NERVE GRAFTING

The use of nerve grafts to bridge a nerve defect has advantages and disadvantages. The most important advantage is that the two nerve repairs, proximal and distal, can be performed under ideal conditions, avoiding tension completely. The most important disadvantage is that regenerating axons have to cross two coaptation sites. For this reason nerve grafts have been regarded as inferior to an

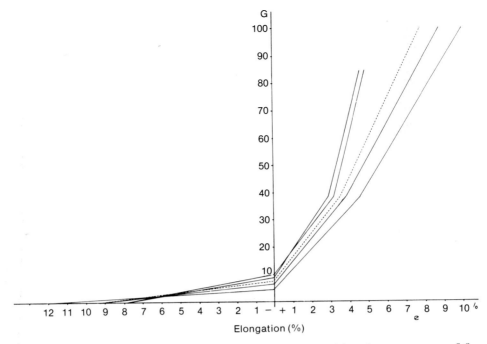

Fig. 37-1. Relation between force (vertical in *G*) and stretching (in percentage of free length) of the extrapelvic sciatic nerve of the rabbit. After transection the two stumps retracted, creating a gap of between 8% and 12% of the free length of the nerve between its exit from the pelvis and its division (left side). A force of between 6 and 10 g was necessary to reunite the two stumps. With an increasing amount of resection, the two stumps had to be stretched to be brought into contact again, because an increasing amount of force had to be applied to achieve this. With a resection of more than 3% to 5%, the force rose rapidly.

end-to-end nerve repair, which is the case if nerve grafts are compared to end-to-end neurorrhaphy in operations performed under ideal conditions. However, it was surprising for us to see that if nerve grafts are performed under ideal conditions, the results can be close to that of end-to-end nerve repairs and are better than end-to-end neurorrhaphies performed under tension.*

Bratton et al.[4] compared nerve grafts with end-to-end nerve repairs without tension to those under slight tension and showed that the nerve grafts were not significantly worse than simple neurorrhaphies. Recovery was slower, but in the final analysis the results were more or less the same. Our experience shows that beyond a certain point of increase in tension, nerve grafts are better than simple repairs. Bratton's experiments were not performed under ideal conditions. In some[34,35] the middle portions of the grafts were compromised by the technique used and they became partially fibrotic; in others[44] the nerve grafts did no better

than neurorrhaphies, but viewed from the opposite standpoint, the nerve grafts did not yield worse results than end-to-end nerve repair.

As far as clinical results are concerned, many papers have been published that support the value of nerve grafts.* Young[88] had only partial success with nerve grafts; he immobilized the extremities with nerve grafts for 72 hours only, and this apparently is not long enough. Martini and Zellner[42] reported unfavorable experience with nerve grafts.

Summary

Nerve grafts are now in widespread use and are of proven value. There are still many unanswered questions, which are discussed next.

NEUROLYSIS

If there is a lesion in-continuity, the chance of spontaneous recovery depends on the amount of damage the nerve tissue has suffered. The classifi-

---

*References 50, 54, 57, 60, 72, 83.

*References 9, 26, 29, 30, 48, 51, 52, 57, 59, 65, 66, 67, 74, 75, 81, 87.

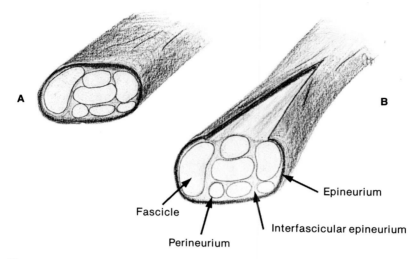

Fig. 37-2. A, Compression by fibrotic epifascicular epineurium. **B,** Relieved by epifascicular epineurotomy.

cation systems of Seddon[70] and Sunderland[79] are well known. Both systems start with the conduction block without morphologic changes (neurapraxia, first degree) and damage of the axons only (axonotmesis, second degree lesion). In Seddon's classification the only alternative to these two types of lesion is neurotmesis. Sunderland differentiates more exactly. A third degree lesion would be a loss of continuity of the nerve fibers inside an intact perineurium. In a fourth degree lesion the perineurium has also suffered, and continuity is preserved by epineurial tissue. The fifth degree lesion defines a complete loss of continuity.

These schemes suggest that the tissue is more sensitive to trauma and reaction from the center to the periphery. In a third degree lesion it is not clear whether the endoneural space has become fibrotic or not or whether the epineural tissue is reactive also. In a fourth degree lesion with the fascicular structure destroyed, it remains unclear whether the epineural tissue is the last intact structure or whether it has also suffered severe damage and continuity is preserved by fibrotic tissue only.

Morphologically a peripheral nerve is designed for optimal protection of its axons. It is true that a conduction block can develop without any morphologic response of other tissues and that axonolysis with wallerian degeneration can occur without involvement of the endoneural connective tissue, the perineurium, or the epineurium. On the other hand, the epineurium readily reacts with fi-

brosis to either trauma or chronic irritation. Such a fibrosis can occur without damage to the perineurium or the intrafascicular structures. It seems that the more superficial layers of the epineurium react more readily and more severely.

Sometimes one encounters fibrosis of the circumferential layers of the epineurium (that is, epifascicular epineurium), which constricts the nerve like a tight stocking (Fig. 37-2). The perineurium and the fascicular structures are intact. The nerve fibers may have suffered a first or second degree lesion, which should regenerate spontaneously but does not do so because of increased pressure within the nerve. In such a case transection of the tight circumferential layer of the epineurium solves the problem *(epifascicular epineurotomy)*. In such a case, if the nerve fibers have sustained a first degree lesion without axonolysis, function might return within a few days of surgery. If the nerve fibers have sustained a second degree lesion with axonolysis, the functional return would take much longer because of wallerian degeneration.

Sometimes the fibrosis of the circumferential epineurium extends somewhat inward, between the groups of fascicles (Fig. 37-3). Here epineurotomy does not provide adequate decompression, and it is necessary to resect part or all of the epifascicular epineurium *(epifascicular epineurectomy)*.

If a greater part of the interfascicular epineurium has become fibrotic, an interfascicular dissection has to be performed to decompress fascicle

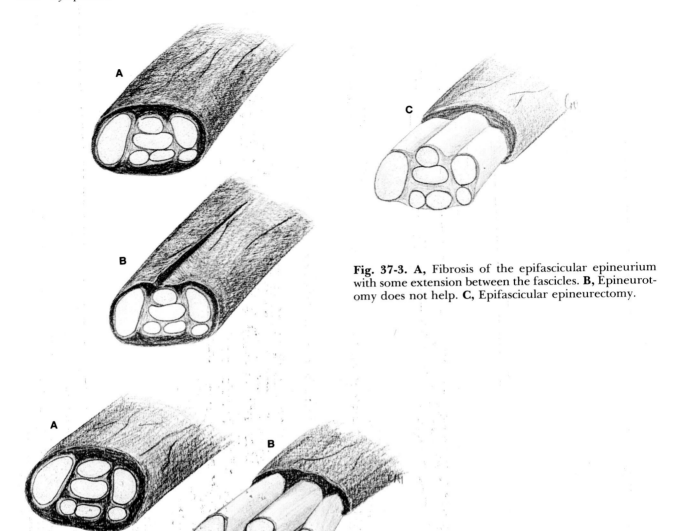

Fig. 37-3. A, Fibrosis of the epifascicular epineurium with some extension between the fascicles. **B,** Epineurotomy does not help. **C,** Epifascicular epineurectomy.

Fig. 37-4. A, Fibrosis of epifascicular and interfascicular epineurium. **B,** Epifascicular and interfascicular (partial) epineurectomy.

groups or larger fascicles (Fig. 37-4). In this case there is, of course, a danger of inadvertently dividing connecting fibers between fascicle groups and injuring vessels within the interfascicular spaces; but these vessels would have been damaged already from the process that caused the fibrosis. An *interfascicular epineurectomy* is always incomplete because it is impossible to excise this tissue completely. Usually the interfascicular epineurium within the fascicle groups remains intact.

If all the endoneural tissue has sustained severe damage and has become fibrotic, the nerve will have been so badly damaged that neurolysis alone will not provide return of function (Fig. 37-5). All

of these different degrees of damage have to be labeled as third degree lesions because of the intact perineurium and the intact fascicular structure. As long as the intrafascicular tissue has not been damaged (except for conduction block or axonolysis with wallerian degeneration), there is a good chance for nerve regeneration if decompression of the fascicles is achieved with neurolysis. However, if the substance of the fascicles has become fibrotic as well, the prospects are poor and resection is the better solution. The chances of spontaneous recovery are nil if the fascicular pattern has been lost and continuity is preserved only by amorphous connective tissue (fourth degree lesion). In this sit-

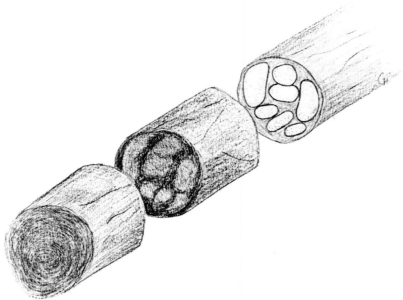

Fig. 37-5. Fibrosis of the whole nerve segment, including perineurium and endoneurium. Resection and restoration of continuity by nerve grafts is indicated.

uation resection and nerve grafting are the treatment of choice.

Before the development of microsurgery, internal neurolysis was generally rejected.[73] Curtis and Eversman[16] could prove that return of function after carpal tunnel release occurred in a high percentage of cases if internal neurolysis was performed. With the use of a meticulous technique under optical magnification, the surgical trauma was appreciably reduced. The advocates of internal neurolysis feel that they can operate within the nerve without eliciting a detrimental amount of tissue reaction. In recent years some objections to internal neurolysis have been put forth: (1) that the effect of the neurolysis will be nullified by the effect of the postoperative fibrosis, (2) that links between fascicles within and outside the fascicle groups are transected, (3) that small neuromas may be formed, causing hyperesthesia, and (4) that the blood supply of the fascicular tissue may be endangered if the neurolysis proceeds over a long distance. These arguments have limited validity. Internal neurolysis is a step-wise procedure. If the fascicles bulge out, showing that the goal—decompression—has been achieved, dissection is discontinued immediately. It is an error to proceed until each individual fascicle is naked. Even in interfascicular epineurectomy, the fascicles of individual groups will remain connected, sparing the vessels that run within the fascicle groups. When an ex-

tended interfascicular epineurectomy is performed, it is done only because of extensive damage, and the next step would be resection with restoration of continuity.

Usually a nerve trunk is not damaged uniformly but rather shows areas of greater damage and, elsewhere, areas of lesser damage. This situation can be identified only by internal neurolysis. In the past the alternatives for a lesion in-continuity have been to perform external neurolysis or to resect. Intraoperative electrostimulation is a source of data for such a decision.[35,37] It is questionable, however, whether these data are valid for the whole cross section. With microsurgical intraneural neurolysis one can decompress the individual fascicle groups and study each of them independently by inspection, palpation, and electric stimulation.[86]

After performing internal neurolysis one must provide an optimal soft tissue bed and an optimal soft tissue cover for the exposed nerve by plastic surgical maneuvers to minimize the potential of postoperative constriction.

Summary

Internal neurolysis, performed by the use of microsurgical techniques, has a secure position in the surgery of peripheral nerves. Dissection must not be excessive and it must be performed as a step-wise procedure.

TIMING

The choice of primary or early secondary repair of peripheral nerves has been a perpetual source of controversy. Because of the variety of lesions and the complexity of the factors influencing nerve regeneration, there is no single answer to this question. The introduction of microsurgery has not resolved the debate. If wallerian degeneration could be avoided by immediate repair as suggested by Schiff,[69] primary surgery would be mandatory, but this is not so. With a single exception,[22] all researchers agree that wallerian degeneration cannot be avoided in mammals, and immediate repair offers no advantage as far as nerve regeneration is concerned. The advantage of a primary repair is a topographic one; minute anatomic landmarks are readily identified, and scarring and retraction are absent. The distal stump is still excitable for identification of motor fibers. Staining techniques can be applied at the distal stump for the same reason. Time is gained; only one operation is necessary. In a clean transection without any complicating injuries, primary repair is clearly indicated if qualified surgeons, modern equipment, and sufficient time are available. Under these circumstances primary nerve repair is performed in connection with global repair of the whole injury, as a primary or delayed primary procedure.[47]

Early secondary or delayed primary repair has the disadvantages of lost time, two operations, scarring, retracted nerve stumps, and the loss of guidance by electric stimulation and axon staining at the distal stump. On the other hand, the neuronal response has its peak in the third week.[17,18] McQuarrie[45] demonstrated that a second cut of a nerve stump initiates a higher number of axon sprouts compared to the first cut. More accurate differentiation between damaged and undamaged parts is possible because of the visible incipient fibrosis of the damaged portions of the nerve stumps.

In primary repair, even with optic magnification, it is impossible to distinguish between damaged tissue (which will become fibrotic) and undamaged tissue (which will become the initial site of regeneration). Therefore, in cases of primary repair, there is sometimes failure to resect all of the damaged tissue. This factor is unimportant in clean transections, but in lacerations it can play a decisive role. The retraction of nerve stumps and the loss of elasticity may increase the difficulty in obtaining end-to-end coaptation of the nerve stumps. This was regarded as one of the major disadvantages of early secondary nerve repair. However, this argument is no longer valid, since by microsurgical grafting techniques, the results of nerve grafts are very close to end-to-end coaptations. The fact remains, however, that in secondary repairs grafts are more frequently indicated than they are in primary repairs. An enormous advantage of the early secondary nerve repair is that the operation can be performed under optimal conditions as far as personnel, equipment, and time are concerned.

Summary

In clean transections, primary nerve repair should be performed if optimal conditions are present. These cases have to be followed by the surgeon to be sure that failures can be recognized in time—that is, before 6 months elapse—to give them a second chance. In the presence of nerve gaps or complicating injuries, late primary or early secondary repairs are recommended.

OPTIMAL TECHNIQUE FOR END-TO-END NEURORRHAPHY

Whether epineural or perineural suture achieves the best result is still a point of discussion. Bora[2] supported the perineural suture. Hakstian[31] attempted to achieve fascicular coaptation by temporary intrafascicular stitches; this technique did not yield satisfactory results.[7,8] Tupper[85] attempted to isolate each individual fascicle in nerve stumps containing many fascicles to perform a fascicular repair. During recent years Bora et al.[3] are again favoring epineural nerve repair, as are Cabaud et al.[14] The survey of recent publications is confusing; it suggests that early expectations from microsurgical end-to-end nerve repair have not been met, and surgeons have returned to conventional epineural nerve repairs. In truth, the problem has been oversimplified. Epineural and perineural (fascicular) repairs are not the only choices available, nor do the terms "epineural nerve repair" or "fascicular nerve repair" describe the surgical procedure sufficiently well. An end-to-end nerve repair consists of the following four basic steps.

Preparation of stumps (Fig. 37-6). The first step is the preparation of the two stumps. This can be performed either by resection of segments or by interfascicular dissection, separating individual fascicles or fascicle groups. The resection is then performed individually for each fascicle or fascicle group. If a nerve consists of one large fascicle or many small fascicles without further arrangement,

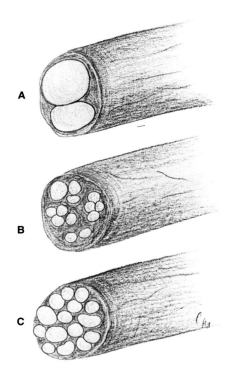

Fig. 37-6. Basic types of fascicular patterns (monofascicular pattern not indicated): **A,** Oligofascicular pattern with two to eight fascicles; **B,** polyfascicular pattern with group arrangement; **C,** polyfascicular pattern without group arrangement.

the stump is best prepared by resection. If the stump consists of a limited number of larger fascicles or of many fascicles arranged in fascicle groups, the interfascicular type of stump preparation is best. Under these circumstances it is possible to resect the epifascicular epineurium and to reduce the amount of interfascicular epineurium, maneuvers that are beneficial because the epineurium is the main source of connective tissue proliferation. The danger of improper alignment (fascicle to nonfascicular tissue) is reduced. Such a capacity to reduce fibroblastic activity—and thus the amount of collagen production—has been a recurring dream of surgeons and favors the ability of the axons to bridge the gap[33] in their competition against the ingrowth of connective tissue. Pleasure et al.[63] tried to reduce connective tissue formation by the use of hydroxyproline analogues. Hastings et al.[32] tried to influence the collagen production by creating a scorbutic state. Meanwhile we have to differentiate between endoneural, perineural, and epineural fibroblasts and that fibroblasts are essential for restoring the continuity of the nerve fibers.[10,11,12,13] Consequently attempts to totally

knock out fibroblastic activity will fail. The only goal we can achieve is a reduction in connective tissue activity. For the present the only effective means of reducing connective tissue proliferation is the resection of epineurium.[47]

Approximation. The two stumps have to be approximated. During this step tension comes into play, as discussed previously. Ideally we would like to be able to approximate the two stumps without any tension.

Coaptation. The term "coaptation" is used for the particular act of bringing into contact the cross-sectional surface of corresponding fascicles. In the presence of tension one stitch provides a point contact only. More stitches are required to obtain complete surface contact. If there is no tension at all, complete surface contact is achieved easily by one stitch. What about the edge of the perineurium? Is it necessary to get firm contact of the perineural edges? Theoretically this could be achieved only by matching stumps of a nerve segment with a limited number of larger or medium sized fascicles. Even in such a case, protruding fascicular contents would have to be trimmed. Our experimental data have suggested that trimming and close contact of the perineural edges are not mandatory to obtain good regeneration. If the number of the fascicles within the two stumps does not correspond, such a coaptation is impossible, and we have to rely on the ability of the axon sprouts to find the correct pathway.[40,41,53]

If we have to deal with stumps of a nerve that consist of one large fascicle, *trunk-to-trunk coaptation* and *fascicular coaptation* are synonymous. In such a case, of course, it is not necessary to resect the epineurium. The same is true with nerve segments containing a few large fascicles with a small amount of interfascicular epineural tissue (*oligofascicular nerve segments* with two to four fascicles) (Fig. 37-6). In this situation an exact coaptation of the fascicles can be achieved and maintained by a few epineural stitches.

In a nerve that contains a greater but still limited number of large fascicles (*oligofascicular nerve segment* with five to ten fascicles; Fig. 37-6), each of them carrying nerve fibers of different quality, the best chance for functional return is provided by separating the fascicles by interfascicular dissection and *fascicular coaptation* of the stumps—provided that identification of the individual fascicles is accurate. The staining technique of Gruber and Zenker,[27] which was used clinically by Freilinger et al.,[25] did not become popular because it required too much time. The future will show whether the different staining technique of Engel et al.,[21] which is based on acetylcholine transferase and which gives results within 60 minutes, will prove its clinical value. Identification of corresponding fascicles or fascicle groups by retrograde tracing is a reliable technique for clinical practice.[49]

If the nerve segment in question consists of many small fascicles *(polyfascicular pattern)*, we have to distinguish between two particular situations: (1) the small fascicles can be distributed diffusely over the cross section without further evidence of a pattern or (2) the small fascicles are arranged in groups of fascicles that are separated from each other by a wider space of interfascicular epineural tissue (Fig. 37-6). In a polyfascicular nerve segment, a fascicular repair can be attempted,[85] but this necessitates extensive surgical trauma. Identification of such a large number of corresponding pairs of fascicles introduces a greater risk of error. In cases of nerve defects, fascicular coaptation is not possible because the stumps do not usually have corresponding pairs of fascicles. If there is *no* grouping and the fascicles are tightly packed with less interfascicular epineurium, *trunk-to-trunk coaptation* using interfascicular guide stitches is still the best technique. If there is *group arrangement*, the individual fascicle groups can be separated by *interfascicular* dissection, identified by retrograde tracing, and coapted with each other *(group-to-group coaptation or interfascicular coaptation)*.

Maintenance of coaptation. If there is no tension at all, minimal efforts are necessary to maintain coaptation; natural fibrin clotting is sufficiently strong to do so. Of course, the surgeon must avoid shearing forces during wound closure and any longitudinal distracting forces during the first few days. Careful handling of the extremity in the final phase of the operation and during dressing is mandatory. The limb is immobilized exactly in the position it had during surgery.

If there is a defect that cannot be overcome by mobilization, an end-to-end nerve repair without tension is not possible and a nerve graft has to be used. If one accepts a certain amount of tension, one has to do more to maintain the coaptation. The tension can be neutralized temporarily by flexion of the adjacent joints; more sutures have to be used or an artificial fibrin clot can be produced, as suggested by Matras et al.[43] The efficiency of these fibrin clots may be reduced significantly by fibrinolytic activity.[38] Duspiva et al.[19] used allogenic fibrinogen solutions in a similar way, but applied, in addition, an antifibrinolytic treatment.

Summary

Microsurgery offers the possibility of operating within the nerve itself. Terms like "epineural" or "perineural" nerve repair do not adequately describe the possible choices of repair available to the surgeon. The technique that is finally chosen will be a sequence of four different steps, each of which can be performed in different ways according to the fascicular pattern of the nerve in question.

INDICATIONS FOR THE USE OF NERVE GRAFT

At present, for nerve defects of more than 6 to 7 cm, everybody uses nerve grafts. For defects of less than 2 to 2.5 cm, everybody uses end-to-end neurorrhaphy. Between these extremes there are different views among different surgeons according to their training, philosophy, and confidence in nerve grafting. Basically one can distinguish two attitudes toward nerve grafting. Some surgeons try to minimize the defects by any means available (mobilization of the nerve stumps, flexion of the adjacent joints, and so on) to be able to use the shortest nerve graft possible.[34] Other surgeons (including me) measure the proposed length of the required nerve graft with the adjacent joints of the limb in neutral position, without mobilization of the nerve stumps, to avoid tension and to have optimal conditions at the two sites of coaptation. The surgeons in this group consistently turn to the use of a nerve graft if approximation of the defect requires tension after slight mobilization of the stumps and without flexion of the adjacent joints. The frequency of nerve grafts performed by this group of surgeons is relatively high. The study of Chanson et al.[15] on secondary end-to-end nerve repairs using microsurgical techniques was disappointing. Consequently the indications for the use of nerve grafts has been expanded[46]; in 1965 this group of surgeons used nerve grafts in one out of ten cases of secondary repairs; now they use nerve grafts in seven out of ten cases.

SELECTION OF TECHNIQUE FOR NERVE GRAFTS (Figs. 37-7 to 37-10)

Free cutaneous nerve grafts are the usual choice. The two stumps are prepared by interfascicular dissections if they consist of several fascicles or of many fascicles arranged in groups. If one cutaneous nerve graft is placed between the two stumps of one fascicle of similar size, we speak of *fascicular grafts*. If one graft is placed between the

Text continued on p. 365.

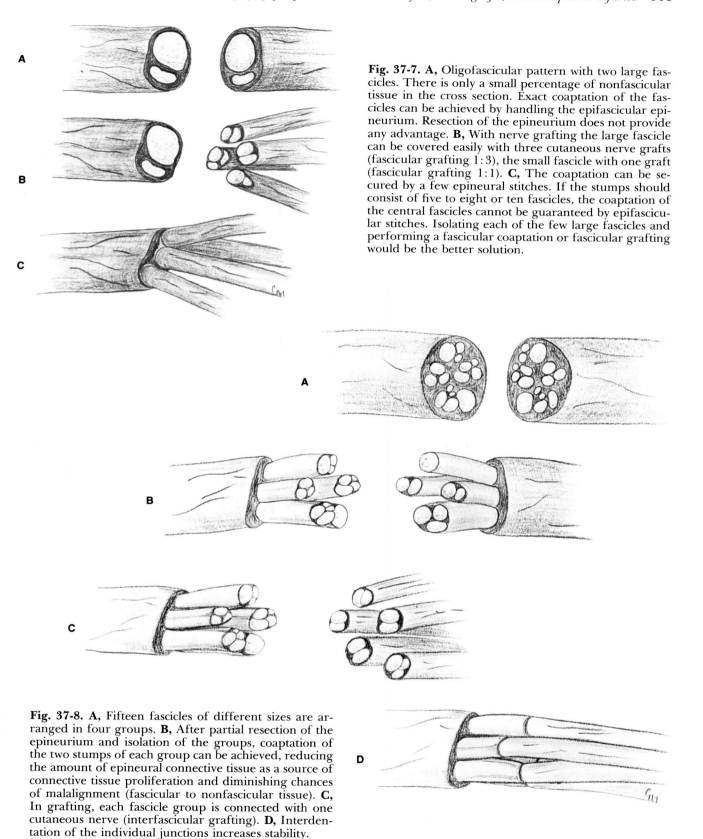

Fig. 37-7. A, Oligofascicular pattern with two large fascicles. There is only a small percentage of nonfascicular tissue in the cross section. Exact coaptation of the fascicles can be achieved by handling the epifascicular epineurium. Resection of the epineurium does not provide any advantage. **B,** With nerve grafting the large fascicle can be covered easily with three cutaneous nerve grafts (fascicular grafting 1:3), the small fascicle with one graft (fascicular grafting 1:1). **C,** The coaptation can be secured by a few epineural stitches. If the stumps should consist of five to eight or ten fascicles, the coaptation of the central fascicles cannot be guaranteed by epifascicular stitches. Isolating each of the few large fascicles and performing a fascicular coaptation or fascicular grafting would be the better solution.

Fig. 37-8. A, Fifteen fascicles of different sizes are arranged in four groups. **B,** After partial resection of the epineurium and isolation of the groups, coaptation of the two stumps of each group can be achieved, reducing the amount of epineural connective tissue as a source of connective tissue proliferation and diminishing chances of malalignment (fascicular to nonfascicular tissue). **C,** In grafting, each fascicle group is connected with one cutaneous nerve (interfascicular grafting). **D,** Interdentation of the individual junctions increases stability.

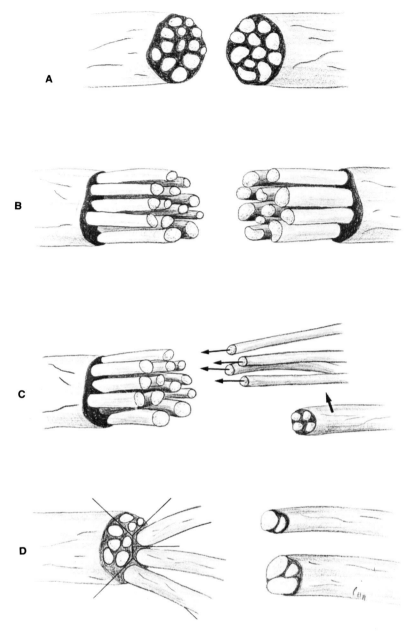

Fig. 37-9. A and **B,** Polyfascicular nerve segment with thirteen fascicles and eleven fascicles in the other stump as a result of a small nerve defect and rapid change of the fascicular pattern along the nerve. If the surgeon attempts to perform a fascicular coaptation after isolation of the individual fascicles, he has to perform extensive dissection and would have a different number of fascicles in each stump. An error in the identification of fascicles would be worse than in stump-to-stump coaptation (which in this case is still the best solution). The alignment of the fascicles can be improved by interfascicular sutures (not shown). **C,** If fascicular grafting is attempted, cutaneous nerves such as the sural nerves have to be split into their individual fascicles, with an increase in surgical trauma. **D,** In such cases we try to connect corresponding sectors of the stumps by individual nerve grafts *(sectoral grafting).*

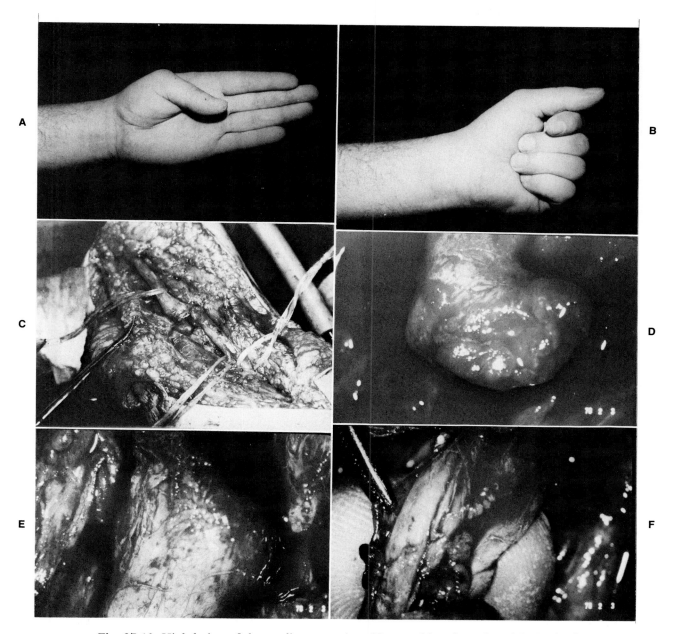

Fig. 37-10. High lesion of the median nerve in a 33-year-old patient. **A** and **B,** Lack of opposition and of full flexion of the index finger, complete loss of sensation. **C,** Site of the lesion, with (**D**) proximal and (**E**) distal stump. **F,** Normal nerve segment to the neuroma. Epifascicular epineurium has been incised and reflected. Note surface of two fascicle groups with interfascicular epineural tissue.

Continued.

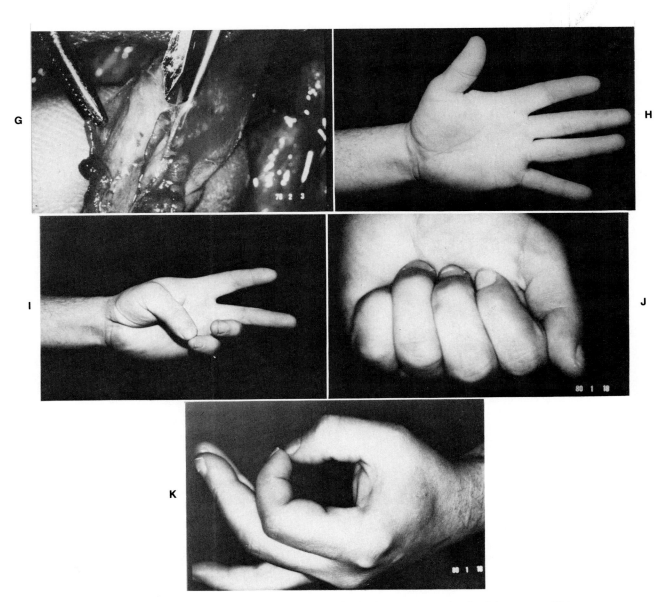

Fig. 37-10, cont'd. G, Dissection is being performed to separate the fascicle groups. **H** to **K,** Nerve grafting is performed as in Fig. 37-8, **B** and **C.** Results after 2 years. Protective sensation is present at the pulp of the index and middle fingers. At the pulp of the thumb two-point discrimination is 10 mm.

two stumps of a group of fascicles, the term *interfascicular grafting* is applied. Covering a large fascicle by two or three cutaneous nerve grafts can be called *fascicular grafting 1:2, 1:3,* and so on. If we have to deal with a polyfascicular nerve segment without group arrangement, each cutaneous nerve graft has to cover a corresponding sector of the stump *(sectoral nerve grafting).*

The main points are that the cutaneous nerve grafts are not packed together and that they have an optimal contact with the recipient bed so that they may be vascularized as soon as possible. If the most direct pathway between the two nerve stumps is scarred, we would accept a longer nerve graft to route it through unscarred soft tissue. At times soft tissue must be provided by plastic surgical procedures. An alternative is offered by the free vascularized nerve graft.[82] Because of the immediate restoration of circulation there is no period of anoxia. It is expected that these nerve grafts are neurotized more rapidly; to date, however, there has been no proof of this hypothesis. If the patient has sustained an amputation, nerve trunks in the stump provide a source for grafts for this procedure. In avulsion of the roots C8 and Th1 after brachial plexus injury, the ulnar nerve could be used as a vascularized nerve graft because we know that regeneration in the ulnar nerve territory is minimal. For other cases the superficial branch of the radial nerve has been used. Recently techniques have been developed to use the sural nerve as a vascularized nerve graft.[23,84]

BRACHIAL PLEXUS SURGERY
(Fig. 37-11)

In the past brachial plexus surgery has been limited for two reasons: (1) Usually long defects have to be repaired, and this has been impossible by end-to-end nerve repair in the majority of cases. Reasonable improvement has been achieved only since microsurgical techniques for nerve grafting have been developed.[48] (2) In many cases of brachial plexus injury the continuity of the nerves is preserved and there is a prospect of spontaneous recovery. Before the introduction of microsurgery, surgeons did not dare to try internal neurolysis, being afraid that intact areas of the nerve (with a chance of spontaneous recovery) might be damaged. Applying microsurgical techniques, this danger has been minimized. Another objection to direct brachial plexus surgery was that the results to be expected are not worth the time-consuming and difficult operations.

From 1963 to 1978 I performed direct brachial plexus surgery in 151 cases. One hundred and four cases are ready for evaluation (Tables 37-1 to 37-4).

In two thirds of these cases useful recovery has been achieved. Useful recovery means that the patient has regained sufficient strength to stabilize the shoulder joint, and subluxation is avoided, and the patient has gained sufficient strength to flex the elbow joint. Combined with the arthrodesis of the wrist joint, the originally useless arm can be transformed into a useful limb. Also in some cases function of the forearm muscles has returned, and this gives the potential for tendon transfers to restore key grip function.

The main point is that direct surgery of the brachial plexus is only one part of a combined treatment that consists of physiotherapy, social services, and palliative surgery. The last point is of particular importance. Palliative surgery consists of arthrodesis of the wrist joint and individual tendon transfers according to the needs of the patient, transfer of the triceps to the biceps tendon in cases of simultaneous innervation of these two antagonistic muscles, transfer of the latissimus dorsi muscle, and so on. If there are three or more avulsions, intercostal nerve transfer is considered. In one third of our cases useful recovery was obtained by these operations. In selected cases branches of the accessory nerve are transferred to the suprascapular nerve.

We have no experience yet with the transfer of the motor part of the cervical plexus to the brachial plexus. We cannot expect to obtain different antagonistic functions by individual intercostal nerves. In our cases that failed we had attempted to neurotize too many nerves by different intercostal nerves. Now we concentrate three intercostal nerves on the musculocutaneous nerve alone, and two or three more intercostal nerves on the median nerve. In contrast to other surgeons, we explore the intercostal nerves at the midaxillary line, transecting and connecting the proximal stump via a nerve graft with the distal stump of the peripheral nerve. Connections between intercostal nerves and parts of the brachial plexus did not lead to a useful recovery.

Summary

Brachial plexus surgery has proved its value. In about two thirds of the patients, sufficient regeneration can be achieved to be regarded as useful and extremely rewarding for the patient.

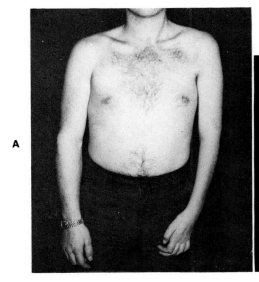
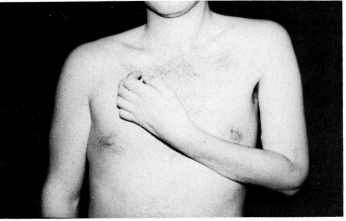

Fig. 37-11. Complete brachial plexus lesion after a motorcycle accident in an 18-year-old patient. The operation revealed a rupture of C5 and C6, an avulsion of C7, and a lesion in continuity of C8 and Th1. The latter roots and the inferior trunk were neurolyzed. Restoration of continuity between C5 and the dorsal cord and C6 and the lateral cord by eleven cutaneous nerve grafts (up to 11 cm long). **A** and **B,** A medium result. There is no longer any subluxation and the shoulder joint can be controlled. The biceps works very well, with good elbow flexion and supination. Protective sensation has returned. There is no useful hand function despite active contraction of finger flexors and wrist extensor. Further improvement would be achieved by arthrodesis of the wrist and a part of the finger joints to use the weak function of the forearm muscles.

Table 37-1. Brachial plexus lesions in 151 patients (1963-1978)

Treatment ongoing	47
Treatment completed	104
Complete palsy	
Root lesion	44
Peripheral lesion	20
Partial palsy	
Root lesion	32
Peripheral lesion	8

Table 37-2. Brachial plexus lesions

Complete palsy	Number	Useful function
Root lesion	44	28
Peripheral lesion	20	18
TOTAL	64	46

Table 37-3. Brachial plexus lesions

Partial palsy	Number	Useful function
Root lesion	32	26
Peripheral lesion	8	7
TOTAL	40	33

Table 37-4. Brachial plexus lesions (palliative surgery)

Triceps to biceps	10
Pectoralis major	2
Pectoralis minor	1
Latissimus dorsi	5
Trapezius	1
Tendon transfer (as for radial nerve palsy)	4
Arthrodesis wrist joint and tenodesis	7
TOTAL	30

CONCLUSION

The introduction of microsurgery has produced a revolution in peripheral nerve surgery. I am quite sure that the process is just beginning and will continue to develop. Nerve grafting procedures performed according to microsurgical principles have produced a significant improvement, especially in cases that in the past had a rather poor prognosis because of the type of the injury, the age of the patient, or the time interval. Tables 37-5 to 37-8 present results of an uninterrupted series of nerve grafts to restore a continuity in cases of defects of the radial nerve, the median nerve, the ulnar nerve, and combined median-ulnar nerve lesions.

Table 37-5. Results of radial nerve repair by nerve grafting according to Highet's scheme (M0-M5)

	M5			M4			M3			M2	
Age	Interval (months)	Defect (cm)	Age	Interval (months)	Defect (cm)	Age	Interval (months)	Defect (cm)	Age	Interval (months)	Defect (cm)
19	18	4.0	8	3	8.5	8	12	12.5	62	3	10.0
30	1	3.0	22	8	6.0	42	29	9.0			
21	11	10.0	53	4	4.0	26	7	6.0			
42	3	3.0	25	5	8.0	16	3	14.0			
25	8	15.0	34	3	12.0						
16	3	6.0	26	18	8.0						
11	2	9.0	63	0	10.0						
22	5	6.0	9	10	7.0						
33	4	8.0	10	29	10.0						
62	6	4.0	18	6	8.0						
25	6	8.0	49	5	12.0						
32	6	11.0	24	7	10.0						
64	1	2.0									

Table 37-6. Results of median nerve repairs by nerve grafting according to Highet's scheme (M0-M5, S0-S4)

	Mixed innervation			M4-5			M3			M2			M1			M0		
	Age	Interval (months)	Defect (cm)	Age	Interval (months)	Defect (cm)	Age	Interval (months)	Defect (cm)	Age	Interval (months)	Defect (cm)	Age	Interval (months)	Defect (cm)	Age	Interval (months)	Defect (cm)
S3+4	21	4	5.0	19	6	2.5				23	4	7.0						
	20	1	2.0	22	8	8.0												
	25	2	3.5	18	7	7.0												
	40	2	2.0	21	2	6.0												
	27	2	3.5	10	9	5.0												
	49	1	6.5	9	2	5.0												
	44	8	5.0	20	3	5.0												
	7	2	2.0	46	5	3.5												
	13	4	4.0	50	2	2.0												
				10	4	4.0												
S3	21	4	4.5	35	6	2.0	43	8	5.0	41	28	15.0						
	21	2	6.0	19	2	4.0	44	36	12.0									
	46	4	2.0	50	2	3.0	48	18	7.0									
	24	4	5.0				25	2	5.0									
	27	2	4.0				6	5	4.0									
	52	12	4.5															
	30	9	10.0															
	23	5	4.0															
	61	3	4.0															
S2	26	11	16.0															
S1																		
S0																		

Thirty-nine cases are represented, with a high percentage of mixed innervation of the thenar muscles.

Table 37-7. Results of combined median and ulnar nerve repair according to Highet's scheme (M0-M5, S0-S4)

	M4-5				M3				M2+				M2				M1				M0			
	M/U	Age	Interval (months)	De-fect (cm)	M/U	Age	Interval (months)	De-fect (cm)	M/U	Age	Interval (months)	De-fect (cm)	M/U	Age	Interval (months)	De-fect (cm)	M/U	Age	Interval (months)	De-fect (cm)	M/U	Age	Interval (months)	De-fect (cm)
S3+-4	M	19	4	5.0	M	15	5	20.0					M	23	6	7.0					M	12	48	19.0
	M	10	4	12.0	M	39	18	13.0					M	10	18	3.0					M	12	49	12.0
	M	13	2	5.0	U	55	10	3.0																
	M	19	7	4.0																				
	U	19	4	5.0																				
	U	10	4	6.0																				
S3	M	51	0	2.0	M	15	5	6.0	U	15	5	20.0	M	69	9	5.0	M	38	8	6.5	U	18	9	15.0
	M	10	29	NS	M	11	2	4.0	U	39	9	7.0	M	18	9	7.0	M	49	11	13.0				
	M	18	6	7.0	M	62	4	3.0	U	18	6	9.0	M	10	3	1.5	U	38	8	4.0				
	M	39	9	5.5	M	46	3	4.0	U	36	3	9.0	U	49	11	4.0								
	U	51	0	2.0	M	55	10	16.0	U	61	16	8.0												
	U	10	29	8.5	M	36	3	13.0	U	59	3	4.0												
	U	18	6	7.0	M	59	3	6.0																
	U	46	3	4.0	U	15	5	7.0																
	U	13	2	5.0	U	11	2	4.0																
	U	23	6	11.0	U	39	18	11.0																
	U	19	2	4.0	U	69	9	5.5																
	U	10	3	9.0	U	39	9	3.0																
					U	10	18	NS																
S2					U	62	4	7.0					M	47	13	7.0					M	61	16	NL
					U	47	13	5.0					M	39	9	8.0								
													M	18	6	18.0								

NS = End-to-end repair; NL = neurolysis.

Twenty-nine patients with thirty involved extremities are represented; in two extremities, after tissue loss by a severe electric burn, the continuity of the median nerve only was repaired. Fifty-five grafting procedures, two end-to-end nerve repairs, and one neurolysis were performed. (Median: twenty-eight grafts, one end-to-end repair, one neurolysis. Ulnar: twenty-seven grafts, one end-to-end repair.)

Table 37-8. Results of ulnar nerve repair by nerve grafting according to Highet's scheme (M0-M5, S0-S4)

	Mixed innervation			M4-5			M3			M2+			M2			M1			M0		
	Age	Interval (months)	Defect* (cm)	Age	Interval (months)	Defect* (cm)	Age	Interval (months)	Defect* (cm)	Age	Interval (months)	Defect* (cm)	Age	Interval (months)	Defect* (cm)	Age	Interval (months)	Defect* (cm)	Age	Interval (months)	Defect* (cm)
S3+4	4	5	2.0	11	2	5.0	13	6	5.0												
	18	10	6.0	11	3	6.0*	55	4	2.0													
				12	2	5.0															
				12	3	3.0*															
				7	4	4.5															
				20	36	7.0															
				23	2	5.0															
				28	9	5.0															
				40	6	3.0															
S3				11	12	5.0	18	3	2.0	27	7	10.0*	31	48	20.0*						
				12	3	10.0*	34	31	20.0*	18	7	13.0*	17	6	6.0*						
				17	5	7.0	39	11	18.0*	37	6	3.0									
				16	6	4.0	40	8	5.0												
				21	4	6.0	48	3	6.0*												
				22	7	2.0*	49	4	4.0												
				19	1	3.0*	45	5	4.0												
				49	2	4.0*	54	8	3.0												
				63	13	3.0*	56	2	3.0												
				64	1	2.0															
				67	13	3.0*															
				25	2	3.0*															
				27	10	4.0															
S2										25	8	6.0*							28	5	15.0*
																			16	4	6.0*
S1										64	2	16.0*									
S0													44	7	11.0				33	6	19.0*

* = High lesion

REFERENCES

1. Ashworth, C.R., Boyes, J.G., and Stark, H.W.: Lecture held at the twenty-sixth annual meeting of the American Society for Surgery of the Hand, San Francisco, March 5-6, 1971.
2. Bora, W.: Peripheral nerve repair in cats, J. Bone Joint Surg. **49A:**659, 1967.
3. Bora, F.W., Pleasure, D.E., and Didzian, N.A.: A study of nerve regeneration and neuroma formation after nerve suture by various techniques, J. Hand Surg. **1:**138, 1976.
4. Bratton, B.R., Kline, D.G., Coleman, W., and Hudson, A.R.: Experimental interfascicular nerve grafting, J. Neurosurg. **51**(3):323, 1979.
5. Braun, R.M.: Comparative studies of neurorrhaphy and sutureless peripheral nerve repair, Surg. Gynecol. Obstet. **122:**15, 1966.
6. Brooks, D.: The place of nerve grafting in orthopaedic surgery, J. Bone Joint Surg. **37A:**299, 1955.
7. Brunelli, G.: Lecture held at the Symposium Mikrochirurgie der peripheren Nerven und Gefässe, Vienna, Austria, October 18, 1972.
8. Brunelli, G.: Indication, technique, and results of nerve grafting, Symposium on Surgery of the Hand, Vienna, May 21-23, 1977. Handchirurgie, Sonderheft No. 2.
9. Brunelli, G., and Brunelli-Monini, L.M.: Long-term results of nerve sutures and grafts, Int. J. Microsurg. **1:**27, 1979.
10. Bunge, M., Williams, A., Wood P., and Jeffrey, J.: Sources of connective tissue components in peripheral nerves. I: Basal lamina and collagen fibril formation by cultured Schwann cells related to neurons, J. Cell Biol. **84:**184, 1980.
11. Bunge, R.P.: Contributions of tissue culture studies to our understanding of basic processes in peripheral nerve regeneration. In Gorio, A., Millesi, H., and Mingrino, S., editors: Posttraumatic peripheral nerve regeneration—experimental basis and clinical applications; International Symposium, Padua, 1980, New York, 1981, Raven Press, p. 105.
12. Bunge, R.P., and Bunge, M.: Evidence that contact with connective tissue matrix is required for normal interaction between Schwann cells and nerve fibers, J. Cell Biol. **78:**943, 1978.
13. Bunge, R.P.: Cytological factors influencing nerve growth and regeneration, Proceedings of the Sixth International Congress of Electromyography, Stockholm, Sweden, 1979, p. 87.
14. Cabaud, H.E., et al.: Epineurial and perineurial fascicular nerve repairs: a critical comparison, J. Hand Surg. **1:**131, 1976.
15. Chanson, L., Michon, J., and Merle, M.: Etude des résultats de la réparation de 85 nerfs dont 49 gros troncs. In Michon, J., and Moberg, E., editors: Monographies du G.E.M.: les lésions traumatiques des nerfs périphériques, ed. 2, Paris, 1979, Expansion Scientifique, Française, p. 139.
16. Curtis, R.M., and Eversmann, W.W.: Internal neurolysis as an adjunct to the treatment of the carpal-tunnel syndrome, J. Bone Joint Surg. **55A:**733, 1973.
17. Ducker, T.B., and Kauffman, C.: Metabolic factors in surgery of peripheral nerves, Clin. Neurosurg. **24:**406, 1977.
18. Ducker, T.B., Kempe, L.G., and Hayes, G.J.: The metabolic background for peripheral nerve surgery, J. Neurosurg. **30:**270, 1969.
19. Duspiva, W., Blümel, G., Haas-Denk, S., and Wriedt-Lübbe, I.: Eine neue Methode der Anastomisierung durchtrennter peripherer Nerven. In Chirug forum, Berlin, 1977, Springer-Verlag, p. 100.
20. Ellis, J.S.: Technical aspects of peripheral nerve surgery, The British Club for Surgery of the Hand, The London Hospital Medical College, **17:**11, 1967.
21. Engel, J., et al.: Choline acetyl transferase for differentiation between human, motor, and sensory nerve fibers, Ann. Plast. Surg. **41:**376, 1980.
22. Erhart, E.A.: Experimental data and practical results which modify concepts of peripheral nerve fibres regeneration. In Gorio, A., Millesi, H., and Mingrino, S., editors: Posttraumatic peripheral nerve regeneration—experimental basis and clinical implications; International Symposium, Padua, 1980, New York, 1981, Raven Press, p. 433.
23. Fachinelli, A., Masquelet, A., Restrepo, J., and Gilbert, A.: The vascularized sural nerve: anatomy and surgical approach, Int. J. Microsurg. **3**(1):57, 1981.
24. Foucher, G., Merle, M., and Michon, J., editors: Manuel technique de microchirurgie vasculaire et nerveuse: Microchirurgie vasculaire et nerveuse. Les Dossiers Persantine 11, Service S.O.S., C.H.U. de Strasbourg et Service Assistance Mains, C.H.U. de Nancy, 1978.
25. Freilinger, G., Gruber, H., Holle, J., and Mandl, H.: Zur Methodik der sensomotorisch differenzierten Faszikelnaht peripherer Nerven, Handchirurgie **7:**133, 1975.
26. Geldmacher, J.: Die Wiederherstellung peripherer Nerven durch Nerventransplantation, Der Chirurg **46:**307, 1975.
27. Gruber, H., and Zenker, W.: Acetylcholinesterase: histochemical differentiation between motor and sensory nerve fibres, Brain Res. **51:**207, 1973.
28. Guegan, Y.: Intérêt du nombre de points de suture dans la réalisation fasciculaires: étude expérimentale. In Michon, J., and Moberg, E., editors: Les lésions traumatiques des nerfs périphériques, Monographie du G.E.M., Paris, 1979, Expansion Scientifique Française, p. 47.
29. Haase, J., Bjerre, P., and Simensen, K.: Median and ulnar transections with microsurgical interfascicular cable grafting with autogenous nerve grafts, J. Neurosurg. **53:**73, 1980.
30. Haftek, J.: Autogenous cable nerve grafting instead of end-to-end anastomosis in secondary nerve sutures, Acta Neurochir. (Wien) **34:**217, 1976.
31. Hakstian, R.W.: Funicular orientation by direct stimulation. An aid to peripheral nerve repair, J. Bone Joint Surg. **50A:**1178, 1968.
32. Hastings, J.C., and Peacock, E.E., Jr.: Effect of injury, repair and ascorbic acid deficiency on collagen accumulation in peripheral nerves, Surg. Forum **24:**516, 1973.
33. Huber, G.C.: A study of the operative treatment for loss of nerve substance in peripheral nerves, J. Morphol. **11:**629, 1895.
34. Kline, D.G.: Discussion. In Gorio, A., Millesi, H., and Mingrino, S., editors: Posttraumatic peripheral

nerve regeneration—experimental basis and clinical implications; International Symposium, Padua, 1980; New York, 1981, Raven Press, p. 322.

35. Kline, D.G., and Hackett, E.R.: Value of electrophysiologic tests for peripheral nerve neuromas, J. Surg. Oncol. **2**:299, 1970.

36. Kline, D.G., Hudson, A.R., and Bratton, B.R.: Use of grafts to repair nerves with serious gaps. In Gorio, A., Millesi, H., and Mingrino, S., editors: Posttraumatic peripheral nerve regeneration—experimental basis and clinical implications; International Symposium, Padua, 1980; New York, 1981, Raven Press, p. 339.

37. Kline, D.G., and Nulsen, F.E.: The neuroma in continuity: its preoperative and operative management, Surg. Clin. North Am. **52**:1189, 1972.

38. Kuderna, H.: Ergebnisse und Erfahrungen in der klinischen Anwendung des Fibrin-Klebers bei der Wiederherstellung durchtrennter peripherer Nerven. Lecture held at the seventeenth annual meeting of the Deutsche Gesellschaft für Plastische und Wiederherstellungschirurgie, Heidelberg, Nov 1-3, 1979.

39. Kurze, T.: Microtechniques and neurological surgery, Clin. Neurosurg. **22**:128, 1964.

40. Lundborg, G., and Hansson, H.A.: Regeneration of a peripheral nerve through a preformed tissue space, Brain Res. **178**:573, 1979.

41. Lundborg, G., and Hansson, H.A.: Studies on the growth pattern of regenerating axons in the gap between the proximal and distal nerve ends. In Gorio, A., Millesi, H., and Mingrino, S., editors: Posttraumatic peripheral nerve regeneration—experimental basis and clinical implications; International Symposium, Padua, 1980; New York, 1981, Raven Press, p. 229.

42. Martini, A., and Zellner, P.R.: Ergebnisse der Nervenwiederherstellung an der oberen Extremität, Der Chirurg. **47**:682, 1976.

43. Matras, H., Dinges, H.P., Lassmann, H., and Mamoli, R.: Zur nahtlosen interfaszikulären Nerventransplantation im Tierexperiment, Wien. Med. Wochenschr. **122**:517, 1972.

44. McCarroll, H.R., Jr., Rodkey, W.G., and Cabaud, H.E.: Results of suture of cat ulnar nerves: a comparison of surgical techniques. In Jewett, D.L., and McCarroll, H.R., Jr., editors: Symposium, San Francisco, 1977, Nerve repair and regeneration: its clinical and experimental basis, St. Louis, 1980, The C.V. Mosby Co., p. 228.

45. McQuarrie, I.G.: The effect of a conditioning lesion on the regenerating motor axon, Brain Res. **152**:597, 1978.

46. Michon, J.: Les techniques modernes de réparation des nerfs périphériques. In Michon, J., and Moberg, E., editors: Monographies du G.E.M.: les lésions traumatiques des nerfs périphériques, Paris, 1979, Expansion Scientifiques Française, p. 115.

47. Michon, J., Merle, M., and Foucher, G.: La microchirurgie de traumatologie de la main, Int. Orthop. **3**(4):245, 1980.

48. Millesi, H.: Zum Problem der Überbrückung von Defekten peripherer Nerven, Wien Med Wochenschr. **118**:182, 1968.

49. Millesi, H.: Fascicular nerve repair and interfascicular nerve grafting. In Daniel, R.K., and Terzis, J.K., editors: Reconstructive microsurgery, Boston, 1977, Little, Brown & Co., p. 430.

50. Millesi, H.: Healing of nerves, Clin. Plast. Surg. **4**(3):459, 1977.

51. Millesi, H.: Wiederherstellung der Kontinuität durchtrennter peripherer Nerven: Überlegungen zur Indikation und Operationstaktik, Zentrabl. Neurochir. **40**:1, 1979.

52. Millesi, H.: Looking back on nerve surgery, Int. J. Microsurg. **2**(3-4):143, 1980.

53. Millesi, H.: How exact should coaptation be? In Gorio, A., Millesi, H., and Mingrino, S., editors: Posttraumatic peripheral nerve regeneration—experimental basis and clinical implications; communication held at Symposium in Padua, 1980; New York, 1981, Raven Press, p. 301.

54. Millesi, H., Berger, A., and Meissl, G.: Experimentelle Untersuchungen zur Heilung durchtrennter peripherer Nerven, Chir. Plast. **1**:174, 1972.

55. Millesi, H., Ganglberger, J., and Berger, A.: Erfahrungen mit der Mikrochirurgie peripherer Nerven, Eighty-third Congress of the Deutsche Gesellschaft für Chirurgie, April 14, 1966.

56. Millesi, H., Ganglberger, J., and Berger, A.: Erfahrungen mit der Mikrochirurgie peripherer Nerven, Chir. Plast. Reconstr. **3**:47, 1967.

57. Millesi, H., Meissl, G., and Berger, A.: Entwicklungstendenzen in der operativen Wiederherstellung durchtrennter peripherer Nerven, Bol. Ozljeda Sake. Med. Naklada (Zagreb) 161, 1970.

58. Millesi, H., Meissl, G., and Berger, A.: The interfascicular nerve-grafting of the median and ulnar nerves, J. Bone Joint Surg. **54A**:727, 1972.

59. Millesi, H., Meissl, G., and Berger, A.: A further experience with interfascicular grafting of the median, ulnar, and radial nerves, J. Bone Joint Surg. **58A**:209, 1976.

60. Miyamoto, Y.: Experimental study of results of nerve suture under tension versus nerve grafting, Plast. Reconstr. Surg. **64**:540, 1979.

61. Miyamoto, Y., Watari, S., and Tsuge, K.: Experimental studies on the effects of tension in intraneural microcirculation in sutured peripheral nerves, Plast. Reconstr. Surg. **63**:398, 1979.

62. Omer, G.E.: Injuries to nerves of the upper extremities, J. Bone Joint Surg. **56A**:1615, 1974.

63. Pleasure, D., Bora, F.W., Lane, J., and Prockop, D.: Regeneration after nerve transection: effect of inhibition of collagen synthesis, Exp. Neurol. **45**:72, 1974.

64. Rushworth, G., Dickson, R.A., O'Hara, J., and Tricker, J.: Nerve gap repair and the quality of regeneration. In Persson, A., editor: Proceedings of the Sixth International Congress of Electromyography, Stockholm, 1979, Symposia, p. 131.

65. Salvi, V.: Problems connected with the repair of nerve sections, Hand **5**:25, 1973.

66. Samii, M.: Modern aspects of peripheral and cranial nerve surgery, In Krayenbühl, H., editor: Advances and technical standards of neurosurgery, Vols. 2 and 3, New York, 1975, Springer.

67. Samii, M., and Kahl, R.I.: Klinische Resultate der autologen Nerventransplantation, Med. Mitt. Melsungen **116**(46):197, 1972.

68. Samii, M., and Wallenborn, R.: Tierexperimentelle Untersuchungen über den Einfluss der Spannung auf den regenerationserfolg nach nervennaht, Acta Neurochir. (Wien) 27:87, 1972.

69. Schiff, M.: Über motorische Lähmungen der Zunge. Heilkunde. Arch Anat. Physiol. (physiol Abt), 10:579, 1851.

70. Seddon, H.J.: Three types of nerve injury, Brain 66:237, 1943.

71. Seddon, H.J.: The use of autogenous grafts for the repair of large gaps in peripheral nerves, Br. J. Surg. 35:151,1947.

72. Seddon, H.J.: Nerve grafting, J. Bone Joint Surg. 45B:447, 1963.

73. Seddon, H.J.: Surgical disorders of the peripheral nerves, Edinburgh, 1972, Churchill Livingstone.

74. Sedel, L.: Traitement par autogreffes des pertes de substance nerveuse, Ann. Chir. Plast. 21:253, 1976.

75. Sedel, L.: Résultats des greffes nerveuses, Rev. Chir. Orthop. (Fr) 64(4):284, 1978.

76. Smith, J.W.: Microsurgery of peripheral nerves, Plast. Reconstr. Surg. 33:317, 1964.

77. Smith, J.W.: Factors influencing nerve repair, I: Blood supply of peripheral nerves, Arch. Surg. 93:335, 1966.

78. Smith, J.W.: Factors influencing nerve repair, II: Collateral circulation of peripheral nerves, Arch. Surg. 93:433, 1966.

79. Sunderland, S.: A classification of peripheral nerve injuries producing loss of function, Brain 74:491, 1951.

80. Sunderland, S.: Nerve and nerve injuries. Baltimore, 1968, The Williams & Wilkins Co.

81. Tallis, R., Staniforth, R., and Fisher, T.R.: Neurophysiological studies of autogenous sural nerve grafts, J. Neurol. Neurosurg. Psychiatry 41:677, 1978.

82. Taylor, G.I., and Ham, F.J.: The free vascularized nerve graft, Plast. Reconstr. Surg. 57:413, 1976.

83. Terzis, J.K., Faibisoff, R., and Williams, H.B.: The nerve gap: suture under tension versus graft, Plast. Reconstr. Surg. 56:166, 1975.

84. Townsend, P.: Microvascular nerve grafts. Personal communication at the Fourth Congress of the European Section of the International Confederation for Plastic and Reconstructive Surgery, Athens, May 10-14, 1981.

85. Tupper, J.W.: Fascicular nerve repair. Communication held at Symposium San Francisco, 1977. In Jewett, D.L., and McCarroll, H.R., Jr., editors: Nerve repair and regeneration: its clinical and experimental basis, St. Louis, 1980, The C.V. Mosby Co., p. 320.

86. Williams, H.B., and Terzis, J.K.: Single fascicular recordings: an intraoperative diagnostic tool for the management of peripheral nerve lesions, Plast. Reconstr. Surg. 57:562, 1976.

87. Yacubovich, F.: Electromyographic follow-up study of fascicular nerve grafts in the upper extremity, J. Hand Surg. 2:162, 1977.

88. Young, V.I., Weeks, P.M., and Wray, R.: The results of nerve grafting in the wrist and hand. Lecture held at the fifty-eighth annual meeting of the American Association of Plastic Surgery, Palm Beach, Florida, April 29-May 2, 1979.

Chapter 38

Microlymphatic surgery

Wayne A. Morrison
Bernard McC. O'Brien

PHYSIOLOGY

The lymph capillaries form the pathway for absorption of colloid and particulate matter from the tissue spaces, whereas the blood capillaries absorb soluble crystalloid substances. Lymphatic capillaries are larger and their endothelial walls are permeable to substances of much greater molecular size; absorption possibly takes place through the phagocytic activity of the endothelial cells. The lymphatic system represents the main pathway by which high molecular weight plasma proteins are returned to the blood circulation.

The movement of lymph is determined by the interstitial pressure in the extracellular space. This is influenced by the resistance of the skin externally and the deep fascial layer internally and by the contraction of the subjacent skeletal muscles, particularly during exercise. Other factors contributing to lymph flow are (1) arterial pulsation near lymphatics, (2) negative respiratory pressure, and (3) contraction of the unstriped muscle of the lymphatic trunk wall just proximal to valves. Although flow is generally slow, it is unidirectional because of the many valves in the lymphatic trunks. The pressure in the lymphatic system under normal circumstances is greater than that in the venous system, so the direction of flow is ultimately from lymphatic to vein.

ANATOMY

Lymphatic capillaries are larger than blood capillaries. They commence blindly and unite to form a system of lymphatic trunks, which run both in the superficial and deep compartments of the limbs. They pass through lymph node systems and ultimately, via the thoracic duct, drain into the inferior vena cava. The superficial lymph vessels generally follow the course of the superficial venous drainage of the limb, the deep lymphatic trunks running with the deep arteries and veins. There are only a few connections between the superficial and deep systems, and in normal circumstances the direction of flow is from the superficial to the deep.

The lymphatic capillary wall consists of a single endothelial cell, and as the capillary enlarges to form trunks, the endothelial cells are coated by a thin connective adventitial layer. The larger connecting trunks consist of three coats with an intermediate muscle layer, the tunica media, made up of unstriped muscle. There are many more valves in the lymphatic system than in veins. Just proximal to each valve there is an expanded sinus that gives the characteristic beaded appearance of lymphatics.[8]

Lymphatic trunks in the limbs are about 0.5 mm in diameter. They can be readily identified on dissection after injection of patent blue dye into the distal subcutaneous tissues. Even when muscle pump action is eliminated by general anesthesia, passage of this dye up the limb is rapid and may be seen in the proximal limb within 5 minutes of distal injection.

LYMPHEDEMA

Lymphedema may be either primary or secondary. Three varieties of primary lymphedema are:

1. Aplasia, in which the main subcutaneous trunks fail to develop and the dermal lymphatic plexus is dilated
2. Hypoplasia, in which the main subcutaneous trunks are few and underdeveloped (most common variety)
3. Dilated and varicose lymphatic trunks

Primary lymphedema, when present at birth, is termed "lymphedema congenita'; if it is familial, it is known as Milroy's disease. When it occurs at puberty it is termed "lymphedema praecox," and when it occurs in adult life, "lymphedema tarda."

Obstructive or secondary lymphedema occurs following trauma (such as surgical ablation of the lymph nodes), but it is rare following simple traumatic division of lymphatic trunks. Following replantation, lymphedema rapidly resolves within a few months, even though the trunks have been totally divided. Obstructive lymphedema also occurs following repeated acute or chronic infections and in malignant disease of the lymph nodes.

The chronic accumulation of protein-rich fluid in the interstitial spaces results in progressive edema; this predisposes the patient to recurrent cellulitis with resultant fibrosis of the interstitial tissues and further obstruction of the lymphatics, so the natural history of the disease is progressive. Lymphatic obstruction, however, is probably never complete, and significant lymph retention does not occur in the deeper muscular compartment of the limb.

Treatment of primary lymphedema

As there is no obstruction in primary lymphedema and because the lymphatics are few in number and hypoplastic, lymphaticovenous bypass has no logical place in management. The mainstay of treatment, although inadequate, must be conservative or ablative measures.

Treatment of secondary lymphedema

The management of mild to moderate obstructive lymphedema, on the other hand, has been managed at St. Vincent's Hospital since 1975 by lymphaticovenous bypass surgery using microvascular techniques.[11] Clinical treatment was preceded by experimental work on lymphaticovenous anastomoses in the nonlymphedematous dog model.[7] This work demonstrated 78% patency at 1 week and 66% patency from 6 to 12 weeks. Laine and Howard[10] reported 40% patency at 3 weeks to 3 months. Yamada[15] reported long-term patency. Clinically, O'Brien,[13] Degni,[6] Fox,[7] and Krilov[9] have reported a significant decrease in lymphedema following lymphaticovenous anastomoses. In a series of 365 cases (100 upper limb and 265 lower limb), Krilov reported 82% good or fair results in the upper limb and 70% good or fair results in the lower limb for obstructive lymphedema. In primary lymphedema the results were 20% good or fair. He classifies good as less than a 2

cm difference in circumference of the limbs, no supportive bandaging, and full use of the limb. Fair is when the difference in circumference is between 2 cm and 5 cm, supportive bandaging is required, and full working capacity of the limb is regained. Up to twenty anastomoses have been performed in one limb. Born et al.[3] and Franklin (see Chapter 10) have demonstrated a significantly increased transit time of radioactive dye from an obstructed limb to the liver following lymphaticovenous repair (Figs. 38-1 to 38-3). Acland,[1] on the other hand, has had poor patency rates following lympho-lymphatic repair and Puckett et al.[14] found that single lymphovenous anastomoses in the lymphedematous dog model did not remain patent for more than 21 days. Baumeister et al.[2] reported good experimental and clinical results after bypassing lymphatic obstruction with lympho-lymphatic grafts and confirmed patency of these anastomoses by radioactive T3 uptake.

Preoperative management

The patient, having been assessed as appropriate for microlymphaticovenous bypass, is admitted to the hospital 3 days before surgery. The limb is maintained in a position of constant elevation and a Jobst pump is applied intermittently to decompress the arm. Volumetric measurements are made by water displacement, comparing the limb to the opposite normal limb. Linear measurements 15 cm above and below the elbow, at the wrist, and at the hand are made at the end of the 3 days, just before surgery.

Lymphangiograms were routinely performed as a preoperative investigation, but it soon became apparent that this was aggravating the edema, and in some cases this deterioration was permanent.[12] Valuable knowledge, however, was gained from these early lymphangiograms regarding the anatomic distribution of the lymphatics in the limb, and now their course can be predicted and incisions made accordingly.

Operating technique

A subcutaneous injection of patent blue dye is injected at the wrist or ankle and the limb is then immediately prepared for surgery. A tourniquet is applied proximal to the incisions to secure hemostasis and to prevent rapid passage of dye from the limb. A transverse incision approximately 6 to 8 cm long is made in the medial aspect of the mid–upper arm or midthigh, as the main superficial lymphatic channels parallel the course of the brachial and femoral vessels.

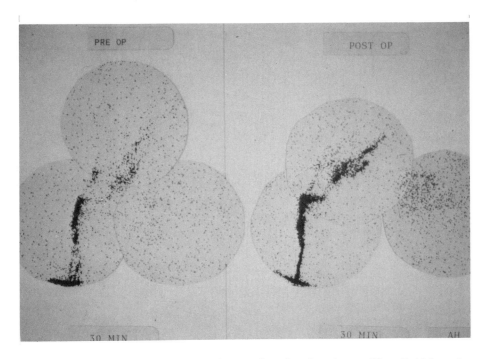

Fig. 38-1. Preoperative and postoperative results of technetium sulfa colloid lymphangiogram at 30 minutes on a patient with upper limb obstructive lymphedema. *Left,* In the preoperative study dye is seen in the forearm lymphatics (lower left circle), but in the upper arm (upper central circle) there is dermal filling only, and no dye is seen in the liver (lower right circle). *Right,* In the postoperative study after eight lymphaticovenous anastomoses have been performed, dye is more clearly seen in both the forearm and upper arm and is present in the liver at 30 minutes. The only satisfactory explanation of dye in the liver is by patent lymphovenous connections. (Courtesy John D. Franklin, M.D., University of Tennessee, Chattanooga, Tennessee.)

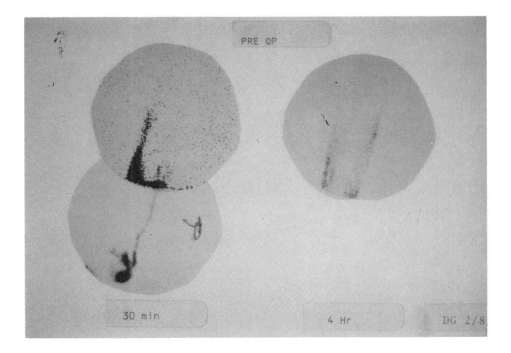

Fig. 38-2. Preoperative scan of another patient with upper limb lymphedema showing lymphatic channels in the forearm (lower left circle) but dermal flow only in the upper arm (upper left circle), which had not cleared after 4 hours (upper right circle). At 4 hours there was uptake in the liver (not shown). (Courtesy John D. Franklin, M.D., University of Tennessee, Chattanooga, Tennessee.)

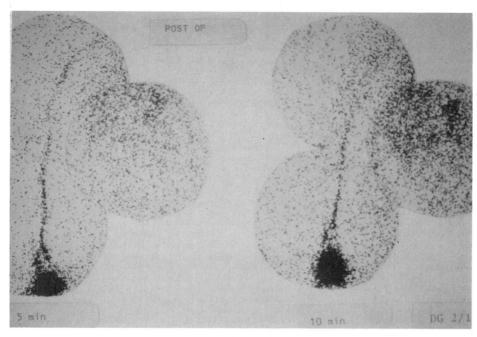

Fig. 38-3. Postoperative following lymphaticovenous bypass. *Left,* Five minutes after injection of dye lymphatic channels are clearly seen in both the forearm and upper arm, presumably in a vein, and a small amount in the liver. *Right,* At 10 minutes channels are still seen in the limb and a large amount of dye is present in the liver, again indicating patent lymphaticovenous channels. (Courtesy John D. Franklin, M.D., University of Tennessee, Chattanooga, Tennessee.)

Once the dermis has been divided, dissection is performed with loupe magnification. Small, blunt scissors are used to separate the tissues in a longitudinal direction, parallel to the expected course of the vessels. Superficial lymphatics may be found at any depth between the dermis and the deep fascia, but usually they lie about midway between the two (Fig. 38-4). The lymphatics have a characteristic beaded appearance and stain green when filled with small amounts of patent blue dye. Branching of lymphatics is rarely seen; this and the beading distinguish them from small veins. Other longitudinal strands found in the dissection are small cutaneous nerve fibers, and distinction among the three structures can sometimes be made only by using the microscope. Lymphatics are often found that are obliterated and do not fill with dye.

Only those lymphatics with a diameter greater than 0.8 mm are worthy of anastomosis to adjacent veins. Frequently one is embarrassed by the number of lymphatics present and is unable to match them to sufficient appropriately sized veins. The tourniquet is usually released after approximately half an hour, when all bleeding will have stopped, and further dye can intermittently be milked from

the wrist up into the upper arm to verify lymphatics.

If no lymphatics (or only one or two) are found at this level, a further exploration is made directly above the elbow or knee, again on the medial aspect of the limb. If nothing is found here, an incision is made below the elbow or knee, again on the medial side. When the hand or foot has significant edema, a further incision may be made on the radial aspect of the wrist or ankle to find vessels that can be anastomosed. Sometimes no adequate lymphatics are found to justify anastomosis, and clinical experience has shown that single lymphaticovenous anastomosis is not worthwhile. The number of lymphatics clinically joined in each case has ranged from two to twelve.

Within the wound the lymphatics are marked with loops of silk and the veins with loops of nylon. The lymphatics are cut as far proximally in the wound as possible and the veins as far distally as possible to gain length for the anastomosis. The technique of anastomosis is akin to small vein repairs. Periadventitial tissue is removed and the lumen irrigated with heparinized saline solution. The lymphatic vessel walls tend to collapse and do

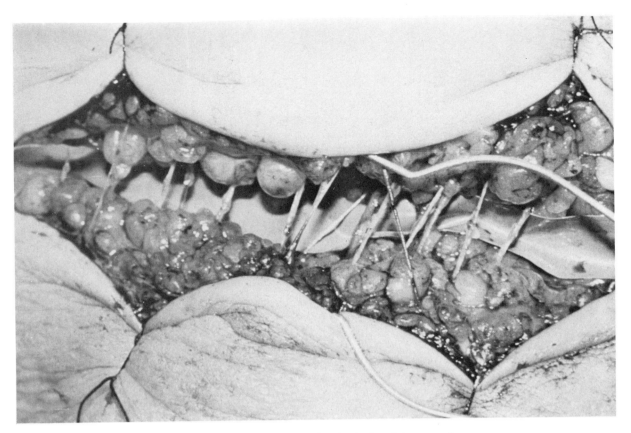

Fig. 38-4. Lymphatics and veins isolated in wound.

not remain open as do veins so that with each stitch the lumen has to be forced open with jeweler's forceps for adequate visualization. No clamps are applied to the lymphatics. The size of the lymphatics joined in obstructive lymphedema have ranged from 0.8 to 2 mm (Fig. 38-5).

Recently, when lymphaticovenous anastomoses have been performed below the elbow or knee only, we have done a simultaneous wedge resection of skin and subcutaneous fat on the lateral aspect of the upper arm or thigh. Occasionally, if no lymphatics are found and the limb size is sufficient to justify a radical ablative procedure, this is performed.

It has been believed that in obstructive lymphedema the deep lymphatic system is occluded first so that the normal direction of flow from superficial to deep lymphatics is reversed.[4] For this reason we have not routinely explored for deep lymphatics, but more recently we have made efforts to find them and have occasionally been greatly rewarded by large patent lymphatics. These have then also been joined to adjacent veins.

Postoperative management

The patient remains in the hospital approximately 4 days, with continued elevation of the extremity. We no longer use postoperative pumping.

Results

From August 1974 to July 1981, 179 cases of lymphedema have been reviewed. Twenty-four of these were primary lymphedema, all in the lower limb, and 155 were secondary or obstructive. Of the obstructive lymphedemas, 128 were upper limb and 27 lower limb.

Of the 155 obstructive cases, 60 were treated by conservative measures alone, 34 were considered too advanced to benefit from lymphatic surgery and were treated by radical reduction, and the remaining 85 were explored with a view to microlymphaticovenous bypass surgery. In 21 of this latter group of 84, insufficient lymphatics were found to justify bypass. In the remaining 64 cases in which microlymphatic surgery was performed, the number of lymphatics joined ranged from two to twelve (Table 38-1).

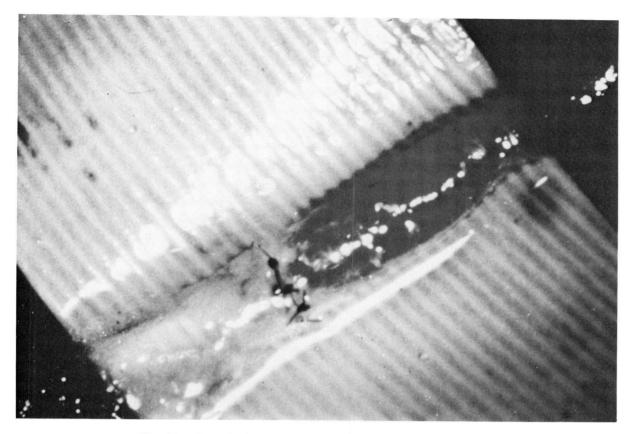

Fig. 38-5. Lymphaticovenous anastomosis (lymphatic, *lower left*).

Table 38-1. Management of cases

Lymphaticovenous anastomoses (LVA)	34
LVA with segmental reduction	26
LVA with segmental reduction as secondary procedure	4
Explored and unsuitable for LVA	21
Reduction alone	34
Conservative treatment	60
TOTAL	179

Fifty-three of these 64 cases involved the upper limb. Fifty-five of the patients were female, because the lymphedema most often followed a radical mastectomy and x-ray therapy to the axilla. The average age was 52.2 years, with a range of 27 to 72. The duration of edema averaged 6.7 years, ranging from 6 months to 21 years. The average preoperative excess volume of the edematous limb over the opposite normal limb in the 64 cases was 1,711 ml.

The subjective and objective results of the sixty-four patients are shown in Table 38-2. Among this group are those who had simultaneous segmental tissue reduction of the limb, and although the volume removed was measured at the time of surgery,

the postoperative evaluation of the benefits derived from the lymphatic bypass alone is obscured as a result. Table 38-3 gives the results for this group, except those patients who had segmental reduction. Again, the degree to which the lymphatic surgery contributed to the improvement is open to question, since some patients in this group had prolonged postoperative conservative measures such as intermittent pumping and stocking bandaging. Table 38-4 analyzes those patients who had neither segmental reduction nor postoperative conservative management or for whom we have now completely stopped conservative management. The mean follow-up period of this group is 28.8 months, and the mean decrease in excess volume is 25%. This includes two patients who objectively worsened following surgery and two who achieved a reduction of almost 70%.

Apart from the objective analysis of decrease in excess volume, the striking feature of the results is the almost universal subjective improvement claimed by the patients. This includes such comments as "The arm feels more comfortable," "It

Table 38-2. Results of LVA—with or without segmental resection or conservative postoperative management (LVA alone, 34—follow-up 30; LVA combined with resection, 30—follow-up 21)

Cases	64
Subjective improvement	88%
Unchanged or worsened	12%
Objective improvement	84%
Average decrease in excess volume	33% (range 11% to 70%)
Unchanged or worsened	16%
Average increase in excess volume	22% (range 12% to 40%)
Overall average decrease in volume	18%

Table 38-3. Results of LVA without segmental reduction but with conservative postoperative treatment

Total cases	34 (follow-up on 30)
Mean time of follow-up	30.7 months
Average decrease in excess volume	15%
Subjective improvement	29 (96%)
Objective improvement (i.e., >10% reduction)	24 (80%)

Table 38-4. Results of LVA alone without segmental reduction or conservative postoperative treatment

Total cases	17
Mean time of follow-up	29 months
Average decrease in excess volume	25% (range −40% to +70%)
Subjective improvement	16 (95%)
Objective improvement	15 (88%)

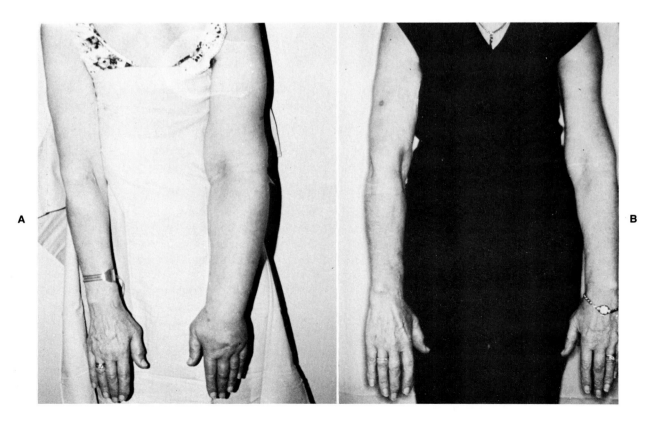

Fig. 38-6. Patient I. **A,** Lymphedema of left arm. **B,** One and a half years postoperatively—six anastomoses.

feels lighter and softer," "Clothes fit better," or "The arm seems smaller and causes less embarrassment," and "The swelling goes down faster when my arm is elevated compared to the way it was before surgery." This subjective improvement, often despite objective reduction in volume, is probably related to decreased tissue tension, and we are now trying to devise a method of tonometry to quantify this.

The other notable feature following surgery is the significant reduction in the incidence of cellulitis.

Some representative cases are shown in Figs. 38-6 to 38-10.

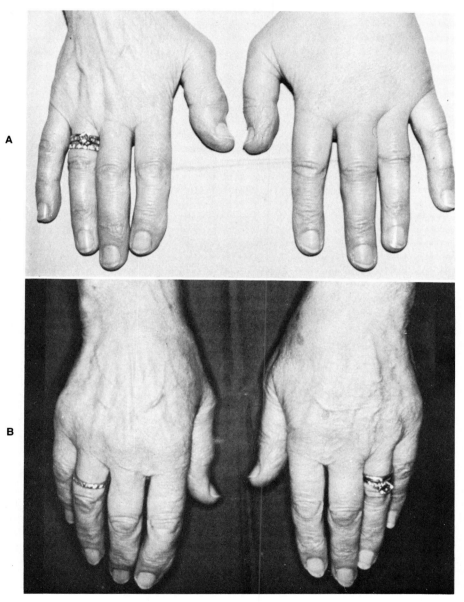

Fig. 38-7. Patient I (same patient). **A,** Hands before surgery. **B,** Hands after surgery.

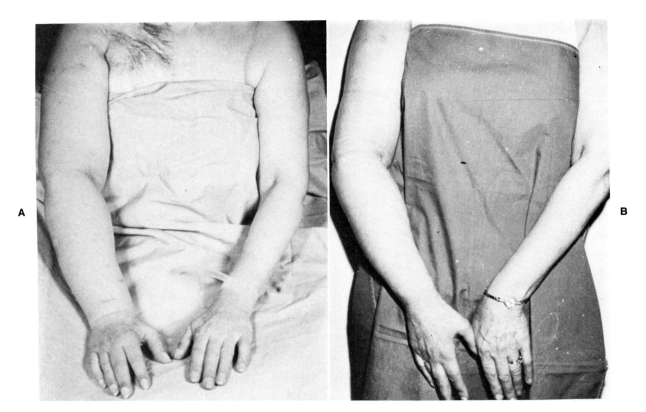

Fig. 38-8. Patient II. **A,** Lymphedema of right arm. **B,** Three years postoperatively, four anastomoses.

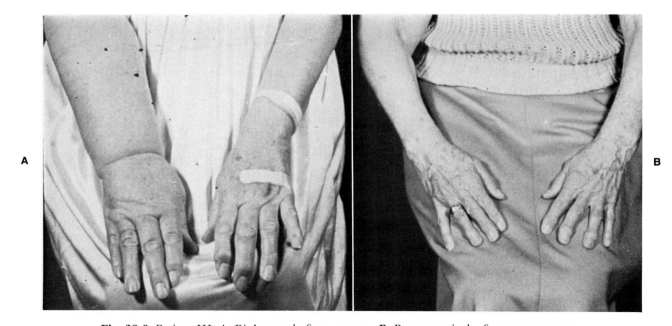

Fig. 38-9. Patient III. **A,** Right arm before surgery. **B,** Postoperatively, four anastomoses.

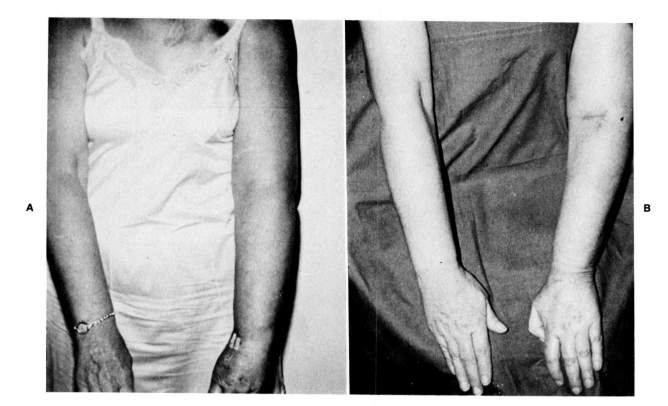

Fig. 38-10. Patient IV. **A,** Left arm before surgery. **B,** Three months postoperatively, five anastomoses.

SUMMARY

Six years of clinical experience with lymphaticovenous bypass surgery for obstructive lymphedema has yielded considerable benefit to many patients with mild to moderate disease. Close analysis of the figures shows that most patients experience significant subjective improvement and a modest objective improvement as well (over 10% reduction in excess volume). On the average the degree of objective improvement is slight. However, as much as a 70% reduction in excess volume has been achieved in individual cases, and for these patients the procedure has been of great benefit. Furthermore, the continued deterioration that might have been expected has not occurred, which in itself constitutes significant gain. In addition, the incidence of cellulitis has been significantly decreased in these patients.

Because the long-term patency of lymphaticovenous anastomoses cannot be confirmed, some writers have been skeptical and have suggested that the improvements achieved could be explained by conservative measures alone.[14] In our series, in two patients 70% reduction in excess volume was achieved with a postoperative follow-up for 4 years and 1½ years, respectively; it would be difficult to explain these results on grounds other than long-term patency, particularly when the natural tendency of the disease is to progress. Postoperative lymphangiograms following lymphaticovenous anastomosis would be unreliable—moreover, it would be deleterious. The reliability of radioactive uptake by lymphatics as a quantitative measurement of flow has been debated; however, it seems that it will prove to be the most satisfactory method of assessment of long-term patency. Tonometry to assess tension in the subcutaneous tissues is also required.

The best results in this series have been obtained when surgery is performed early after the onset of lymphedema, before the remaining lymphatics become sclerosed. Lymphangiograms should be avoided. Small and single lymphatic anastomoses are not worthwhile, and segmental reduction of the upper portion of the limb can be effectively combined with lymphaticovenous anastomoses.

The patient stands a good chance of achieving

subjective improvement and a modest chance of achieving very significant objective improvement. At worst, the morbidity he suffers is a small transverse scar on the limb.

ACKNOWLEDGMENT

My thanks to John D. Franklin, M.D., Vanderbilt University, Nashville, Tennessee, whose cases are discussed in Figs. 38-1, 38-2, and 38-3.

REFERENCES

1. Acland, R.: Personal communication, 1980.
2. Baumeister, R.G., Seifert, J., and Wiebecke, B.: Homologous and autologous experimental lymph vessel transplantation: initial experience, Int. J. Microsurg. **3:**19, 1981.
3. Born, M.L., et al.: Lymphoscintigraphic evaluation for upper extremity microlymphaticovenous anastomoses, Clin. Nucl. Med. **5:**95, 1980.
4. Clodius, L.: The experiemental basis for the surgical treatment of lymphedema, Stuttgart, 1977, Georg Thieme-Verlag.
5. Davies, D., and Davies, F., editors: Gray's anatomy of the human body, ed. 33, London, 1962, Longman's Green & Co.
6. Degni, M.: New technique of lymphatic-venous anastomosis (buried type) for the treatment of lymphedema, Vasa **3**(4):479, 1974.
7. Fox, U., and Romagnoli, G.: Lymphatic-venous shunts for treatment of limb lymphedema (film), Sixth Symposium of the International Society of Reconstructive Microsurgeons, Melbourne, Australia, February, 1981.
8. Gilbert, A., O'Brien, B.M., Vorrath, J.W., and Sykes, P.J.: Lymphaticovenous anastomosis by microvascular technique, Br. J. Plast. Surg. **29:**355, 1977.
9. Krilov, V.: Personal communication, 1981.
10. Laine, J., and Howard, J.: Experimental lymphaticovenous anastomosis, Surg. Forum **14:**111, 1963.
11. O'Brien, B.M.: Microvascular reconstructive surgery, London, 1977, Churchill Livingstone.
12. O'Brien, B.M., Das, S., Franklin, J., and Morrison, W.: Effect of lymphangiography on lymphedema, Plast. Reconstr. Surg. **68:**922, 1981.
13. O'Brien, B.M., Sykes, P.J., Threlfall, G.N., and Browning, F.S.: Microlymphaticovenous anastomoses for obstructive lymphedema, Plast. Reconstr. Surg. **60:**197, 1977.
14. Puckett, C., et al.: Evaluation of lymphovenous anastomoses in obstructive lymphedema, Plast. Reconstr. Surg. **66:**166, 1980.
15. Yamada, Y.: Studies on lymphatic venous anastomosis in lymphedema, Nagoya J. Med. Sci. **32:**1, 1969.

Part XIII

Complications

Chapter 39

Vascular complications in free flap transfer

Rollin K. Daniel
Disa Lidman

Vascular complications are a major risk in free skin flap transfers. Despite recent emphasis on the end-to-side anastomosis and introduction of additional donor sites whose vessel length and diameter are quite large, free flaps are still lost as a result of vascular thromboses. In contrast to the partial loss of conventional flaps, free flaps usually undergo total necrosis, with catastrophic consequences. In this chapter we will attempt to document the incidence, etiology, and treatment of vascular complications.

REVIEW OF THE LITERATURE

Success rates vary enormously among large series of free flap transfers for several reasons[2]: (1) case composition—indication, recipient site, and donor site, (2) experience of the surgical team, (3) frequency of reexploration, and (4) prospective versus retrospective analysis. Harii experienced an 8% complete failure rate in his initial 100 free flaps. The failure rate was higher with free groin flaps (11%) than with free scalp flaps (4%), which probably reflects the latter's simplicity of dissection and ideal recipient bed.

Serafin et al.[6] reported a 23% (4/17) failure rate with free groin flaps to the lower extremity. In a subsequent analysis the complication rate had dropped dramatically to 4% (23/25), with the improvement attributed to these factors: (1) preoperative arteriography, (2) latissimus dorsi donor site, and (3) end-to-side anastomosis.[7] Obviously additional experience had led to refinement of the surgical technique—an important consideration for the beginning surgeon. Also, the period at which one commences clinical cases has an impact on the success rate—that is, the "pioneering groin flap era" or the "maturing latissimus dorsi decade."

Goodstein and Buncke[4] presented an intriguing study of the relationship between the pattern of vascular anastomoses and the success rate of free groin flaps. In a retrospective analysis of forty cases, failures were associated with long vein grafts (greater than 5 cm) and transfers to the lower extremity. Godina[3] attributed his initial 38% failure rate with free flap transfers to the end-to-end anastomosis and a subsequent 0% failure rate to the end-to-side anastomosis. A detailed analysis of his series indicated that many factors influenced the change; the astute microsurgeon should analyze the series carefully before accepting any single factor as the cause of success.[1]

PERSONAL SERIES

In 1977 a prospective study of free skin flap transfers was initiated at the Royal Victoria Hospital. Preoperatively a detailed physical examination of each patient was done, photographs were taken, and arteriograms were obtained of the recipient site but not the donor site. Intraoperatively all microvascular anastomoses were performed by a single surgeon (R.K.D.). A detailed flow sheet with drawings of the anastomoses was made and the operative record was dictated immediately. Postoperatively all patients were monitored in the recovery room for the first 24 hours. The basic parameters were flap color and bleeding on incision; fluorescein staining was reserved until definite indications of failure were present.

During a 3-year period a total of forty-two free flaps from multiple donor sites were transferred to a wide variety of recipient sites (Table 39-1). A total of eleven vascular complications occurred, two intraoperatively and nine postoperatively; none occurred more than 15 hours postoperative-

Table 39-1. Vascular complications of free flaps (1977-1979)

Donor sites	
Cutaneous	
Groin	11
Foot	4
	15
Osteocutaneous	
Groin	8
Foot	4
	12
Neurovascular	
Foot	4
Web space	1
Intercostal	1
	6
Myocutaneous	9
TOTAL	42
Recipient sites	
Lower extremity	16
Head and neck	15
Upper extremity	7
Torso	4
TOTAL	42

Table 39-2. Vascular complications

Incidence	26%	(11/42)
Occurrence		
Intraoperative	2	
Postoperative	9	
Etiologic origin		
Artery	63%	(7/9)
Vein	37%	(2/9)
Salvage	75%	(6/8)
Vein graft	5	
New vessel	2	
Revision	1	
Results		
Success	93%	(39/42)
Failure	7%	(3/42)

ly. Most problems were arterial; revisions required vein grafts, and salvage was possible in most cases (Table 39-2).

The diverse reasons for these vascular complications may be divided into three groups: (1) errors in technique, (2) errors in judgment, and (3) unrecognized errors. Assignment to a category is arbitrary, but a worthwhile exercise.

Errors in technique (Fig. 39-1)

The most common technical errors for the neophyte are related to the vascular anastomoses, but as the surgeon gains experience, other aspects of the operative procedure influence the result.

Patient I

A 15-year-old female was initially seen with an 8-year history of bilateral facial atrophy secondary to Romberg's disease. Because of the severity of the deformity, we selected reconstruction with a deepithelialized groin flap. Following isolation of the recipient vessel and dissection of the pocket, we isolated an 18 by 8 cm groin flap. A large cheek pocket was created and the flap inserted with transcutaneous anchoring sutures. The superficial circumflex iliac artery was anastomosed to the facial artery and the superficial circumflex iliac vein to the facial vein. The facial flap was replaced and the wound closed over Hemovac drains. On the third postoperative day the facial flap became necrotic and serosanguineous drainage was present. The flap had obviously failed, and it was debrided.

The error in technique was a tight closure and inability to monitor the flap. In five subsequent dermafat flaps for facial atrophy we have solved these problems by incorporating a skin graft in the closure and by retaining a small visible "monitor" on the flap. Six months later the patient is seen on an outpatient basis, local anesthetic is administered, and the scar is revised.

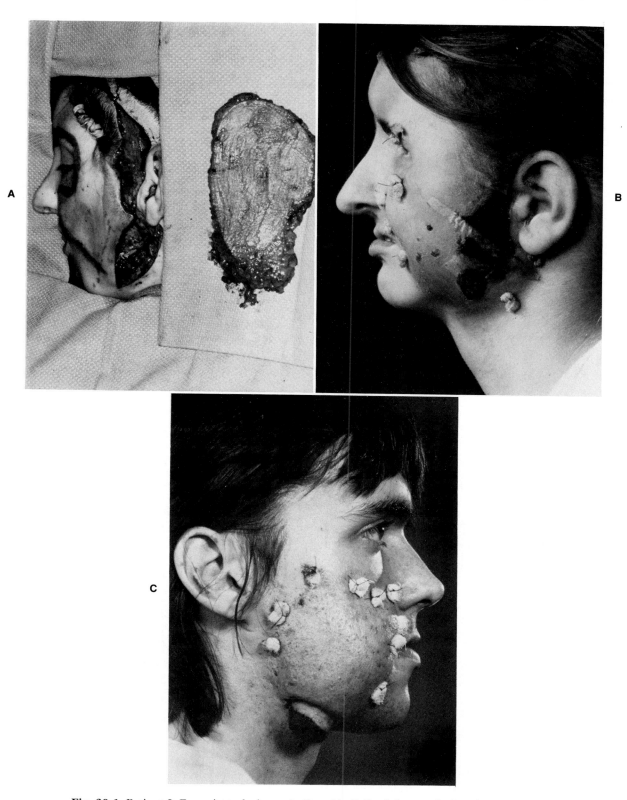

Fig. 39-1. Patient I. Error in technique. **A,** Deepithelialized free groin flap for correction of Romberg's disease. **B,** Flap loss and skin slough from tight closure. **C,** Another patient with modification of technique by incorporating a skin graft to decrease tension, and exposure of a portion of the flap for monitoring.

Errors in judgment (Fig. 39-2)

Throughout the perioperative period numerous decisions are made that influence the final outcome. Perhaps the most critical judgment is selection of the recipient vessels, especially intraoperative evaluation of their quality. It is generally agreed that the artery must possess a strong, spurting, pulsatile flow with no visible intimal damage.

Patient II

A 56-year-old male had been seen 5 years before for a $T_4N_1M_0$ squamous cell carcinoma of the anterior mouth and was treated with surgery and radiation therapy. When seen in plastic surgery consultation, the patient had an orocutaneous fistula with a protruding K-wire aligning his mandibular rami. After extensive evaluation, we elected to restore bony continuity and tongue mobility with an osteocutaneous flap from the foot.

Following isolation of the recipient vessels and preparation of the mandibular remnants, we transferred an 8 by 8 cm square dorsalis pedis flap with a 4.5 cm segment of second metatarsal. The bone was fixed with a compression plate and the vascular anastomoses were performed. Patency tests demonstrated excellent flow beyond the arterial anastomosis, but the flap did not turn pink, nor was outflow present in the vein. The dorsalis pedis artery was dissected 3 cm toward the flap and a strong flow remained present. After considering several possibilities, we decided that nonperfusion of the flap resulted from anatomic vascular variation within the flap, and thus the problem was not correctable.

The flap was removed on the fourth postoperative day. The arterial anastomosis was still patent and blood flow continued beyond the anastomosis. Dissection of the vascular stalk indicated a retrograde clot from a side branch that obstructed the main lumen of the dorsalis pedis artery.

In retrospect, we had made an error in judgment. The flap should have been completely exteriorized and the dorsalis pedis artery dissected well into the flap. It is better to be definitive than to temporize in the hope that blood flow will magically reappear; it never does.

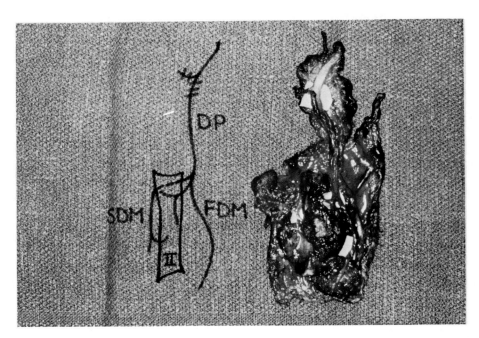

Fig. 39-2. Patient II. Error in judgment. Retrograde clot 5 cm distal to the anastomosis.

Unrecognized errors (Fig. 39-3)

Many free flaps have been lost by unforeseen errors that were induced by tight tracheostomy tapes, avulsion of the vascular pedicle while obtaining the "perfect photograph," early mobilization by well-intentioned nurses, and various "acts of God," as insurance companies refer to natural disasters.

Patient III

A 23-year-old female had a $T_2N_1M_0$ squamous cell carcinoma of the oral cavity resected following failed radiation therapy.[8] Immediate reconstruction was achieved with an 8 by 8 cm dorsalis pedis flap, revascularized by anastomosis of the dorsalis pedis artery to the external maxillary artery. The flap turned pink and had bright red bleeding on incision. Six hours postoperatively the flap turned pale, did not bleed on incision, and did not fluoresce. The patient was immediately returned to the operating room and the neck wound was opened. We found that the arterial anastomosis had been sucked into the drain. A 4 cm reverse interposition vein graft reestablished flap perfusion and there were no further complications.

The patient's head had been turned in the opposite direction at the time the drain was shortened, and unknowingly, we had left a dangerous excess in length. A dramatic change in relative length occurred when, postoperatively, the patient turned her head toward the operative site. The drain had been quite short and had been sutured posteriorly.

Thus a certain number of vascular complications are unforeseen and are best diagnosed early. An intraoral color change is indeed difficult to detect but can be observed by frequent inspection during the first 24 hours.

Several interesting observations can be drawn from this series: (1) all vascular complications occurred within the first 24 hours, (2) there were no partial failures, (3) the incidence of vascular complications did not reflect frequency of donor site use (no significant difference between groin flaps and latissimus flaps), (4) rapid reoperation was successful in most cases, (5) the clinical diagnosis correlated with the findings at reoperation, and (6) temporizing measures were of no value.

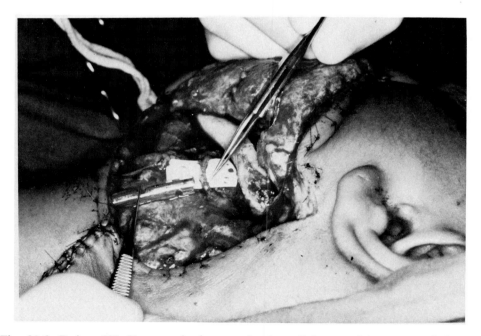

Fig. 39-3. Patient III. Unrecognized error. Suction of the arterial anastomosis into a drainage catheter.

CURRENT CLINICAL PROBLEMS

As reconstructive microsurgery evolves, the types of vascular complications will change and new difficulties will arise. Currently most problems occur in transfers to the lower extremities. The following three cases demonstrate the difficulty in judgment and technique required when dealing with latissimus dorsi flap transfers to one-vessel lower extremities.

The recipient vessel may be either the only healthy vessel that supplies the foot or a previously damaged artery (proximally or distally via retrograde flow). The anastomosis to the only patent artery can be either an end-to-side anastomosis, including an interposition vein graft, or an end-to-end anastomosis, including an interposition T-shaped graft. Despite numerous claims for the end-to-side anastomosis, one must approach the one-vessel extremity carefully. Based on our experience with five of these cases, we offer the following recommendations or observations:

1. Preoperatively it is important for the patient to accept that an amputation may be necessary if the flap fails.
2. The anastomoses should be placed proximally, and access to the popliteal fossa should be discussed.
3. Healthy recipient veins are often a major problem, with the deep venous system the usual selection.
4. The arterial anastomosis should be located proximal to the "zone of injury."
5. An end-to-side anastomosis to the dominant artery is justifiable.

It should be remembered that experience with single-vessel extremities is limited. In Serafin's series only four of fifty free flaps to the lower extremities were done under these conditions. The following three cases illustrate some of the vascular complications one can expect to encounter.

Patient IV

A 42-year-old female had suffered from cavitary osteomyelitis of the distal tibia for 8 years (Fig. 39-4). Numerous skin grafts had been attempted without successful wound closure. Preoperative arteriograms demonstrated a patent posterior tibial artery, with all other vessels transected in the upper third of the tibia. At operation the posterior tibial artery was isolated and pulsation was noted. The bony cavity was curetted down to bleeding bone. A 12 by 10 cm latissimus dorsi flap was harvested, with preservation of the T-shaped take-off of the thoracodorsal artery. The flap was sutured into place and the vessels were approximated. A clamp approximator was applied to the posterior tibial artery and the vessel was transected. The proximal clamp was released, but there was no flow. Dissection proximally failed to demonstrate any significant pulsation. Therefore a Fogarty catheter was inserted until bleeding occurred. Under careful control, the catheter was removed with the balloon partially inflated. Moderate blood flow was obtained, and two end-to-end anastomoses were performed. The flap survived completely, and the patient remained symptom free 5 years later. This case emphasizes that vascular spasm is the primary cause of vascular complications in free flap transfers. Would this problem have been avoided by an end-to-side anastomosis?

Patient V

A 19-year-old female suffered an avulsion of the right heel, with subsequent skin grafting. Over a 1-year period she developed numerous ulcerations and could not walk about easily. A second full-thickness skin graft did not endure. After repeated evaluation, an 8 by 8 cm neurovascular dorsalis pedis flap transfer was planned. A preoperative arteriogram demonstrated patency of only the posterior tibial artery.

At operation the posterior tibial artery was exposed and excellent pulsation was noted. The dorsalis pedis flap was then harvested from the opposite foot and was anchored into place. A clamp approximator was placed on the recipient artery and an elliptical excision was made for the end-to-side anastomosis. The proximal clamp was released, but no arterial perfusion occurred, despite a transmitted pulsation. The posterior tibial artery was then dissected proximally for 8 cm and another elliptical excision was made. A strong pulsatile arterial spurt occurred, but there was no bleeding through the distal ellipse.

We postulated that the intervening artery, which had been shown to be patent on arteriogram, was undergoing severe spasm and that the proximal opening had been made beyond the zone of injury. The flap was successfully vascularized by an interposition vein graft, while the distal ellipse was closed with a venous patch graft. This case emphasizes that an end-to-side anastomosis is not a universal solution and that the problem is usually in the recipient artery.

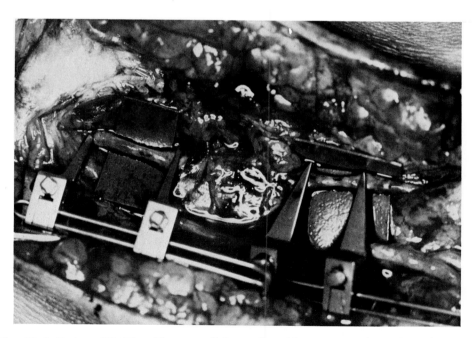

Fig. 39-4. Patient IV. The dilemma of the end-to-side anastomosis no-flow despite a transmitted pulsation. An elliptical excision does not guarantee flow from a vessel in refractory spasm.

Patient VI

A 35-year-old male had sustained severe injuries to the right leg in a car accident 7 years earlier (Fig. 39-5). The patient had undergone six skin grafts for a chronic ulcer over the Achilles tendon area. A preoperative arteriogram demonstrated patency of the posterior tibial artery, with occlusion of all other vessels. A 15 by 10 cm latissimus dorsi flap was transferred with end-to-side anastomosis of the thoracodorsal artery to the posterior tibial artery. The flap was immediately vascularized, and no further problems were encountered until 11 hours postoperatively. At this point an obvious arterial failure was present; the patient was returned to the operating room. The wound was opened and a thrombus was found at the arterial anastomosis extending into the posterior tibial artery, both proximally toward the knee and distally into the foot. The anastomosis was resected, and a Fogarty catheter was inserted to break the spasm in the posterior tibial artery. However, repeated resection of the recipient artery was necessary before pulsatile blood flow could be sustained. Eventually a 10 cm long interpositional vein graft was placed between the posterior tibial and thoracodorsal artery. As a result of stagnation the venous anastomosis had thrombosed, requiring resection and insertion of a 3 cm long vein graft. Despite the prolonged ischemic time, the flap survived completely.

This case demonstrated convincingly that a thrombus can propagate from the anastomosis into the recipient artery and along the donor artery. Fortunately the foot survived on its collateral circulation. Furthermore, the flap's origin—whether groin, latissimus, or scapula—is irrelevant.

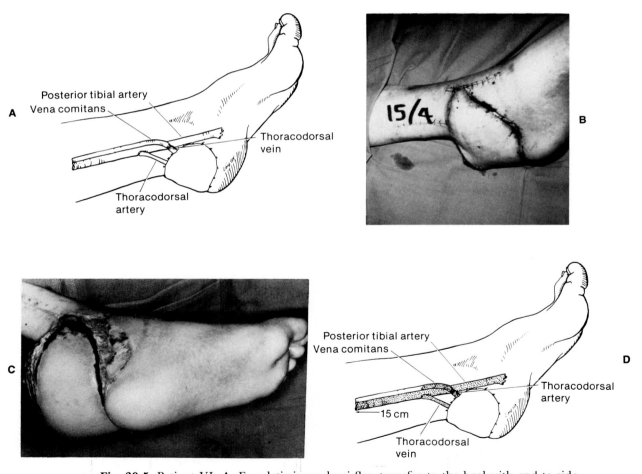

Fig. 39-5. Patient VI. **A,** Free latissimus dorsi flap transfer to the heel with end-to-side anastomosis of the thoracodorsal artery to the posterior tibial artery. **B,** Arterial failure began 11 hours postoperatively. **C,** Extensive thrombosis in all vessels with loss of the only vessel to the foot. **D,** Eventual salvage of the flap by insertion of a vein graft with end-to-end anastomoses.

DISCUSSION

Most case series give retrospective analyses of statistical data and conclude with a postulation of the cause of the problems. In 1979 we began a 1-year prospective study to determine the cause of vascular complications in microvascular procedures.[5] The factors that cause failure can be divided into extravascular and intravascular (Table 39-3). From our previous experience we believed that the most probable causes were either anastomotic problems resulting from suture error or use of a damaged recipient vessel. At the initial operation, biopsies were taken routinely of both the recipient and donor vessels. If a vascular complication occurred, the failed anastomoses were excised and biopsies of both vessels were repeated. In fifteen free tissue transfers there were four reoperations, which provided forty-five biopsies and ten anastomoses for analysis. Initial biopsies disclosed significant intimal hyperplasia in 75% (9/12) of recipient arteries with significant damage of the internal elastic lamina. Thus, despite a *patent arteriogram* and good spurting flow on transection, these vessels had evidence of previous trauma. Among the ten anastomoses there were no suture errors, which contrasts with our replantation cases. The cause of failure in the four cases were both external (a vein compressed by hematoma) and internal (two cases of a damaged recipient artery and one case of severe spasm). The latter case consisted of an architecturally normal vessel at the anastomotic site, but with extensive intimal hyperplasia more proximally, corresponding with the level of a tibial fracture. Since none of these cases was performed following acute trauma, nor were any suture errors discernible, one must conclude that a previously damaged artery is prone to severe spasm; this results in slow flow and ultimately thrombosis at the vulnerable anastomosis. Future research must be directed toward methods of intraoperative identification of damaged vessels and treatment of refractory vascular spasm.

Table 39-3. Etiologic factors in vascular complications

Intravascular	
Local	
Anastomosis	Suture error
Vessel damage	Acute trauma
	Previous trauma
	Radiation
	Atherosclerosis
Systemic	
Reduced blood flow	Vascular spasm
	Generalized ASCVD
Extravascular	
Vessel compression	Hematoma
	Tight skin closure
	Suction drains

PREVENTION

The ultimate goal is to avoid vascular complications. Its attainment is a constant challenge to the reconstructive microsurgeon throughout the perioperative period. Preoperatively one should perform an arteriogram of the recipient site and select the ideal recipient vessels. Combining this with radiographs and inspection of the wound, one should determine the zone of injury. A detailed operative plan is made, problems are anticipated, and solutions are held in readiness or sought with dispatch.

Intraoperatively the procedure is broken down into a sequence of steps, each of which must be completed successfully before the surgeon proceeds to the next. We routinely isolate the recipient vessels and perform any reconstructive procedures first, then harvest the donor tissue, and finally perform the microvascular anastomoses. We try to obtain wide exposure of healthy recipient vessels and evaluate them under the microscope. Patency tests are performed on all the microvascular anastomoses, and a second vein or artery is anastomosed whenever possible.

The patient is kept in a recovery room adjacent to the operating room for the first 24 hours. The free flap is checked every 30 minutes by a specially trained nurse, and the flap is inspected personally by a microsurgery fellow every 4 hours throughout the night. Once a vascular complication is suspected, the patient is immediately returned to the operating room.

With unrelenting attention to these details in care, we were able to achieve over fifty consecutive successful free tissue transfers. When the work load dictated an increase in staff and additional surgeons were trained, vascular complications began to reappear and basic concepts had to be relearned. There is little doubt that a 95% success rate is realistic, provided a commitment to excellence and attention to detail is maintained.

REFERENCES

1. Daniel, R.K.: Preferential use of end-to-side arterial anastomoses in free flap transfers (letter) Plast. Reconstr. Surg. **65:**849, 1980.
2. Daniel, R.K., and Terzis, J.K.: Reconstructive microsurgery, Boston, 1977, Little, Brown & Co.
3. Godina, M.: Preferential use of end-to-side arterial anastomoses in free flap transfers, Plast. Reconstr. Surg. **64:**673, 1979.

4. Goodstein, W.A., and Buncke, H.J.: Patterns of vascular anastomoses vs. success of free groin flap transfers, Plast. Reconstr. Surg. **64:**37, 1979.

5. Lidman, D., and Daniel, R.K.: Evaluation of clinical microvascular anastomoses—reasons for failure, Ann. Plast. Surg. **6:**215, 1981.

6. Serafin, D., Georgiade, N.G., and Smith, D.H.: Comparison of free flaps with pedicled flaps for coverage of defects of the leg or foot, Plast. Reconstr. Surg. **59:**492, 1977.

7. Serafin, D., Sabatier, R.E., Morris, R.L., and Georgiade, N.G.: Reconstruction of the lower extremity with vascularized composite tissue: improved tissue survival and specific indications, Plast. Reconstr. Surg. **6:**230, 1980.

8. Taylor, G.I., and Daniel, R.K.: Aesthetic aspects of microsurgery: composite tissue transfer to the face, Clin. Plast. Surg. **8:**333, 1981.

Part XIV

Monitoring

Chapter 40

Monitoring the circulation in the free flap transfer

Douglas H. Harrison
Marjorie Girling
Godfrey Mott

The success of a free flap transfer depends on revascularizing an area of skin and fat, possibly containing bone, by small vessel anastomoses to recipient vessels. In the human subject it is not known how long this anastomosis must remain patent before the surrounding tissue will support the flap by small vessel ingrowths. Animal experiments suggest that it takes at least 8 days before the surrounding tissue will maintain the viability of the flap.[2] It has also been noted that if the small vessel anastomosis becomes thrombosed, there is a time limit after which the blood flow into the flap cannot be successfully reestablished. The permissible delay period in the human is not known, but again, in animal expriments the upper limit would appear to be approximately 12 hours.[3,7] In view of the considerable investment in surgical effort that is required for a free flap transfer, it is essential to have positive confirmation of vascular thrombosis as soon after it develops as possible so that the patient may be quickly returned to the operating room and blood flow reestablished.

CLINICAL OBSERVATION

All experienced plastic surgeons would have little difficulty in confirming that a pink flap with rapid capillary return following local exsanguination is evidence of good blood flow within the skin. However, there are occasions when clinical observations can be misleading. A groin flap with excellent blood flow may be white. The test of local exsanguination is meaningless, since it remains white after pressure. Alternative clinical methods of ascertaining flow within the flap are to plunge a knife directly through the skin and observe dermal bleeding or to remove stitches from the edge of the flap and again observe dermal bleeding from its edge. These invasive tests are hardly suitable for frequent observations.

A flap may develop congestion, with its typically mottled appearance, during the postoperative period. Peripheral vasoconstriction seen early after the operation may prove difficult to differentiate from a venous thrombosis. Not only may clinical interpretation be difficult for the experienced surgeon, but also the nurse who is observing it throughout the night may well miss the subtle change in color. Therefore there is a place for a reliable instrument that can confirm whether or not blood flow into the flap has been maintained. In principle such a monitoring device should be noninvasive, should indicate pathologic changes that can be easily interpreted by both the nursing and medical staff, and should provide a continuous reading for at least 48 hours. In a series of over sixty free flaps we have not seen any vascular thrombosis develop after this 48-hour period.

METHODS AVAILABLE

In our search for a suitable instrument to measure blood flow within a flap we have explored the values of a number of machines. We have not found the following four methods to be very successful.

Radioisotope clearance

A radioactive tracer such as sodium 22 is introduced into the skin subcutaneously, and its disappearance is monitored with an appropriate radiation detector.[1] The rate of clearance, which is exponential, depends on blood flow, although a value of the partition coefficient must be assumed before the flow can be expressed in terms of volume per unit time. The disadvantages with this technique are that it is too localized and the chosen area may show evidence of no blood flow, whereas the rest of the flap may be entirely viable. Also it does not yield a continuous reading and only measures for about 1 hour. It cannot be repeated frequently because of the radiation hazard and the accumulation of background activity.

Doppler ultrasound probe

The Doppler ultrasound probe is suitable for measuring blood flow within a large-caliber vessel but cannot reflect blood flow within the small vessels in the dermal plexus. Clinically it is often difficult to ascertain whether or not the point of sudden cessation of sound may signify a point of obstruction or an increase in the depth of the blood vessel relative to the surface. Moreover, assumptions of blood vessel size and geometry must be made to convert flow into absolute values.

Percutaneous oxygen tension monitor

The percutaneous oxygen tension monitor, which is commonly used in neonatal units, would seem to have considerable advantages in measuring the viability of a flap. Svedman[10] showed that skin flaps could be monitored with this technique and that the tissue Po_2 decreased from the base of a flap to its distal extremity. Serafin[9] has demonstrated that free flap viability may be monitored with this instrument. Unfortunately, in a series of six free flap transfers that we observed in which this technique was employed, we found that during the first 48 hours postoperatively the instrument tended to record 50 mm Hg above the preoperative value; there is then a steady decline to normality after this period. The fact that the machine reads high may suggest good viability in the flap. This can be confirmed by having the patient inhale oxygen and then observing whether there is a further increase in Po_2 values. However, the high value is unsatisfactory, since it may reflect the presence of anesthetic gases retained within the circulation or the effects of sympathectomy.

Temperature

The absolute temperature of the skin does indicate the state of perfusion, and its measurement may be made noninvasively and continuously. However, it is affected by many other factors, and consideration must be given to environmental conditions and control areas must be monitored for comparison. Although it is quantifiable, absolute changes in temperature are small, and surface temperature is relatively slow to respond to changes in perfusion.

PHOTOPLETHYSMOGRAPHY

Photoplethysmography has been used for several decades as a means of assessing blood flow by measuring either transmitted or reflected light.* Like all noninvasive methods it has the disadvantage of not providing an absolute measure of blood flow in terms of volume per unit time, but under controlled conditions it can be used to monitor changes in perfusion at a single site. The principle underlying the use of photoplethysmography is skin transillumination. A pulsatile change in tissue blood volume produces a corresponding change in the amount of light reflected. These changes may be detected, amplified, and displayed on an oscilloscope. The exact depth of light penetration is probably no more than 2 mm and therefore reflects changes in subdermal circulation. We have developed a probe that is stable and considerably more sensitive than transducers previously described. It consists of multiple infrared light sources surrounding a single detector (Fig. 40-1). The light sources produce a radiation of 940 nm, which optimizes the depth of light penetration. It has been miniaturized, employing fiberoptics, for use in replantation and toe-to-thumb transfers (Fig. 40-2).

Interpretation of the signal

Our results show that a reproducible, consistent wave pattern can be produced when monitoring normal circulation and that in the presence of a vascular problem, distinction may be made between arterial and venous obstruction.

Fig. 40-3 illustrates the waveform associated with each cardiac cycle; ΔP represents the small fluctuation in reflected light that occurs with pulsatile blood flow. It is characterized by a sharp up-

---

*References 4, 5, 6, 8, 11, 12, 13.

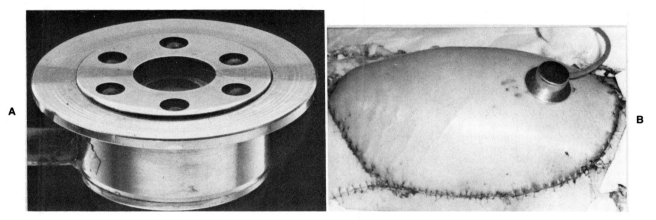

Fig. 40-1. A, Undersurface of the modified photoplethysmograph probe, showing the central light sensor surrounded by six infrared light sources. The metal flange is for the application of double-surface adhesive. **B,** Photoplethysmograph probe applied to a free flap transfer. (From Harrison, D.H., Girling, M., and Mott, G.: Experience in monitoring the circulation in free-flap transfers, Plast. Reconstr. Surg. **68**(4):543, 1981.)

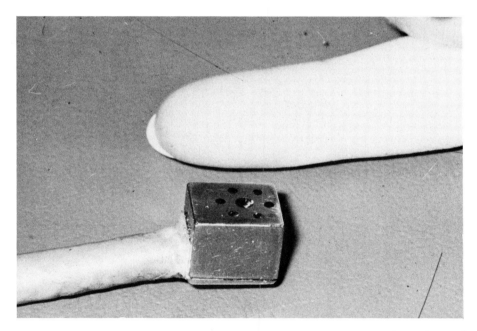

Fig. 40-2. Miniaturized probe for use in replants and toe-to-thumb transfers. The configuration of the light source remains the same and is achieved with the use of fiberoptics.

Simulation

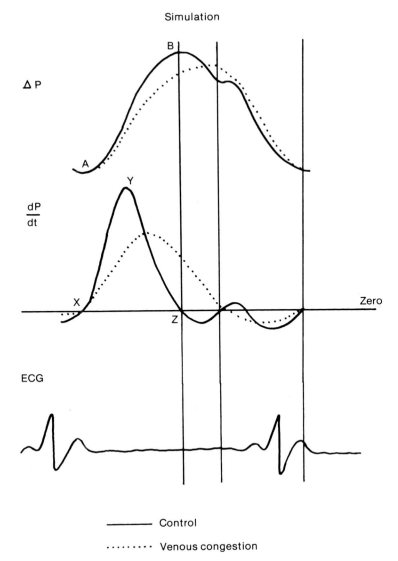

ΔP

$\dfrac{dP}{dt}$

Zero

ECG

——— Control

········· Venous congestion

Fig. 40-3. The upper waveform depicts the fundamental signal ΔP; beneath this dP/dt is the electronically attained first derivative. The dotted line represents the changes seen in venous congestion. (From Harrison, D.H., Girling, M., and Mott, G.: Experience in monitoring the circulation in free flap transfers, Plast. Reconstr. Surg. **68**(4):543, 1981.)

stroke as the blood pulse arrives at the capillary bed, followed by a more gradual return to its original level. It is possible to examine the upstroke of the signal ΔP and express it as a waveform. This electronically attained first derivative of ΔP, designated dP/dt, is similarly recorded. It is a more stable waveform, since it is less influenced by lower frequency respiratory fluctuations. It also emphasizes the main characteristics of the signal. In the normal waveform (solid lines) a sharp upstroke XY and a good peak height indicate good arterial inflow, while a steep downstroke YZ indicates adequate venous outflow. In the presence of venous congestion (dotted lines) the downstroke YZ is prolonged and the peak is reduced and delayed.

Abnormal blood flow—animal experiments

To confirm our clinical findings we chose an axial pattern flap on a rabbit flank as a suitable model. A series of twenty rabbits was examined. It was possible to raise the axial pattern flaps, place them on a cork plinth in such a way that they were not sensitive to respiratory movements, and apply the photoplethysmograph probe (Fig. 40-4). The axial vessels were then carefully dissected under the microscope in such a way as to avoid spasm. A

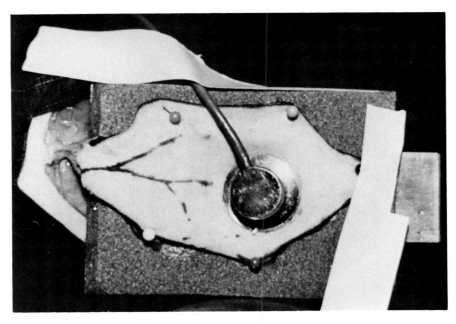

Fig. 40-4. Axial pattern flap raised on the flank of a rabbit and pinned out on a cork plinth. Photoplethysmograph probe may be seen applied to its surface. (From Harrison, D.H., Girling, M., and Mott, G.: Experience in monitoring the circulation in free flap transfers, Plast. Reconstr. Surg. 68:1, 1981.)

A

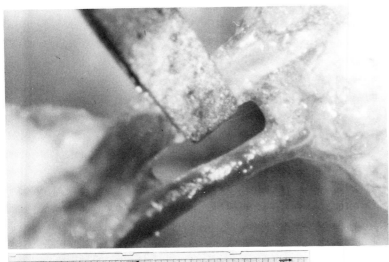

B

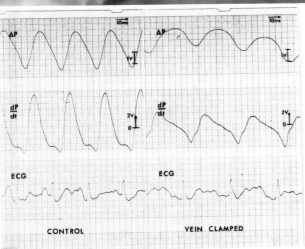

Fig. 40-5. A, Photomicrograph of the dissected axial vessels with a clamp applied to the vein. B, Waveform produced by clamping the vein shows a depressed amplitude in dP/dt and a prolonged downstroke. (From Harrison, D.H., Girling, M., and Mott, G.: Experience in monitoring the circulation in free flap transfers, Plast. Reconstr. Surg. 68(4):543, 1981.)

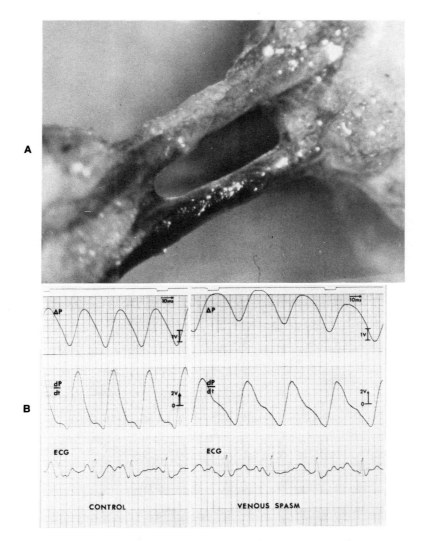

Fig. 40-6. A, The superior vessel; the axial vein is in spasm. **B,** The venous spasm causes depression in the amplitude of dP/dt and there is a delayed downstroke, but this is not as profound as seen in venous obstruction. (From Harrison, D.H., Girling, M., and Mott, G.: Experience in monitoring the circulation in free flap transfers, Plast. Reconstr. Surg. **68**(4):543, 1981.)

stable reading was achieved and then fine vascular clamps were applied to each of the vessels. Complete obstruction of the vein produced the expected reduction in amplitude of dP/dt, and the downstroke (YZ) was prolonged (Fig. 40-5). Venous spasm was produced by manipulation of the vein, causing a reduction in the amplitude of dP/dt with a prolonged downstroke, but it was not so profound as when the vein was totally obstructed (Fig. 40-6). A vascular clamp applied to the artery eliminated the signal entirely and reflected no blood flow within the flap (Fig. 40-7). Spasm in both the artery and vein could be produced and was reflected by a short upstroke in dP/dt with a very delayed downstroke (Fig. 40-8).

CLINICAL EXPERIENCE

In the plastic surgery unit at Mount Vernon Hospital a series of fifty free flap transfers has been monitored by various methods. The last thirty were monitored with the modified photoplethysmograph. Two of the flaps failed while being monitored. In the first failure, which occurred early in the study, a groin flap was thought to be viable clinically but had an asynchronous, irregular waveform unrelated to the electrocardiogram; this was clearly suggestive of arterial obstruction but unfortunately was ignored. Obvious clinical necrosis was not apparent for 3 days. The second failure was in an osteocutaneous free groin flap to the leg. Spasm that could not be reversed developed in the recipi-

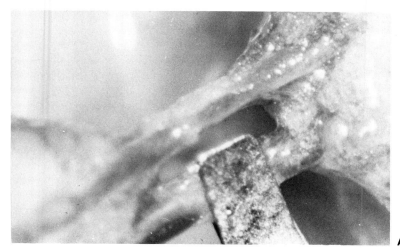

A

Fig. 40-7. A, The artery is clamped. B, The waveform produced by arterial obstruction is flat, since there is no blood entering the flap. (From Harrison, D.H., Girling, M., and Mott, G.: Experience in monitoring the circulation in free flap transfers, Plast. Reconstr. Surg. **68**(4):543, 1981.)

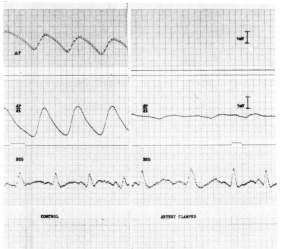

B

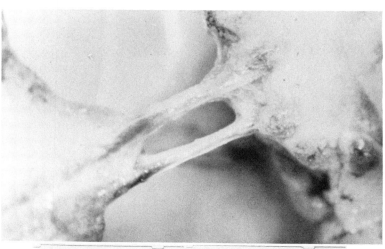

A

Fig. 40-8. A, Spasm produced in both artery and vein. B, The waveform seen in dP/dt shows a low wave amplitude and a very prolonged downstroke, suggesting that little blood is entering the flap. (From Harrison, D.H., Girling, M., and Mott, G.: Experience in monitoring the circulation in free flap transfers, Plast. Reconstr. Surg. **68**(4):543, 1981.)

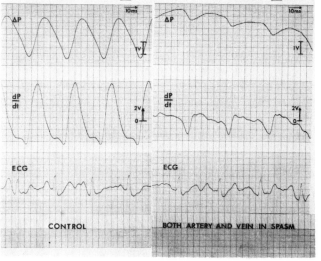

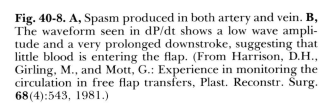

B

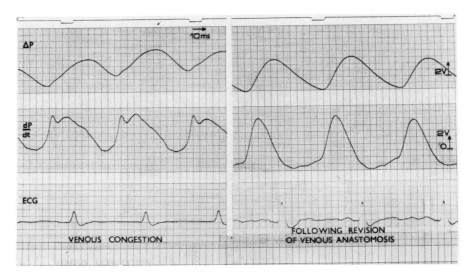

Fig. 40-9. Clinical case in which the patient was returned to the operating room because a waveform suggested venous obstruction. Following revision of the venous anastomosis, the waveform returned to normal. (From Harrison, D.H., Girling, M., and Mott, G.: Experience in monitoring the circulation in free flap transfers, Plast. Reconstr. Surg. **68**(4):543, 1981.)

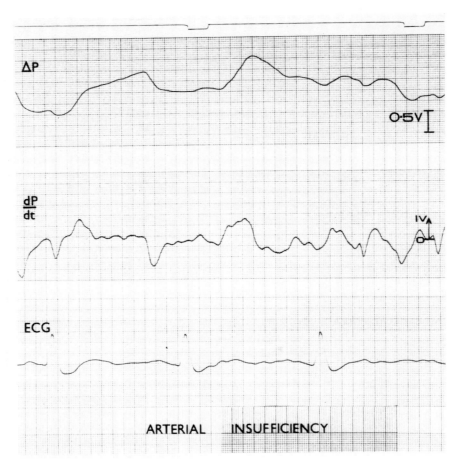

Fig. 40-10. A waveform that may trap the unwary is "background noise," seen in cases of arterial insufficiency. Note that the electrocardiogram tracing is unrelated to the wave patterns. (From Harrison, D.H., Girling, M., and Mott, G.: Experience in monitoring the circulation in free flap transfers, Plast. Reconstr. Surg. **68**(4):543, 1981.)

ent anterior tibial artery. In five other cases the wave pattern on the photoplethysmograph clearly showed evidence of abnormalities in the circulation. These patients were returned to the operating room for reexploration of the transfer site, and all proceeded to a satisfactory outcome. One of those reexplored had an arterial obstruction and four had venous obstruction (Fig. 40-9). In arterial obstruction a flat tracing is not always obtained, and some "background noise" may be reflected. Therefore, it is important to confirm that the electrocardiographic complex relates to the wave pattern (Fig. 40-10). One factor that has become apparent clinically and has been confirmed experimentally is that if there is venous obstruction but compensatory hemorrhage occurs either from the edge or from beneath the flap, the photoplethysmograph will respond by producing a virtually normal wave pattern. However, once the hemorrhage ceases, the venous thrombosis is revealed on the monitor by the typical alteration in the wave pattern.

SUMMARY

The modified photoplethysmograph, with the special configuration of the monitor head and the use of the first derivative of the fundamental signal, has provided an entirely reliable method of monitoring free flaps and toe-to-thumb transfers—a method that is noninvasive and easily understood. It may also be easily programmed to sound an alarm if various electronically arranged criteria are not achieved. In our hands it has proved the most reliable method of monitoring free flap transfers.

REFERENCES

1. Barron, J.N., Laing, J.E., Colbert, J.G., and Veall, N.: Observations on the circulation of tubed skin pedicles using the local clearance of radioactive sodium, Br. J. Plast. Surg. **5:**171, 1952.
2. Black, M.J., et al.: How soon may the axial vessels of a surviving free flap be safely ligated: a study in pigs, Br. J. Plast. Surg. **31:**295, 1978.
3. Chait, L.A., May, J.W., Jr., O'Brien, B.M., and Hurley, J.V.: The effects of the perfusion of various solutions on the no-reflow phenomenon in experimental free flaps, Plast. Reconstr. Surg. **61:**421, 1978.
4. Hard, J.D., and Muschenheim, C.: Radiation of heat from the human body. V: The transmission of infrared radiation through skin, J. Clin. Invest. **15:**1, 1936.
5. Hayes, J.E., Robinson, D.W., and Masters, F.W.: A simple inexpensive method of evaluating circulation in pedicled tissues, Plast. Reconstr. Surg. **42:**141, 1968.
6. Hertzman, A.: Photoelectric plethysmography of the nasal septum in man, Proc. Soc. Exp. Biol. Med. **37:**290, 1937.
7. May, J.W., Jr., Chait, L.A., O'Brien, B.M., and Hurley, J.V.: The no-reflow phenomenon in experimental free flaps, Plast. Reconstr. Surg. **61:**256, 1978.
8. Ramirez, Z.M.A., et al.: Reimplantation of limbs, Plast. Reconstr. Surg. **40:**315, 1967.
9. Serafin, D., Lesesne, C.B., Mullen, R.Y., and Georgiade, N.G.: Transcutaneous Po$_2$ monitoring for assessing viability and predicting survival of skin flaps: experimental and clinical correlation, J. Microsurg. **2:**165, 1981.
10. Svedman, P., Jacobsson, S., Lindell, S.E., and Ponnert, L.: Measurement of transcutaneous oxygen tension: a method for studying the blood supply to the skin, I.R.C.S.J. Med. Sci. **6:**339, 1978.
11. Thorne, F.L., Georgiade, N.G., Wheeler, W.F., and Mladick, R.A.: Photoplethysmography as an aid in determining the viability of pedicle flaps, Plast. Reconstr. Surg. **44:**279, 1969.
12. Webster, M.H.C., and Patterson, J.: The photoelectric plethysmograph as a monitor of microvascular anastomoses, Br. J. Plast. Surg. **29:**182, 1976.
13. Weinman, J., and Manoach, M.: A photoelectric approach to the study of peripheral circulation, Am. Heart J. **63:**219, 1962.

Chapter 41

Assessing skin flap viability and predicting survival using the transcutaneous PO$_2$ monitor

Donald Serafin
Carroll B. Lesesne
Vincent E. Voci
R. Yaeger Mullen
Nicholas G. Georgiade

Early postoperative assessment of skin flap viability and prediction of survival may be difficult.[2] There are several methods of assessing viability and perfusion, including saline, atropine, epinephrine, or radiographic dyes, but these are invasive and may cause tissue injury.[12,15,16,20,21] Injection of fluorescein or radioactive tracers assesses perfusion and viability at that instant, but cannot be repeated for many hours and does not predict survival.[19]

A method of determining oxygen delivery in the microcirculation of cutaneous tissue that is accurate, rapid, repetitive, and noninvasive would give information that could provide assessment of viability and perhaps predict survival.[7,8,9]

Continuous noninvasive measurement of skin oxygen tension levels can be done with a transcutaneous oxygen tension (TcPo$_2$) monitor.[3] A Clark polarographic electrode records the level of oxygen diffusing through the skin. This requires a maximally dilated capillary bed beneath the electrode; therefore a heating coil is incorporated into the TcPo$_2$ probe, which is set to a specified temperature to maintain a state of constant local hyperemia directly under the probe (Fig. 41-1). Hach and his colleagues have shown that local hyperemia accelerates O$_2$ transport.[4,5] Oxygen transport can be increased sufficiently that oxygen tension in the skin can approximate arterial Po$_2$ and can rapidly respond to changes in the concentration of inspired oxygen.[13]

A study was designed both in laboratory animals and in clinical cases to assess the use of a transcutaneous oxygen tension monitor. Its reliability, response to changes in inspired oxygen, and ability to predict survival of flaps were assessed.[18]

LABORATORY SERIES

Rectangular skin flaps based on the right superficial epigastric vessels were designed on thirty-six Sprague-Dawley rats. Group A and group B rats had simple 2 by 8 cm rectangular flaps outlined (Fig. 41-2). Group C had a distal horizontal extension that would predictably undergo necrosis (Fig. 41-3). Group A served as a control; the flaps were not raised. Transcutaneous Po$_2$ values were recorded. Preoperative, intraoperative, and postoperative readings of oxygen tension were made in all groups at proximal, central, and distal sites on the flaps (as well as on a control area on the abdominal wall) under various conditions of inspired oxygen.

Baseline TcPo$_2$ values on room air (20% O$_2$) at control sites and proximal sites preoperatively were not significantly different. After elevation of

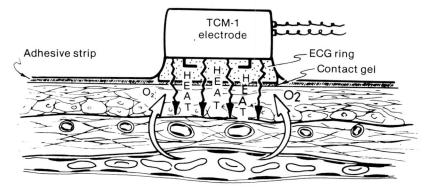

- Heat causes local capillary dilatation
- O₂ diffuses through skin, contact gel, and into the electrode

Fig. 41-1. Process by which oxygen and heat readily diffuse through the contact gel. Vascular dilatation occurs only under probe. (From Serafin, D., Lesesne, C., Mullen, R.Y., and Georgiade, N.G.: Transcutaneous Po_2 monitoring for assessing viability and predicting survival of skin flaps: experimental and clinical correlations, J. Microsurg. **2:**165, 1981.)

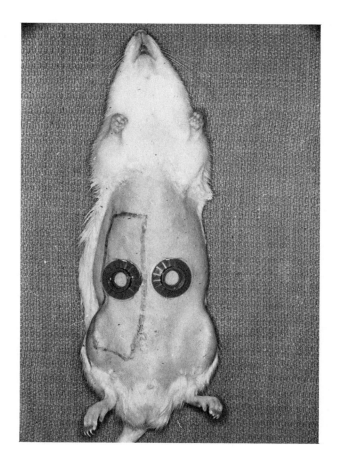

Fig. 41-2. Group A rat (control). A 2 by 8 cm groin flap is outlined but not raised. The $TcPo_2$ probe contact rings are applied to the recording sites. (From Serafin, D., Lesesne, C., Mullen, R.Y., and Georgiade, N.G.: Transcutaneous Po_2 monitoring for assessing viability and predicting survival of skin flaps: experimental and clinical correlations, J. Microsurg. **2:**165, 1981.)

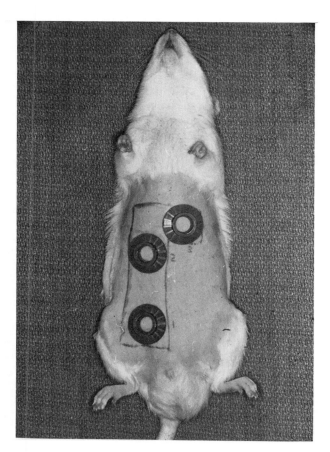

Fig. 41-3. Group C rat. A 3 by 9 cm groin flap is outlined before elevation. The contact rings are on the experimental preoperative and postoperative sites. The control site on the left midabdomen does not have a ring. (From Serafin, D., Lesesne, C., Mullen, R.Y., and Georgiade, N.G.: Transcutaneous Po_2 monitoring for assessing viability and predicting survival of skin flaps: experimental and clinical correlations, J. Microsurg. **2:**165, 1981.)

Table 41-1. Comparison of transcutaneous oxygen tension (TcPo₂) values (in mm Hg) in undisturbed control skin, proximal sites preoperatively, and after elevation of the flaps, in three groups of rats breathing room air, pure oxygen, or pure nitrogen.

Skin flap group	Room-air baseline (20% O_2)	100% O_2	100% N_2 (0% O_2)
Control sites (preoperative)			
Group A	86.8 ± 3.0		
Group B	84.5 ± 2.1		
Group C	84.0 ± 3.7		
Proximal sites (preoperative)			
Group A	84.4 ± 3.5	151.7 ± 11.0	21.3 ± 5.2
Group B	83.8 ± 3.2	166.7 ± 14.7	20.0 ± 4.2
Group C	74.3 ± 4.9	155.3 ± 7.3	20.5 ± 6.4
Proximal sites (flaps elevated)			
Group A	54.7 ± 10.7	105.0 ± 13.1	6.0 ± 4.2
Group B	55.1 ± 2.8	95.8 ± 13.6	14.4 ± 6.8
Probability	$P<0.001$	$P>0.05$	$P>0.0$

From Serafin, D., Lesesne, C., Mullen, R.Y., and Georgiade, N.G.: Transcutaneous Po₂ monitoring for assessing viability and predicting survival of skin flaps: experimental and clinical correlations, J. Microsurg. **2**:165, 1981.

the flaps in groups B and C, TcPo₂ values dropped significantly (Table 41-1).

In group C the TcPo₂ monitor also recorded a progressive decrease in postoperative room air values (20% O₂) at proximal, central, and distal sites. The readings at proximal and central sites varied but were always above 36 mm Hg and 25 mm Hg respectively. Distal site measurements in group C, however, were uniformly 0 mm Hg (Fig. 41-4). The results were reliable.

The response time to changes in concentrations of inspired oxygen and to application of a tourniquet were rapid—and statistically significant—both before and after flap elevation. The response time of the skin to changes in the concentration of oxygen was rapid (less than 15 seconds) (Fig. 41-5). The response time to application of a tourniquet was even more rapid, with TcPo₂ readings falling within 5 seconds after occlusion.

The transcutaneous oxygen tension monitor (TCM-1) accurately predicted skin survival or necrosis at all sites except two that had been abraded. Any flap site with a TcPo₂ reading greater than 25 mm Hg survived. Any flap site with a reading of 0 mm Hg eventually became necrotic (Table 41-2).

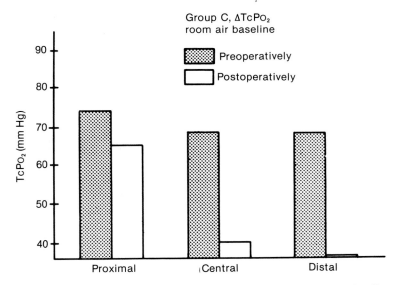

Fig. 41-4. Progressive fall in the room-air baseline values from sites proximally, centrally, and distally. (From Serafin, D., Lesesne, C., Mullen, R.Y., and Georgiade, N.G.: Transcutaneous Po₂ monitoring for assessing viability and predicting survival of skin flaps: experimental and clinical correlations, J. Microsurg. **2**:165, 1981.)

Table 41-2. Predictions of flap viability by measurements of transcutaneous oxygen tension (TcPo₂) in experimental studies in rats

TcPo₂ reading	Number of sites	Surviving flaps	Necrotic flaps
25 mm Hg	42	42	0
0 mm Hg	18	2*	16

From Serafin, D., Lesesne, C., Mullen, R.Y., and Georgiade, N.G.: Transcutaneous Po₂ monitoring for assessing viability and predicting survival of skin flaps: experimental and clinical correlations, J. Microsurg. **2:**165, 1981.
*Two sites that were abraded when they were shaved gave TcPo₂ readings of 0 mm Hg but survived.

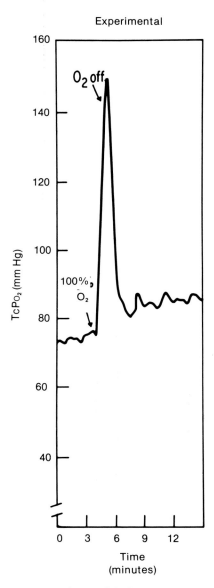

Fig. 41-5. An experimental TcPo₂ response curve following administration of 100% O₂ for 1 minute in one of the rats. The initial response time is 15 seconds. The TcPo₂ continued to rise for 20 seconds after the oxygen was discontinued. (From Serafin, D., Lesesne, C., Mullen, R.Y., and Georgiade, N.G.: Transcutaneous Po₂ monitoring for assessing viability and predicting survival of skin flaps: experimental and clinical correlations, J. Microsurg. **2:**165, 1981.)

The monitor successfully demonstrated its usefulness in assessing viability and in predicting skin flap survival in the laboratory animal. A clinical evaluation was then carried out.

CLINICAL SERIES

Eighteen flaps in sixteen patients were selected for evaluation with the TcPo₂ monitor (Table 41-3). When possible, preoperative, intraoperative, and postoperative measurements were obtained from proximal, central, and distal sites on the flaps. The infraclavicular region was used as a control. The TcPo₂ measurements, again, were significant and reproducible. Variations in core temperature, systemic blood pressure, and pulse did not significantly affect TcPo₂ values. The response to changes in the concentration of inspired oxygen, as in the experimental series, was rapid (approximately 15 seconds) (Fig. 41-6).

Control TcPo₂ measurements from the infraclavicular region approximated arterial Po₂ values but were often 10 to 15 mm Hg lower. These control measurements were essential in evaluating changes in flap TcPo₂ readings. Control values were significantly influenced by the ventilatory exchange of the patient. Preexisting pulmonary disease, changes in the level of consciousness, and the concentration of inspired oxygen influenced the TcPo₂ readings the most. Variation in an individual's hematocrit level also had some effect.

Flap measurements were also altered by these systemic factors. In addition, factors influencing local blood flow, such as vascular insufficiency, thrombosis, edema, abrasions at the probe site, and wound infection, altered TcPo₂ measurements in the flaps. Such local changes, of course, were not reflected in control readings.

In most patients early postoperative measurements in control and flap sites were lower than

Table 41-3. Breakdown of eighteen flaps in sixteen patients selected for monitoring of transcutaneous oxygen tension (TcPo$_2$)

Type of flap	Number
Vascularized latissimus dorsi musculocutaneous	13
Vascularized groin	1
Island latissimus dorsi musculocutaneous	3
Random cutaneous	1

From Serafin, D., Lesesne, C., Mullen, R.Y., and Georgiade, N.G.: Transcutaneous Po$_2$ monitoring for assessing viability and predicting survival of skin flaps: experimental and clinical correlations, J. Microsurg. **2:**165, 1981.

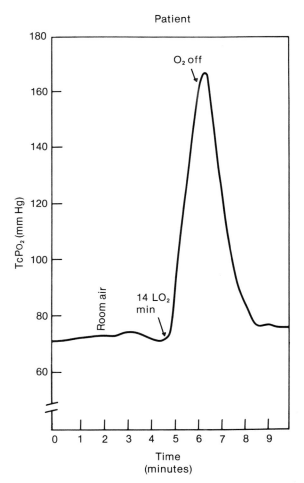

Fig. 41-6. A clinical TcPo$_2$ response curve to the administration of 14 liters of oxygen for 1 minute. (From Serafin, D., Lesesne, C., Mullen, R.Y., and Georgiade, N.G.: Transcutaneous Po$_2$ monitoring for assessing viability and predicting survival of skin flaps: experimental and clinical correlations, J. Microsurg. **2:**165, 1981.)

Table 41-4. Serial measurements of transcutaneous oxygen tension (TcPo$_2$) in mm Hg in patients who had vascularized latissimus dorsi flaps and who were breathing room air (20% O$_2$)

	TcPo$_2$ reading					
	Preoperative		Intraoperative		Early postoperative	
Case number	Flap site	Control site	Flap site	Control site	Flap site	Control site
7	87	92	58	49*	55	65
8	88	95	45	70	76	83
9	63	60	54	76	68	79
12	70	63	46	54	29	59
13†		46	37		60	41

From Serafin, D., Lesesne, C., Mullen, R.Y., and Georgiade, N.G.: Transcutaneous Po$_2$ monitoring for assessing viability and predicting survival of skin flaps: experimental and clinical correlations, J. Microsurg. **2:**165, 1981.
*This was the only control site not in the infraclavicular region.
†This patient received bilateral latissimus dorsi musculocutaneous flaps and was suffering from chronic pulmonary disease.

preoperative values; this probably represented a change in ventilation. Transcutaneous Po$_2$ values were lowest in patients who had chronic pulmonary disease or in patients with probable decreased chest wall compliance (i.e., secondary to a latissimus flap donor site) (cases 1, 2, and 13).

Intraoperative measurements taken from vascularized latissimus dorsi musculocutaneous flaps were also lower than the control and the preoperative measurements (Table 41-4). This may be explained by surgically induced vasoconstriction and consequently decreased blood flow.

Early postoperative TcPo$_2$ values were generally higher than intraoperative measurements but lower than postoperative controls (Fig. 41-7). This may reflect alterations in blood flow secondary to sympathectomy. All patients in this subgroup underwent complete interruption of the neurovascular pedicle of the latissimus dorsi musculocutaneous flap with revascularization at the recipient site.

Postoperative measurements were taken at proximal, central, and distal flap sites. Proximal values were obtained from an area immediately above the entrance of the neurovascular pedicle into the muscle or subcutaneous tissue of the flap. The proximal site TcPo$_2$ values were the highest, approximating control values on the first postoperative day. A progressive decrease in TcPo$_2$ values was seen at the central and distal sites (Fig. 41-8).

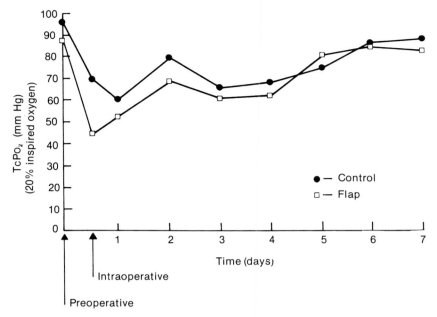

Fig. 41-7. Decrease in intraoperative TcPo_2 values (case 8). Note that the intraoperative measurements were obtained on this vascularized musculocutaneous flap before division of the neurovascular pedicle. (From Serafin, D., Lesesne, C., Mullen, R.Y., and Georgiade, N.G.: Transcutaneous Po_2 monitoring for assessing viability and predicting survival of skin flaps: experimental and clinical correlations, J. Microsurg. **2:**165, 1981.)

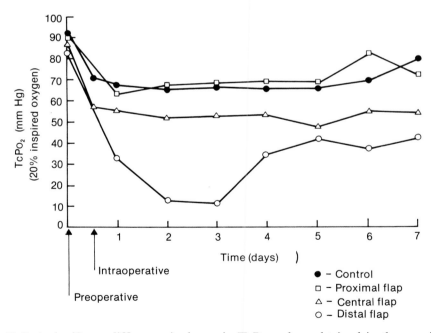

Fig. 41-8. A significant difference is shown in TcPo_2 values obtained in the proximal, central, and distal portions of a flap (case 7). (From Serafin, D., Lesesne, C., Mullen, R.Y., and Georgiade, N.G.: Transcutaneous Po_2 monitoring for assessing viability and predicting survival of skin flaps: experimental and clinical correlations, J. Microsurg. **2:**165, 1981.)

Table 41-5. Results of the monitoring of transcutaneous oxygen tension (TcPo₂) in eighteen flaps in sixteen patients, all of whom were breathing room air (20% O₂)

Case number	Type of flap*	Control TcPo₂ reading (mm Hg)	Central flap TcPo₂ reading (mm Hg)	Time when measurement was taken postoperatively	Fate of flap
1	VLDMC (LLE)	72	66	4 days	Survived
	VLDMC (RLE)	72	71	2 mo	Survived
2	VLDC	72†	58†	1 hr	Survived
3	ILDMC	91	93	3 hr	Survived
4	VLDMC	126†	110†	1 hr	Survived
5	R	68	47	8 hr	Survived
6	VLDMC	67	75	1 hr	Survived
7	VLDMC	103†	92†	3 hr	Survived
8	VLDMC	83	76	1 hr	Survived
9	VLDMC	62	52	1 hr	Survived
10	VGr	109†	0†	1 hr	Distal necrosis
11	VLDMC	80†	80	6 hr	Survived
12	VLDMC	74	43	2 hr	Survived
13	ILDMC	46	0	3 days	Necrosis
	VLDMC	41	60	1 hr	Survived
14	VLDMC	75	50	1 hr	Survived
15	ILDMC	86	0	3 days	Necrosis
16	VLDMC	47	40	1 hr	Survived

From Serafin, D., Lesesne, C., Mullen, R.Y., and Georgiade, N.G.: Transcutaneous Po₂ monitoring for assessing viability and predicting survival of skin flaps: experimental and clinical correlations, J. Microsurg. **2:**165, 1981.
*Abbreviations for types of flaps: VLDMC = vascularized latissimus dorsi musculocutaneous flap; ILDMC = island latissimus dorsi musculocutaneous flap; R = random flap; VGr = vascularized groin flap.
†These readings were taken with the patient breathing 40% O₂.

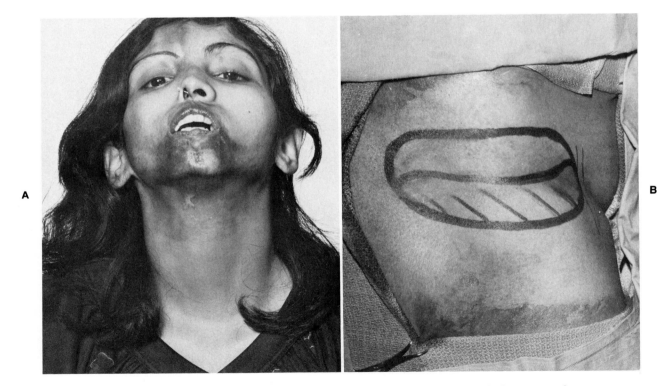

Fig. 41-9. A, Preoperative view of a patient with scleroderma (case 10). **B,** Intraoperative view demonstrating deepithelialized vascularized groin flap (slashed lines). Note cutaneous island to be used for monitoring. (**A** to **E** from Serafin, D., Lesesne, C., Mullen, R.Y., and Georgiade, N.G.: Transcutaneous Po₂ monitoring for assessing viability and predicting survival of skin flaps: experimental and clinical correlations, J. Microsurg. **2:**165, 1981.)

Transcutaneous Po₂ measurements accurately predicted the survival of fifteen flaps and necrosis in the remaining three (Table 41-5). In one of these patients (case 10), central and distal necrosis of a vascularized groin flap was accurately predicted (Fig. 41-9). Progressive clinical deterioration of two island latissimus dorsi musculocutaneous flaps prompted a request for a TcPo₂ evaluation on the third postoperative day. Readings of 0.0 mm Hg were obtained at all sites on these flaps. Exploration revealed venous thrombosis in the vascular pedicles, probably secondary to excessive tension (cases 13 and 15). However, exploration on the third postoperative day was too late and necrosis supervened. One patient (case 13) with exposed

dura had cutaneous cover provided by a vascularized latissimus dorsi musculocutaneous flap taken from the contralateral chest (Fig. 41-10). The other patient underwent reconstruction with a conventional deltopectoral flap.

Another patient (case 5), 12 hours after undergoing division and insetting of a Tagliacozzi flap for nasal reconstruction, developed signs of vascular insufficiency (Fig. 41-11). A TcPo₂ recording at the distal, discolored portion of the flap was 44 mm Hg, with a control of 68 mm Hg. The flap was detached from its insertion and placed in its original site. The flap was successfully reinset 1 week later; no necrosis occurred.

A patient with recurrent vulvar carcinoma and

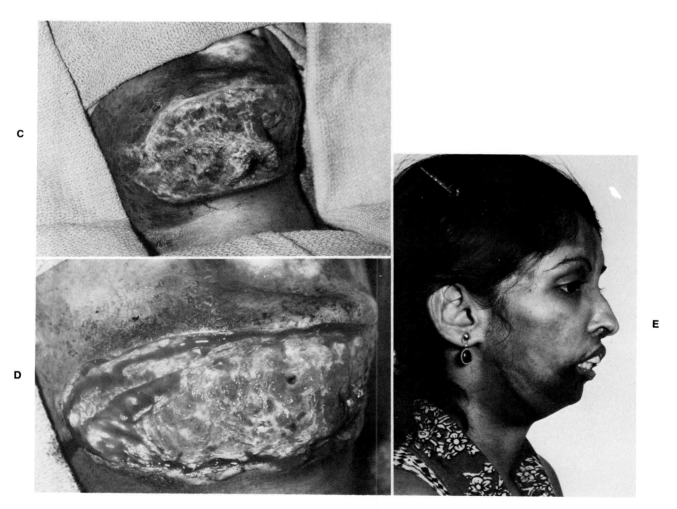

Fig. 41-9, cont'd. C, Early postoperative view demonstrating vascular insufficiency with distal flap necrosis; TcPo₂ recording 0.0 mm Hg. **D,** Superficial portion of flap excised; note bleeding from deep dermis and subcutaneous fat. **E,** Postoperative result following revised split-thickness graft.

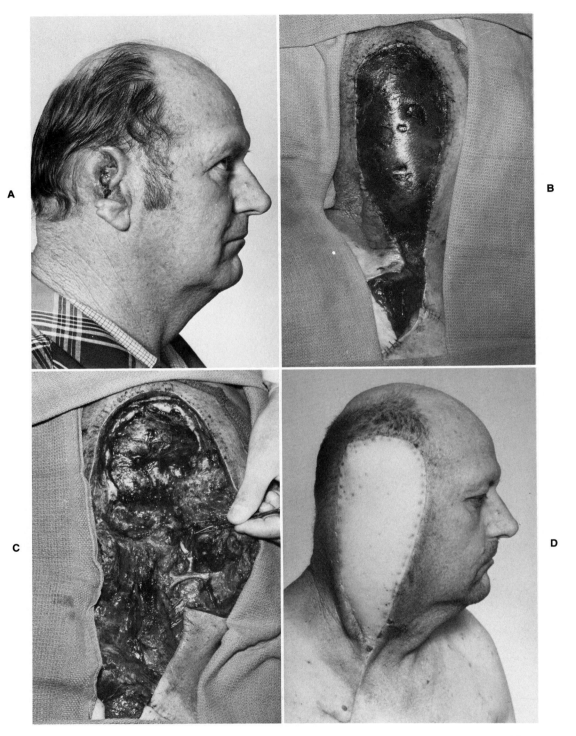

Fig. 41-10. A, Preoperative view demonstrating auricular malignancy requiring wide excision and temporal bone resection (case 13). **B,** Early postoperative view demonstrating vascular insufficiency of island latissimus dorsi musculocutaneous flap. Note $TcPo_2$ recordings of 0.0 mm Hg. **C,** Intraoperative view demonstrating exposed dura following removal of nonviable flap. **D,** Postoperative view after successful wound closure with a vascularized latissimus dorsi musculocutaneous flap from the contralateral chest. $TcPo_2$ recordings on the seventh postoperative day with 20% O_2: flap 49 mm Hg, control 42 mm Hg. (From Serafin, D., Lesesne, C., Mullen, R.Y., and Georgiade, N.G.: Transcutaneous Po_2 monitoring for assessing viability and predicting survival of skin flaps: experimental and clinical correlations, J. Microsurg. **2:**165, 1981.)

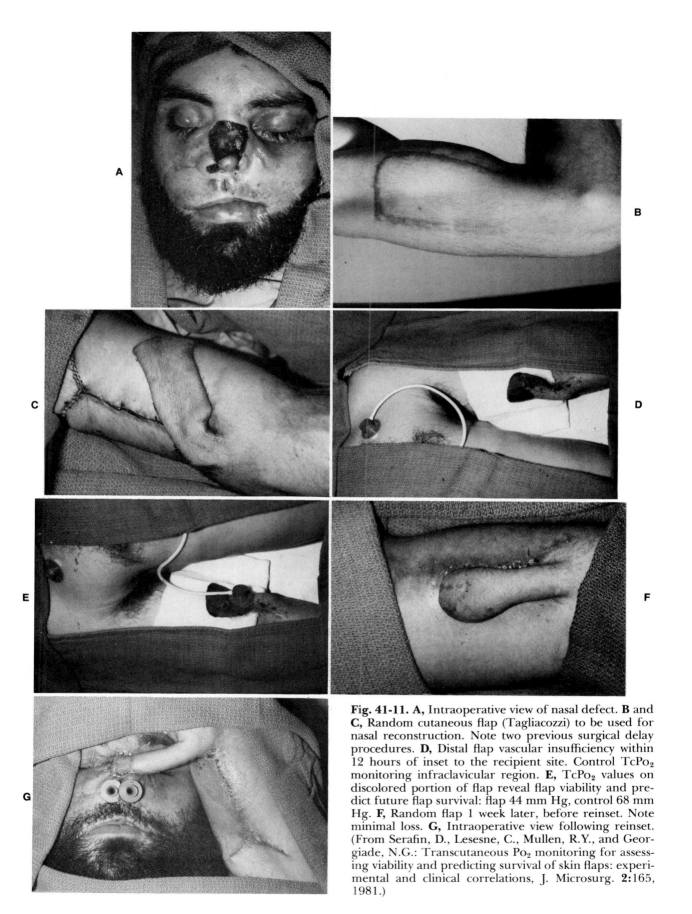

Fig. 41-11. A, Intraoperative view of nasal defect. **B** and **C,** Random cutaneous flap (Tagliacozzi) to be used for nasal reconstruction. Note two previous surgical delay procedures. **D,** Distal flap vascular insufficiency within 12 hours of inset to the recipient site. Control $TcPo_2$ monitoring infraclavicular region. **E,** $TcPo_2$ values on discolored portion of flap reveal flap viability and predict future flap survival: flap 44 mm Hg, control 68 mm Hg. **F,** Random flap 1 week later, before reinset. Note minimal loss. **G,** Intraoperative view following reinset. (From Serafin, D., Lesesne, C., Mullen, R.Y., and Georgiade, N.G.: Transcutaneous Po_2 monitoring for assessing viability and predicting survival of skin flaps: experimental and clinical correlations, J. Microsurg. **2:**165, 1981.)

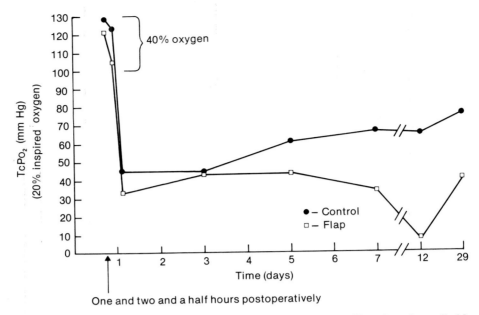

Fig. 41-12. Low control and flap TcPo$_2$ recordings in seriously ill patient (case 4). Note decrease in flap TcPo$_2$ readings on seventh postoperative day. A significant wound infection became clinically apparent 2 days later. (From Serafin, D., Lesesne, C., Mullen, R.Y., and Georgiade, N.G.: Transcutaneous Po$_2$ monitoring for assessing viability and predicting survival of skin flaps: experimental and clinical correlations, J. Microsurg. **2**:165, 1981.)

unsuccessful bilateral island gracilis musculocutaneous flaps (case 4), underwent radical extirpation and high dose irradiation. Pelvic reconstruction was accomplished with a vascularized latissimus dorsi musculocutaneous flap. The TcPo$_2$ monitor was employed postoperatively to measure flap viability (Fig. 41-12). Both control and flap sites had low values on the first postoperative day. These values reflected, in part, a low hematocrit level (21%) and poor pulmonary function in a seriously ill patient following surgery. Control values improved with transfusion and improved pulmonary function; however, flap readings remained low and continued to fall. On the ninth postoperative day a wound infection became clinically apparent. After adequate drainage and administration of systemic antibiotics, the patient recovered and the entire flap survived.

DISCUSSION

The TcPo$_2$ monitor has been useful in diagnosing neonatal disease,[6,10,14,17] and recently Achauer et al.[1] and Matsen et al.[11] have reported that the monitor may be useful in assessing the viability of skin flaps and replanted parts.

In our study, experimentally and clinically, the TcPo$_2$ monitor has demonstrated its value in accurately measuring capillary oxygenation. Its potential is unlimited as a clinical monitoring tool and as a valuable instrument to collect physiologic data. Many studies are being conducted in our laboratory, using the TcPo$_2$ monitor to assess the effects of drugs and other factors on microcirculation.

Studies are also being done to accurately determine the intimal TcPo$_2$ values predicting flap survival. Investigations are also underway to develop the capability of diagnosing selective venous or arterial occlusion. Important data have already evolved on the timing of different delay, division, and insetting procedures on a variety of conventional skin flaps. Finally, TcPo$_2$ monitoring is being used to look at changes in oxygenation at the electron transport system level.

Lower TcPo$_2$ values, noted clinically in the intraoperative period, were also seen experimentally (see Table 41-1). The TcPo$_2$ values were lowest immediately after elevation of the flaps. Within 24 hours the flap values approximated control values; in 1 week both flap and control measurements reached preoperative levels (Fig. 41-10). More information is needed to better define the local factors responsible for vasoconstriction and alteration of capillary flow in flaps. Further work is also needed to define the effects of surgical sympathectomy on the microcirculatory flow of free vascularized flaps. These studies will be forthcoming.

SUMMARY

The $TcPo_2$ monitor is a safe, reliable instrument that provides accurate, rapid, continuous, and noninvasive measurement of the oxygen level in the microcirculation of skin. These measurements can be used to monitor flap viability and to predict flap survival as well as to monitor systemic factors that influence oxygen transport in general. The simultaneous measurement of control and flap $TcPo_2$ levels can provide continuous monitoring of the status of the microcirculation, thus improving the postoperative management of the patient by detecting vascular occlusion or other difficulties early, allowing the prompt institution of appropriate therapy. It may also provide a very important method for investigating the known and unknown factors that influence cutaneous circulation.

REFERENCES

1. Achauer, B.M., Black, K.S., and Litke, D.K.: Transcutaneous Po_2 in flaps: a new method of survival prediction, Plast. Reconstr. Surg. **65**:738, 1980.
2. Creech, B.J., and Miller, S.H.: Evaluation of circulation in skin flaps. In Grabb, W.C., and Myers, M.B., editors: Skin flaps, Boston, 1975, Little, Brown & Co., p. 21.
3. Gothgen, I., and Jacobsen, E.: Transcutaneous oxygen tension measurement, I: Age variation and reproducibility, Acta Anaesthesiol. Scand. (Suppl.) **67**:66, 1978.
4. Hach, A., Hach, R., Arner, B., and Rooth, G.: Continuous transcutaneous oxygen tension measured with a heated electrode, Scand. J. Clin. Lab. Invest. **31**:269, 1973.
5. Hach, R., Hach, A., and Lubbers, D.W.: Transcutaneous measurement of blood Po_2 ($TcPo_2$)—method and application in perinatal medicine, J. Perinat. Med. **1**:183, 1973.
6. Jacobson, L., and Löfgren, O.: Transcutaneous monitoring of Po_2 in different skin areas in the neonate and in the scalp of the fetus during labor: methodological and physiological observations, Acta Obstet. Gynecol. Scand. (Suppl.) **66**:55, 1977.
7. Jöbsis, F.F.: Basic processes in cellular respiration. In Fenn, W.O., and Rahn, H., editors: Handbook of physiology, Vol. 1, Washington, D.C., 1964, American Physiological Society.
8. Jöbsis, F.F., editor: Oxygen and physiological function, Dallas, 1977, Professional Information Library.
9. Jöbsis, F.F., Boyd, B., and Barwick, W.J.: Metabolic consequences of ischemia and hypoxia: effects on transplant survival. In Serafin, D., and Buncke, H.J., Jr., editors: Microsurgical composite tissue transplantation, St. Louis, 1979, The C.V. Mosby Co., p. 47.
10. Löfgren, O., and Jacobson, L.: Monitoring of transcutaneous Po_2 in the fetus and mother during normal labor, J. Perinat. Med. **5**:252, 1977.
11. Matsen, F.A., Bach, A.W., Wyss, C.R., and Simmons, C.W.: Transcutaneous Po_2: a potential monitor of the status of replanted limb parts, Plast. Reconstr. Surg. **65**:732, 1980.
12. McClure, W.B., and Aldrich, C.A.: Time required for disappearance of intradermally injected salt solution, JAMA **81**:293, 1923.
13. Peabody, J.L., Willis, M.M., and Severinghaus, J.W.: Characteristics of non-aqueous electrolytes for transcutaneous oxygen electrodes, Acta Anaesthesiol. Scand. (Suppl.) **68**:49, 1978.
14. Pollitzer, M.J., et al.: Continuous comparison of the vitro and in vivo calibrated transcutaneous oxygen tension ($TcPo_2$) with arterial oxygen tension (PaO_2) in infants with respiratory illnesses. Pediatr. Res. **13**:81, 1979.
15. Prather, A., Blackburn, J.R., Williams, R.T., and Lynn, J.A.: Evaluation of tests for predicting the viability of axial pattern skin flaps in the pig. Plast. Reconstr. Surg. **63**:250, 1979.
16. Reisin, J.H., Guthrie, R.H., Jr., and Goulian, D., Jr.: Timing of pedicle flap delays by measurements of flap oxygen carbon dioxide, J. Surg. Oncol. **6**:79, 1974.
17. Rooth, G.: Transcutaneous oxygen tension measurements in newborn infants. Pediatrics **55**:232, 1975.
18. Serafin, D., Lesesne, C., Mullen, R.Y., and Georgiade, N.G.: Transcutaneous Po_2 monitoring for assessing viability and predicting survival of skin flaps: experimental and clinical correlation, J. Microsurg. **2**:165, 1981.
19. Sejrsen, P.: Measurement of cutaneous blood flow by freely diffusable radioactive isotopes, Dan. Med. Bull. (Suppl. III) **18**:1, 1971.
20. Starr, I.: Change in the reaction of the skin to histamine as evidence of deficient circulation in lower extremities, JAMA **90**:2092, 1928.
21. Toomey, J.M., and Wilson, W.R.: Mass spectrometric observations of skin flap physiology, Laryngoscope **83**:559, 1973.

Chapter 42

Transcutaneous oxygen: past, present, and future

Bruce M. Achauer
Kirby S. Black

In an attempt to monitor arterial O_2 tension by noninvasive means, transcutaneous oxygen sensors were developed. During the 1970s the Huchs of Germany were pioneers in modifying the Clark electrode for this purpose in neonates.[7] The Clark electrode consists of an anode and a cathode surrounded by a KCl electrolyte and a mylar membrane into which oxygen can diffuse. Current flow between the anode and cathode is proportional to the oxygen concentration within the electrolyte.[6]

Although it was first demonstrated in 1851 that oxygen can diffuse through intact skin,[3] virtually no oxygen diffuses under normal conditions.[6] Oxygen does diffuse readily through the skin when heated to 42° C.[5] Therefore local hyperemia is created by a thermostatically controlled heating coil to increase the amount of oxygen coming through the skin to a measurable level. Close correlation of transcutaneous Po_2 ($TcPo_2$) to arterial Po_2 was the major goal of early workers and has been realized for neonates (Fig. 42-1). However, this has not been true for adults. $TcPo_2$ is a function of skin condition and skin thickness. Therefore a $1:1$ correlation of $PaO_2:TcPo_2$ was not found in adults because of the increased skin thickness and increased oxygen consumption.[13]

With the increasing use of monitoring in different areas of medicine, it was realized that $TcPo_2$ was an entity of its own, not just a reflection of arterial oxygen. $TcPo_2$ is very dependent on adequate skin blood flow, as we saw in rabbits that were bled and then transfused (Fig. 42-2). This was also observed in intensive care units for adults.[15] The dependence of $TcPo_2$ on peripheral blood

flow is one of its major drawbacks, but we and others have found a silver lining in this dark cloud.

We first used $TcPo_2$ to predict flap survival on rabbits and pigs[1] and continued our work clinically,[2] as did others.[10,11,14] From these studies it was concluded that the presence of a $TcPo_2$ response to increased FiO_2 (oxygen tension of inspired air) indicated adequate flap circulation and therefore tissue survival. A simple diagnostic observation also correlated with the readings: a flap with close to normal $TcPo_2$ levels (normal being a control site nearby) and a relatively fast response to increased FiO_2 also exhibited improved healing. Poor healing and a negative clinical course correlated with low readings and a sluggish response to increased FiO_2. Highly vascular flaps such as the dorsalis pedis flap demonstrated unusually high $TcPo_2$ levels with a very fast response to increased oxygen and, again, an excellent clinical course. In an effort to clarify the diagnostic value of the $TcPo_2$ measurements, we developed a method to quantify the rate of response to oxygen.

Previous work by Hoopes and colleagues[4,8,9] gave convincing evidence of an alternating metabolism in flaps. It was suggested that when a flap is ischemic there is a shift to an anaerobic metabolism for energy production. When the blood supply returns to normal levels, the skin reverts to its normal metabolism.

It seemed logical that this shift could be detected by measuring oxygen utilization rates by means of $TcPo_2$ values of the skin. This was tested in rabbits by occluding a tubed flap at its base with a sphygmomanometer; the resultant drop-off rate

420

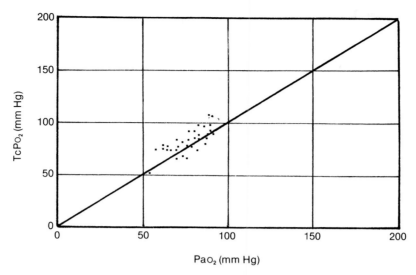

Fig. 42-1. Scatter diagram demonstrating good correlation between transcutaneous Po_2 values and arterial Po_2 values obtained from blood samples in neonates. Diagonal line represents what would be perfect correlation. (From Huch, A., and Huch, R.: Transcutaneous noninvasive monitoring of Po_2, **11**(6):43, 1976.)

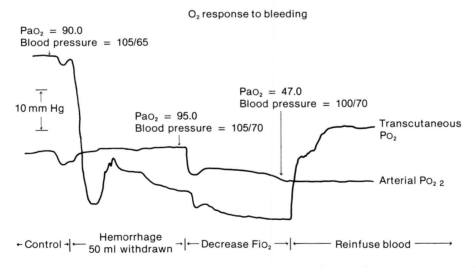

Fig. 42-2. Rabbit experiment correlating transcutaneous and arterial Po_2 at various blood pressures. Change in blood pressure was produced by withdrawing 50 ml of blood and then reinfusing it. Although the arterial oxygen did not change, the skin oxygen changed dramatically in response to peripheral vasoconstriction. This effect proved to be reversible.

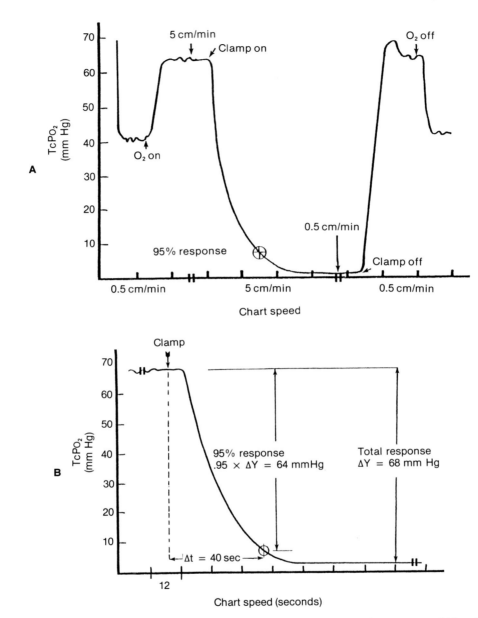

Fig. 42-3. A, Transcutaneous oxygen measurements on tubed skin flaps on rabbits. A response to increased oxygen is seen. When a maximum effect has been obtained, the base of the tube is clamped and the disappearance rate noted. The 95% response time is noted. This produces the number Δt from the time of clamping until 95% disappearance of oxygen. Δt then reflects the efficiency of the metabolism of the flap. **B,** Diagram of the derivation of Δt. The total change in transcutaneous oxygen was 68 mm of mercury; 95% of this equals 64 mm, which then determines the 95% response point. In this example Δt is 40 seconds, which is the normal value.

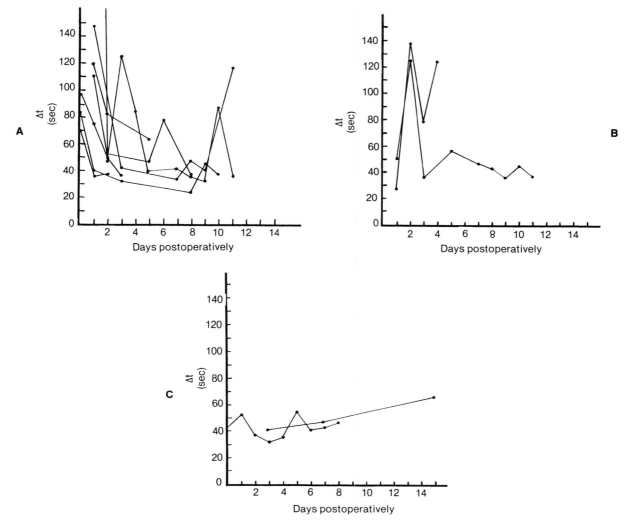

Fig. 42-4. Δt responses were found to fall within three groups. **A,** Most flaps were mildly ischemic immediately following surgery and returned to a normal reading 3 to 8 days postoperatively. **B,** Some flaps were unaffected by a surgical procedure. Theoretically the skin circulation was not significantly altered by the surgery. **C,** Some flaps were profoundly disturbed by the surgical procedure and suffered severe metabolic changes. This may be reflected in free flaps in which the time to clear oxygen from the clamped flap increases over threefold immediately postoperatively.

of $TcPo_2$ was calculated and recorded on each postoperative day (Fig. 42-3, *A* and *B*). Again, three types of flaps were found—the mildly ischemic flap (Fig. 42-4, *A*), the nonischemic flap (Fig. 42-4, *B*), and the very ischemic flap (Fig. 42-4, *C*)—each with its distinct signature.

The clinical use of $TcPo_2$ for monitoring flaps and replantations has been initiated by several centers.[2,10,11,14] A number of problems still exist: the cost and availability of equipment, the need for calibration and maintenance, skin fixation, and the speed of measurement. Interpretation of data is

also difficult because of the paucity of clinical reports. Is a low reading the result of edema, electrode malfunction, or true vascular compromise of the flap? The machines are becoming more widely available, less expensive, and more reliable. With increasing clinical experience and new methods of interpretation of the data provided, the widespread use of $TcPo_2$ in plastic surgery is anticipated.

Another technique used to reflect tissue perfusion is the laser Doppler.[12,16] The laser Doppler, employing the same principle as the acoustic Doppler, measures the frequency shift of the laser light instead of the frequency shift of the acoustic signal. This allows the measurement of the velocity of the red cells in superficial capillaries. Measurements from this device seem to correlate with tissue survival, but a full clinical study has yet to be done. It would have the advantage of a very quick response time.

The future of flap monitoring may well involve all of these devices and concepts, in addition to newly emerging technologies. This will give the plastic surgeon a noninvasive means of obtaining the quantitative data needed to make correct clinical decisions.

REFERENCES

1. Achauer, B.M., Black, K.S., Beran, A.V., and Huxtable, R.F.: Transcutaneous Po_2 monitoring of flap circulation following surgery, Birth Defects **15**(4): 517, 1979.
2. Achauer, B.M., Black, K.S., and Litke, D.K.: Transcutaneous Po_2 in flaps: a new method of survival prediction, Plast. Reconstr. Surg. **65**:738, 1980.
3. Gerlach, J.V.: Uber das hautothmen, Arch. Anat. Physiol. Lpz. 431-455, 1851.
4. Hoopes, J.E., Su, C.T., and Im, M.J.: Enzymatic response to skin flap elevation following a delay procedure, Plast. Reconstr. Surg. **66**:369, 1980.
5. Huch, A., and Huch, R.: The development of the transcutaneous Po_2 technique into a clinical tool. In Continuous transcutaneous blood gas monitoring, Birth Defects **15**(4):5, 1979.
6. Huch, R., Lubbers, D.W., and Huch, A.: Quantitative continuous measurement of partial oxygen pressure on the skin of adults and newborn babies, Pfluegers Arch. **337**:185, 1972.
7. Huch, H., Lubbers, D.W., and Huch, A.: Reliability of transcutaneous monitoring of arterial Po_2 in newborn infants, Arch. Dis. Child. **49**:213, 1974.
8. Im, M.J., and Hoopes, J.E.: Distribution of glucose in the pedicle skin of guinea pigs, J. Surg. Res. **25**: 269, 1978.
9. Im, M.J., and Hoopes, J.E.: Enzyme activities in experimental skin flaps, J. Surg. Res. **25**:465, 1978.
10. Keller, H.P., Flave, P., and Lubbers, D.W.: Transcutaneous Po_2 measurements for evaluating the oxygen supply of skin allo and autograft, Eur. Surg. Res. **10**:272, 1978.
11. Matsen, F.A., Bach, A.W., Wyss, C.R., and Simmons, C.W.: Transcutaneous Po_2: a potential monitor of the status of replanted limb parts, Plast. Reconstr. Surg. **65**:732, 1980.
12. Powers, E.W., and Frazer, W.W.: Laser Doppler measurement of blood flow in the microcirculation, Plast. Reconstr. Surg. **61**:250, 1978.
13. Rooth, G., Hedstrand, U., and Ogren, C.H.: Interpretation of the $TcPo_2$ curve in adult patients in an intensive care unit, Birth Defects **15**(4):557, 1979.
14. Serafin, D., Lesesne, C.B., Mullen, R.Y., and Georgiade, N.G.: Transcutaneous Po_2 monitoring for assessing viability and predicting survival of skin flaps: experimental and clinical correlations, J. Microsurg. **2**:165, 1981.
15. Tremper, K., et al.: Transcutaneous oxygen during respiratory failure, cardiac decompensation, cardiac arrest and CPR, AAMI Fifteenth Annual Meeting, San Francisco, p. 219, 1980, Arlington, Va., AAMI.
16. Watkins, D., and Holloway, G.A.: An instrument to measure cutaneous blood flow using the Doppler shift of laser light, IEEE Trans. Biomed. Eng. BME **25**:28, 1978.

Part XV

Pharmacologic treatment

Chapter 43

Pharmacologic agents in microvascular surgery

Philip M. Hendel

In microvascular surgery, two types of complications can potentially benefit from pharmacologic intervention: (1) complications at the anastomosis site, resulting in thrombosis and occlusion, and (2) those beyond the anastomosis site, resulting in insufficient capillary blood flow and tissue death.

This chapter will review pharmacologic studies at these two levels and rationalize a clinical program based on present knowledge.

PHARMACOLOGY AT THE ANASTOMOTIC LEVEL

There are no figures to indicate the frequency with which problems occur at the site of microvascular anastomoses in clinical practice. The only figures at this time are those of Converse et al., which show an overall success rate of 93.3% in microvascular surgery (see Chapter 1). This figure refers to the ultimate success rate without consideration of the number of repeat procedures that were needed for success. As a rough estimate, one can assume that the anastomotic failure rate—temporary or permanent—was twice that of the final failure rate. The expense of these failures in lost time and hospital resources is sufficient to warrant a search for pharmacologic means of reducing such complications to a minimum.

The use of pharmacologic agents has frequently been advocated.* At first materials and methods were crude and drugs were often reported to be beneficial. Then, as materials and methods improved, it was apparent that refinement of microsurgical technique was the key to success.[8-10,16] Today some surgeons even advocate the use of no drugs at all. However, most authors now support

the use of anticoagulants for cases in which endothelial damage has occurred, such as in the replantation of digits.[21,25,27] The rationale for this practice is supported by laboratory studies.[17]

Certain deleterious factors beyond the surgeon's control may be successfully treated by nonsurgical means. This appears to be true of endothelial damage. Not only does endothelial damage occur with accidental trauma, it has also been found to be an inevitable part of the operative procedure itself.[3,4,34] Endothelial damage is caused by clamping, dilating, irrigation, countertraction, needle perforations, anoxia, and introduction of foreign material (sutures). Usually the damage is insufficient to cause thrombosis, but problems do occur in a significant number of cases.

Until now the beneficial effects of pharmacologic agents have not been supported by convincing clinical evidence, and their use has been empirical. Inasmuch as these drugs are not innocuous but can cause complications such as oozing, hematoma, or vascular headaches, many surgeons have tended to withhold this form of therapy, awaiting more compelling evidence of their efficacy.

Survey of a series of failed clinical anastomoses

For this reason we have attempted to determine whether pharmacologic agents are indeed useful in clinical microvascular surgery. To avoid engaging in clinical experimentation, we studied a series of failed clinical anastomoses to determine what events led to failure. The center chosen was Jewish Hospital in Louisville, Kentucky, because of the large volume of microsurgery performed there.

Method. A survey of the records of digital replantations at Jewish Hospital showed that between 1975 and 1979 anastomotic failure occurred

---

*References 2, 5, 14, 22, 30, 33.

in fifty patients after they left the operating room. A retrospective review was done to determine what events were associated with the onset of failure. Factors studied included drug therapy up to the time of failure, onset and duration of the anesthetic (all patients in this group had been given an axillary block), time elapsed after surgery, and the time of day. We also searched for specific factors that led to the decision to reexplore.

The time of onset of failure was determined from temperature probe records and from clinical notes. All patients in this group had hourly digital temperature recordings by thermistor. Digits that were reexplored and that subsequently failed were also included in this study. This gave a total of seventy unsuccessful reanastomoses.

Result. The patients were divided into five groups according to the time of failure (Table 43-1):

1. Immediately after surgery
2. Following cessation of the axillary block
3. Following cessation of heparin
4. Between midnight and dawn
5. Unclassifiable

The first category, immediately after surgery, covered the first 2 hours after surgery, while the patient was still in the recovery room. This group was felt to represent a technical error during surgery that had not been immediately recognized, such as a backwall stitch, inclusion of adventitia in the suture line, or failure to resect sufficient damaged epithelium.

The second category was failure of the anastomosis within 2 hours of cessation of the axillary block (i.e., within 2 hours of the time indicated in the records for the onset of pain in the anesthetized limb). Two significant events occur at this time: (1) loss of vasodilation in the limb caused by the axillary block, and (2) the onset of pain and the associated release of catecholamines, which cause vasoconstriction. In either event, loss of vasodilation with the resultant loss of flow velocity across the anastomosis could precipitate thrombosis and anastomotic failure.

The third category included failures within 4 hours of discontinuing heparin. Usually this was on the third or fourth postoperative day and was seen as early as 1½ days and as late as 7 days postoperatively. The mechanism here appeared to be loss of the protective effect of heparin.

In the fourth category failure occurred between midnight and 8 AM, a period of reduced cardiac output. Examination of digital temperature records of all replants in this group and of records of replants that did not fail showed that in the majority of replanted digits (80%) a cycling of digital temperature of 0.5° C occurred each day. The lowest part of the cycle was seen between 2 AM and 8 AM, while the highest part was seen between 2 PM and 8 PM (Fig. 43-1). This temperature cycle is only rarely seen in normal digits, thus incriminating vascular compromise as a probable cause. This diurnal variation was seen in 80% of the replanted digits, whether or not there were problems with the anastomosis. However, it was noteworthy that the 20% of replanted digits that did not show this

Table 43-1. Causes of anastomotic failure in seventy patients

Recovery room		Discontinuance of axillary block		Discontinuance of heparin		Midnight to dawn		Other	
LM*	OR2†	BP		CF	OR1 POD3	CT	OR1 POD3	CF	OR2 1°
ER		PB	OR2	RM	OR2 POD2	DM	OR1 POD3½	JC	POD5
AC		CR	OR1	LM	OR1 POD4½	PB	OR1 POD3	RA	POD1½
DJ	OR1	WM	OR1	JS	POD3½	RM	OR1 POD1	JS	1°
HH		DD	OR1	KB	POD1	RE	POD2	MW	POD4
CW		CL	OR1	B	OR1 POD1½	CR	OR2 POD5	AC	OR1 POD1½
RR	OR1	AS	OR1	B	OR3 POD2½	CL	OR1 POD4	MB	POD½ W/NV
LM	OR1	TT	OR2	MD	OR2 POD7	MD	OR1 POD1½	WM	OR1 Palmar hematoma
PL	OR1	DP	III	DG	POD1½	MD	OR1 POD1½	SP	OR2 POD4
TM	OR1	DP	IV	DG	OR1 IV POD1½	BR	OR1 POD1	TT	1st POD1
DG	OR1	DG		SP	POD4	AW	POD¼	MD	3rd 1°
GJ	OR1			WL	POD4			L	POD 5
GJ	OR2							BP	POD½ Skin too tight
SC	DM, ASO							EB	Combination
HB								DG	OR2 IV POD2
RW	OR1							DG	OR3 IV POD6
WM	OR2							DG	OR1 III 5 weeks
								AF	Hematoma

*Identifies patient.
†*DM*, diabetes mellitus; *ASO*, atherosclerosis; *OR* (number), procedure number; *III*, middle finger; *IV*, ring finger; *POD* (number), postoperative day number; *1°*, failure to establish anastomosis during primary procedure; *W/NV*, failure associated with systemic illness.

pattern were consistently the most vigorous replants. The diurnal variation also tended not to occur if the patient was in a hypermetabolic state as a result of systemic fever.

In the final group there was no single precipitating factor leading to the failure. Nineteen digits (27% of the anastomosis failures) were in this group. Two were so badly damaged that flow was never established, two developed a hematoma while receiving heparin (these were evacuated and the finger survived), one resulted from infection, and one from a tight skin closure. Four occurred subsequent to a repeat operation that had been done to correct a failure associated with other causes (e.g., cessation of heparin). Eleven cases underwent reexploration procedures that yielded five ultimate successes. One failure occurred 5 weeks after replantation because of fibrosis around the entire length of a vein graft used to replace a digital artery.

Discussion. It appears from this review that two forms of nonsurgical therapy favorably influence microvascular patency rates in humans.

The first is the use of heparin. Of all failures, nearly 20% occurred within 4 hours of discontinuing heparin. All patients in this group were receiving dextran (l.m.d., at least 500 ml/day) and aspirin (4 to 6 tablets, 300 mg/day) at the same time, indicating that the action of heparin is separate from the other two agents. These failures usually occurred at 3 to 4 days postoperatively but were also seen as early as 1½ days and as late as 7 days. We interpret this association between the cessation of heparin and anastomotic failure as evidence that heparin is of benefit to anastomotic patency in microvascular surgery in humans.

The second is vasodilation. Of all failures, 17% occurred within 2 hours of the termination of the axillary block. An axillary block causes vasodilation and increases flow rates in the limb; loss of these beneficial effects apparently tipped the balance on borderline anastomoses, and failure resulted. Another group of failures (also 17% of the total) occurred during the period from midnight to dawn, a period of reduced cardiac output and flow rates. We found that during this period the majority of replanted digits (80%) showed a fall in temperature of 0.5° C. This gave a diurnal temperature curve with the time of lowest temperature (2 AM to 8 AM) corresponding to a period of failure.

To investigate this diurnal variation further, a preliminary trial was performed on an additional group of ten patients who showed this pattern after undergoing successful replantation. Administration of prazosin, a long-acting vasodilator (1 mg p.o.), eliminated this cycling in the majority of patients (Fig. 43-1). With the more potent vasodilator terbutaline, a beta-2 adrenergic (0.5 to 1 mg intramuscularly), not only was the cycle eliminated, but also an increase in digital temperature of up to 0.75° C was observed. This rise was attributed to an adrenergic (beta-1) effect, which increased cardiac output (Fig. 43-1). The short-acting vasodilators chlorpromazine HCl (Thorazine) and isoxsuprine HCl (Vasodilan) were also studied. They were less effective in altering the diurnal cycle.

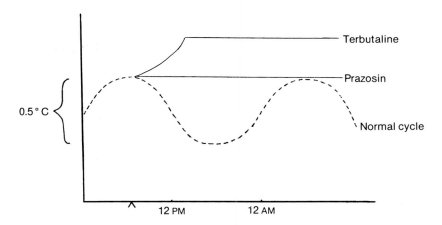

Fig. 43-1. Daily xenon washout studies on axial pattern flaps show increase in capillary circulation beginning proximally.

Four patients who had undergone replantation were coincidently receiving phenytoin (Dilantin sodium) for other problems. Examination of the temperature charts of these patients showed absence of cycling, provided the daily dose was at least 400 mg p.o. Besides its anticonvulsant properties, phenytoin is also a potent alpha-blocker and vasodilator.[16]

Conclusion. This study demonstrates a strong association between microvascular failure and the discontinuance of heparin, the loss of vasodilation (axillary block), or a period of reduced flow rates. This is interpreted to mean that the use of heparin and the use of vasodilators are beneficial to anastomotic patency in humans.

PHARMACOLOGY AT THE CAPILLARY LEVEL

The complication rate resulting from vascular insufficiency in pedicled skin flaps has been reported to be about 14%.[33] Most microvascular surgeons using free flaps have also experienced cases of partial flap necrosis despite a functioning anastomosis, which would be an analagous situation.

This laboratory study was undertaken to analyze pharmacologic effects on flaps at the capillary level and to try to give a rationale for pharmacologic enhancement of both capillary and anastomotic circulation. This is part of a series of related studies carried out at the Ralph K. Davies Medical Center with Drs. H.J. Buncke, Jr., and L. Lilien.

Because the understanding of the difference between acute and delayed flaps was considered the key to clinical control of capillary circulation, the focus of this study was the control mechanism responsible for increase in blood flow from the

delay phenomenon. We compared the effects of vasoactive drugs on an acute flap and with the effects on a delayed flap in the same animal. The delayed flap was raised and replaced 3 weeks before the acute flap. In its distal segment, normally supplied by the lateral thoracic artery, this flap would be "delayed" (Fig. 43-2).

With this model any difference in the response of blood flow between the two flaps would result from events occurring within the delayed flap that would change its circulatory dynamics. The manner in which vasoactive drugs affected this delayed flap would, we postulated, shed light on the mechanism of the delay phenomenon. Because only the relative differences in response was sought and because any systemic changes in blood flow would effect both flaps equally, no cardiac monitoring was performed. Monitoring of blood flow was by xenon washout[7,19,20,28] using the local deposition method.

The role of the sympathetic nerve terminal in the delay phenomenon

In the past the sympathetic nerve terminals and receptors have been implicated as playing a role in the "delay phenomenon." In this section we compare the sensitivity of the acute and delayed flaps to exogenous alpha adrenergic drugs. After performing the experiment with the sympathetic nerve terminals intact, we repeated the experiment in a second group of animals in whom the terminals had been previously chemically destroyed. In this way both the change in sensitivity of the sympathetic receptors and the role of the sympathetic nerve terminals in the delay process could be determined.

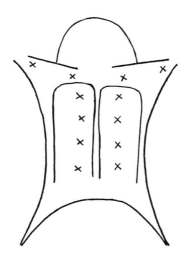

Fig. 43-2. Ventral schematic drawing of laboratory rat. Flaps based on inferior epigastric vessels.

Method. The animal model (Fig. 43-2) used for this study contained an acutely raised flap (1 to 2 hours postoperatively, right side) and an anatomically identical flap that had been raised 3 weeks earlier (left side). Both flaps were based on the inferior epigastric vessel system, and both extended as far as the clavicle. The delayed flap was first elevated and then resutured. Three weeks later the acute flap was elevated and the delayed flap was reraised. Both flaps were then resutured in their original positions.

Baseline measurements of blood flow on both the acute and delayed flaps were made starting 1 to 2 hours after surgery. Intraperitoneal drug injection followed immediately thereafter. Thirty minutes elapsed between the intraperitoneal drug injection and the trial blood flow measurements (except with adrenaline—15 minutes).

Each drug trial was designed as a dose response matrix and was run twice on two separate groups of four animals. Changes in blood flow were considered valid if a significant difference between trial and control readings could be shown by Student's *t* test. Results were plotted as a percent change, with a control value of 100%. For purposes of the graphs, the average of the distal two sites in each flap on each animal was used for plotting the curves.

Sprague-Dawley rats of the same weight (within 25 g) were used for each matrix. Sedation for the xenon studies and surgery was achieved with pentobarbital sodium (Nembutal). A deeper level of anesthesia for the surgery itself was achieved with halothane.

Xenon washout by the local disposition method was used to monitor blood flow. Sites to be studied were injected with a tuberculin syringe through a 30-gauge needle. Each site was given 0.5 ml of 0.9% sodium chloride containing 25 to 150 μCi of Xe-133. Disappearance of activity was monitored using a gamma scintillation camera (Ohio Nuclear Model 410 or Model 420) on-line with a microprocessor-based nuclear medicine data system (ADAC Clinical Data System). Injection sites were placed 3 to 4 cm apart to prevent contamination of one region by counts from an adjacent region. When repeat experiments in the same animal were performed, increasing the injected dose of Xe-133 or changing collimation was used to avoid the effect of residual background counts.

Cutaneous blood flow was calculated by the computer, using washout curves obtained by monitoring the first 7 minutes of xenon disappearance. Two groups of animals were tested for sensitivity to alpha agonist drugs. In one group there was no modification of the sympathetic nerve terminals. In the other group the sympathetic terminals were previously destroyed by giving 100 mg/kg of 6-hydroxydopamine hydrobromide intravenously[23] 24 hours before the drug trials. Because methoxamine causes core vasoconstriction, an initial rise in cutaneous blood flow was expected with this agent.[18]

Result. In animals with the sympathetic nerve terminals intact, both noradrenaline and methoxamine caused a decrease in blood flow to the acute flap at a lower dose than the delayed flap (Figs. 43-3 and 43-4). In animals with the sympathetic nerve terminals destroyed, blood flow to the delayed flap fell more rapidly than to the acute flap (Fig. 43-5). Control skin in both groups paralleled the response of the delayed flap.

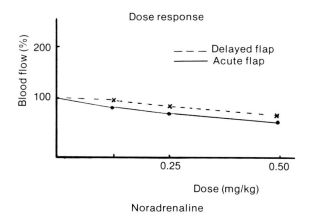

Fig. 43-3. Points represent average of eight xenon readings. Dose response adjusted so 100% represents the initial baseline blood flow.

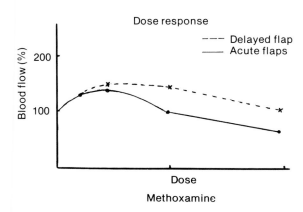

Fig. 43-4. Ventral schematic drawing of laboratory rat. Flaps based on inferior epigastric vessels.

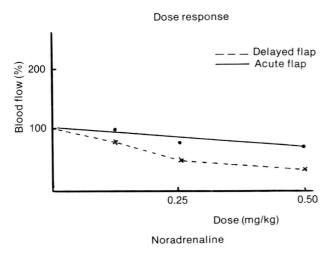

Fig. 43-5. Ventral schematic drawing of laboratory rat. Flaps based on inferior epigastric vessels.

Table 43-2. Catecholamine content (pg/g)

Rat	Acute flap	Delayed flap
1	40.71	0.91
2	96.62	4.65
3	91.41	1.24
4	88.08	2.94
5	56.58	14.30
6	40.26	2.19

Determination of catecholamine content by radioimmune assay

Before trying to draw any conclusions from the results of the previous section, we attempted to analyze what happens to the sympathetic nerve terminals during the delay phenomenon. Since catecholamine stores are found almost exclusively in the sympathetic nerve terminals, a good way of monitoring their existence is by radioimmune assay of tissue catecholamine content. Again, an animal model containing both an identical acute and delayed flap was used.

Method. Six animals, each with an identical acute and delayed flap, were tested. The same approach as described previously was used to generate this model. One hour after developing the acute flap (second surgery), tissue samples were taken from the distal aspect of both flaps just proximal to the distal suture line.

Results (Table 43-2). The catecholamine content[29] was significantly decreased in the distal portion of delayed flaps as compared to acute flaps. The results are statistically significant (t − 5.86, df = 5) by Student's *t* test.

Discussion. These two parts of the study indicate that the sympathetic nervous system is at least partly responsible for the mechanism of the delay phenomenon.

In the first experiment xenon washout monitoring demonstrated that if the sympathetic nerve terminals were intact, the acute flap is more sensitive to systemic alpha agonists than the delayed flap. This is the reverse of what was expected; it was expected that the delayed flap would be more sensitive because of denervation hypersensitivity. This was seen only in the second group of animals in which the sympathetic terminals had been previously destroyed. Here the delayed flap was the most sensitive. From these studies it appears that in the acute period after surgery the sympathetic nerve terminals are involved in a process that increases receptor site sensitivity.

In the second experiment, radioimmune assay showed significant decrease in tissue catecholamine stores during the delay period. As these stores exist mainly in the sympathetic terminals, raising a flap seems to cause the sympathetic terminals to release their stores without replacement.

Together these two experiments indicate that changes related to the sympathetic nerve terminals are occurring during the delay process. They appear to be losing their catecholamine stores, and they appear to be causing a transient increase in sensitivity of the alpha receptors after surgery.

Theoretically these two findings are consistent with a picture of wallerian degeneration of the cut sympathetic fibers. With degeneration the terminals would release their catecholamine stores onto adjacent alpha receptors, lowering their threshold to further stimulation. This would also be accompanied by loss of the amine-pump, the process normally responsible for clearing the receptors. With time this process would end and the vessels would relax. With the resulting dilation of the vessels, blood flow would increase to the now "delayed flap."

A search for a second component to the delay phenomenon

On reviewing the results of the previous section, we noticed that destruction of the sympathetic nerve terminals did not fully equalize blood flow to the acute and delayed flaps in any animal tested. This section was included, therefore, to search for the characteristics of any second component to the delay phenomenon beyond vasoconstriction caused by release of catecholamine from the degenerating sympathetic nerve terminals.

First, any component caused by the sympathetic nerve terminals was eliminated by pretreating the animals with 6-hydroxydopamine hydrobromide.[23] Then, using the previous animal model containing an identical acute and delayed flap, we searched for further differences in the response of these two flaps.

The systemic drug chosen for this section was the beta agonist terbutaline, for two reasons: (1) to demonstrate any increase in sensitivity of the beta receptors in the delayed flap, and (2) to demonstrate any lag in response of the acute flap, indicating the presence of a second vasoconstrictor mechanism within the acute flap in competition with the exogenous vasodilator.

Again, no cardiac monitoring was performed, since only the relative difference in response of the two flaps was looked for.

Method. The animal model (Fig. 43-2) was prepared as described on pp. 430-431. Twenty-four hours before the second surgery all sympathetic terminals were destroyed by administering to each animal 100 mg/kg of 6-hydroxydopamine hydrobromide intravenously.

Control xenon washout measurements were made 1 to 2 hours postoperatively. Drug trials were begun immediately afterward. Terbutaline doses used were 0.05 mg/kg, 0.10 mg/kg, and 0.15 mg/kg. Other aspects of the method in this section are the same as those described earlier.

Result. Blood flow to the acute flap steadily increased with increasing doses of the vasodilator (Fig. 43-6). Blood flow to control skin paralleled this pattern. Blood flow to the delayed flap showed a relative decrease. Control readings of blood flow in the acute flap and the delayed flap were not equal in any of the eight rats.

Discussion. Two important observations were seen in the results of this experiment. The first was that elimination of the sympathetic terminals did not equalize blood flow to the acute and delayed flaps in any animal. A similar finding was seen in the previous section. This indicates that changes occurring in the sympathetic terminals are not the only mechanism differentiating acute and delayed flaps. At least one other component exists in the delay phenomenon.

The second observation was that after destruction of the sympathetic terminals, the response of the acute flap to terbutaline was a direct increase in blood flow paralleled in the control skin. No initial lag or dip occurred. At the highest level, blood flow surpassed the delayed flap by an average of 50%.

The observation of an increase in blood flow

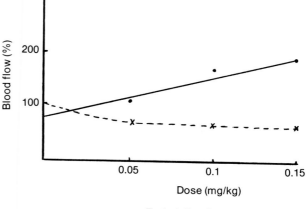

Terbutaline in rats
pretreated with 6-hydroxydopamine

Fig. 43-6. Ventral schematic drawing of laboratory rat. Flaps based on inferior epigastric vessels.

without an initial lag or dip in the acute flap suggests that no vasoconstrictor mechanism exists after elimination of the sympathetic terminals. It appears that the second component is not the loss of a second vasoconstrictor substance. If one did exist, it would be expected to compete with the action of the exogenous vasodilator terbutaline within the acute flap in comparison to the rest of the vasculature, causing an initial lag or dip in the response of the acute flap.

Theoretically at this point only a limited number of possibilities remains for the mechanism of action of the second component. These include either a vasodilator event within the delayed flap acting at the receptor site level or a vasodilator event acting beyond the receptor site level. The fact that the delayed flap was less responsive to terbutaline than the acute flap indicates that the event is not sensitization of the beta receptors; rather it appears to be a mechanism acting beyond the level of the beta receptors at the smooth muscle or vascular architecture level.

The possibilities include an unidentified vasodilator that acts directly on the vascular smooth muscle (e.g., a prostaglandin) and bypasses the beta receptors or a structural change such as a vessel remodeling or denervation smooth muscle atrophy.

Summary. These experiments indicate that there are two components to the delay phenomenon:

1. Passive vasodilation caused by loss of tone in the acute flaps originating from release of

catecholamine from degenerating sympathetic nerve terminals

2. Active vasodilation not involving loss of a second vasoconstrictor mechanism or sensitization of the beta receptors

While the second component could not be identified, its characteristics suggest that its site of action is directly at the smooth muscle or vascular architecture level without involving the beta receptors for vasodilation.

All together these experiments are consistent with the predictions of Finseth[13] that vessels in the acute flap are under the influence of vasospastic forces and that vasodilator drugs are of benefit to flap circulation. Theoretically it would appear that initially these forces should be greater in a free flap than in a pedicled flap, since a higher percentage of sympathetic nerve terminals are cut.

THEORETICAL CONSIDERATIONS

At this point it appears that one can accept the basic premise that pharmacologic agents are beneficial in microvascular surgery. Heparin is useful at the level of the anastomosis in preventing clot formation, at least in the case of damaged endothelium, and vasodilation is useful at both the anastomosis level and at the peripheral levels of flap nutrition. Rather than advocate a blanket application to all cases, however, one should examine the modes of action and theoretical implications in the use of these agents and use them according to a specific program.

Heparin. In the Louisville study it was found that heparin has a beneficial effect in humans separate from that of aspirin or dextran. Since neither dextran nor aspirin was discontinued in any of the patients before heparin was discontinued, no conclusions regarding the efficacy of these two drugs could be drawn. In animal studies other anticoagulants and antiplatelet agents have been reported to be of benefit in the past, and, since clot formation is the crux of the problem, it would seem that any agent capable of inhibiting it should be of benefit. Theoretically, however, heparin may be the best of all. The reason lies in its other modes of action beyond simple anticoagulation. These other actions appear to be specific to damaged endothelium.

Chemically, commercial heparin consists of a mixture of linear carbohydrate chains of varying lengths called linear anionic polyelectrolytes. There are twenty-one separate components ranging in weight from 3,000 to 37,000.[14] The chains are characterized by the presence of acid radicals

at intervals along their length. In solution these radicals create an envelope of strong negative charges that prevent coiling and crosslinkage. On neutralization of the negative charges with a positive charge, the chains fold and coil, bringing more negative charge into the vicinity. The result is that heparin has many actions, including the activation or blockage of several "lock and key" receptor mechanisms. These actions include activation or inhibition of hormones, protection against toxins, protection against sensitivity reactions, and cellular effects such as inhibition of osteoblasts and lymphocytosis. Chemically, the strong negative charges on the heparin molecule can neutralize the strong base histamine. The anticoagulant property of heparin does not appear to be one of its primary physiologic functions.

Heparin has two effects on the blood stream that are of benefit to the microvascular surgeon. The first is the activation of antithrombin III (AT-III). This protein inhibits thrombin and other enzymes of the coagulation pathway. The other effect is to lower blood viscosity.[11,33] This effect occurs at very low doses and is the result of surface binding to red blood cells. The resulting negative charge decreases aggregation of red blood cells and lowers shear forces, decreasing viscosity. This is felt to be the mechanism of action of low-dose heparin.

Of greater importance to microvascular surgery, however, is the fact that heparin preferentially binds to endothelial cells, giving concentrations of 100 times the plasma concentration.[25] This reinforces the normal negative charge of the endothelial cells that is lost whenever there is damage or inhibition of metabolism. This superconcentration at the site of the problem also inhibits platelet accumulation, reduces fibrinogen clotting, and activates local AT-III.

While this ability of heparin to concentrate at the endothelial level makes it particularly attractive to microvascular surgery, it must be remembered that it is also associated with complications. Excessive oozing (which makes nursing care difficult) is well known, as is hematoma formation. (Two of the seventy failures in the Louisville study resulted from hematoma. These went on to ultimate success after evacuation.)

Vasodilators. Both studies indicate that vasodilators can be beneficial both to anastomotic patency and to peripheral nutrient blood flow. Many regimens for vasodilation have been described, including axillary block, local irrigation by catheter, regional intraarterial instillation, or systemic vasodilation. The question we pose is: which regimen is the best to use clinically?

To answer this question, one must first remember that the goal is continuous vasodilation throughout the period of endothelial regeneration, local edema, and inflammation. Since most failures in the Louisville study occurred at 3 to 4 days postoperatively, it would appear that vasodilation to protect the anastomosis should be continuously given for 5 to 7 days. Vasodilation to increase nutrient blood flow should be given longer. Neither repeated axillary blocks nor local instillation by an indwelling catheter is suitable for this length of time. In addition, the agents usually advocated for catheter instillation can themselves cause endothelial damage.

Regional intraarterial instillation is also best avoided at this time.

The problem is twofold. First, intraarterial drugs, with few exceptions,[1] are not confined to the arterial territory but rapidly become systemic. Second, agents that do become bound to local tissue can all cause endothelial damage. This was seen to cause very serious problems in animal trials with guanethidine and reserpine. In addition, reserpine is not water soluble, which means that once it is diluted by blood it precipitates into a shower of crystals.[15]

It appears that in humans, for the present, it is most prudent to use only systemic agents until the question of endothelial damage has been studied further. Ideally the agent should be powerful but not cause a fall in blood pressure and should be long acting to maximally protect against the nocturnal drop in peripheral circulation during the 8-hour period from midnight to dawn.

CLINICAL APPLICATION
Clinical principles

Vascular pharmacology, like all other forms of treatment, should only be administered according to a definite clinical strategy. Without this, patients will receive a melange of therapy with inconsistent results and complications. In microvascular surgery the following principles are evident at this time:

Surgery versus pharmacology. Despite the fact that pharmacology has been shown to be of benefit in microvascular surgery, it should never be considered as more than an adjuvant. Surgical principles for good anastomosis and avoidance of tension must never be ignored.

Patient selection. Not all patients should be treated, since all pharmacologic agents can cause

unwanted complications. Patients should be classified as routine or problem cases. Routine cases should receive either no drug therapy or therapy associated with the fewest side effects. Problem cases should receive all therapy known to be of benefit. The problem case classification should include all patients with endothelial damage. Normally this will include all but the sharpest amputations and all elective cases in which there was difficulty with the anastomosis. Withholding protective therapy from serious problems cannot be justified.

When to start. For maximum benefit any drug therapy should start as early as possible, before problems appear. Clinical experience in both San Francisco and Louisville showed that once problems were clinically recognized, drug therapy could rarely reverse it. Not only do the drugs not perfuse into an obstructed area, but once thrombosis has started, conventional pharmacologic agents will not resolve it. Prophylaxis is the approach to take. For maximum impact the agents should be started intraoperatively or as soon as technically possible.

When to stop. The duration of drug therapy will depend on the reasons they are given. One must always be careful not to stop the therapy before the reasons for starting it have passed.

Protection of anastomosis. Heparin or vasodilators, given to protect the anastomosis, should always be given for the entire period of danger (5 to 7 days). In the Louisville study most discontinuance failures occurred at 3 to 4 days, but failures have also been seen 7 days after stopping heparin.

Augmentation of nutrient blood flow. Once starting vasodilator therapy to augment capillary blood flow in a flap that clinically caused concern at surgery, one should continue the therapy long enough for peripheral capillaries to grow in and augment blood flow. Normally this would be the same length of time that you would wait to divide a pedicled flap (14 to 21 days).

What to use
Anticoagulants. There are several anticoagulants that may be used.

Heparin. In the Louisville study only full heparinizing doses were found to make a difference; 1250 U/hr low-dose regimens do not seem to be indicated.

Antiplatelet agents. Antiplatelet agents have not specifically been found to be of benefit in these studies but theoretically should be helpful and have minimal side effects. Full antiplatelet doses are recommended.

Dextran. While dextran's mode of action is not totally understood, it appears to be a heparinoid. Part of its action may also result from release of endogenous heparin from mast cells. Generally it has been preferred by microvascular surgeons, since it is more gentle-acting than heparin. This may be just an illusion. At the present time no good evidence exists to support the use of this agent. It appears that the best approach is to heparinize the patient if this effect is needed (i.e., do not rely on dextran) and to inhibit the platelet action with specific antiplatelet agents.

Vasodilators. The ideal agent should be powerful, long lasting, and yet should not lower blood pressure. Finseth has recently shown that isoxsuprine HCl (Vasodilan) in 20 mg doses increases blood flow to free flaps in humans (see Chapter 44). In the Louisville study this dose was not quite high enough to guarantee protection against the diurnal dip in temperature in replanted digits. Two other powerful agents that are available are discussed below.

Terbutaline. Terbutaline is a beta agonist[15] suitable for intramuscular use, with a 12-hour duration of action; the effective dose is 1 mg/q. 12 hours intramuscularly. (Caution—terbutaline is very stimulating, making it difficult for patients to sleep.)

Prazosin (Minipres). Prazosin is an alpha-blocker and antiphosphodiesterase agent[6] suitable for p.o. use only; it has a 12-hour duration of action, and the effective dose is 1 mg/q. 12 hours. (Caution—ambulatory patients will often complain of vascular headaches that usually respond to perphanizine [Trilafon].)

Isoxsuprine (Vasodilan). Isoxsuprine is a beta agonist and alpha-blocker, suitable for intramuscular or p.o. use. It has a 4-hour duration of action, and the effective dose is 40 to 60 mg/q. 4 hours.

Practical considerations

Dressings. Because the sites of anastomosis in heparinized patients ooze more, it is necessary to alter the type of dressing used. The general principle should be to expose the part and cover the suture line with an antibiotic cream. It has been found that if the part is covered with gauze, the dressing will cause pressure on the anastomosis when the clotted blood dries and contracts.

Discontinuing drugs. Never discontinue drug therapy in the evening before the period of reduced blood flow, and never discontinue it on a "struggling" digit or flap to see if it will survive. Chances are it will not.

The anesthetist. If possible, try to convince the anesthesiology department to avoid the use of vasoconstrictor agents as much as possible during microvascular surgery cases.

Remember surgical priority. Pharmacologic agents must never be used in place of good surgery. A perfect anastomosis and closure without tension, even if it means grafting exposed fat in an unsightly position, must always be given the highest priority.

ACKNOWLEDGMENT

This project was funded by grants from the Research Committee of the American Association of Plastic Surgeons, the Hearst Foundation, and the Office of Naval Research. Research facilities were generously provided by the Ralph K. Davies Medical Center, Letterman Army Hospital, and the Department of Anesthesiology and the Department of Nuclear Medicine at the University of California, San Francisco. Dr. M.F. Roisen provided facilities for catecholamine assay.

REFERENCES

1. Aauts, H.F.: Regional intravascular sympathetic blockade for better results in flap surgery: an experimental study of free flaps, island flaps and pedicle flaps in the rabbit ear, Plast. Reconstr. Surg. **66**:690, 1980.
2. Acland, R.: Prevention of thrombosis in microvascular surgery by the use of magnesium sulphate, Br. J. Plast. Surg. **25**:292, 1972.
3. Acland, R.D., and Trachtenberg, L.: The histopathology of small arteries following experimental microvascular anastomoses, Plast. Reconstr. Surg. **59**:868, 1977.
4. Baxter, T.J., O'Brien, B.M., Henderson, P.N., and Bennett, R.C.: The histopathology of small vessels following microvascular repair, Br. J. Surg. **59**:617, 1972.
5. Buncke, H.J., and Blackfield, H.M.: The vasoplegic effects of chlorpromazine Plast. Reconstr. Surg. **31**:353, 1963.
6. Cohen, M.L., Wiley, K.S., and Slater, I.H.: In vitro relaxation of arteries and veins by prazosin: alpha adrenergic blockage with no direct vasodilation, Blood Vessels **16**:144, 1979.
7. Daley, M.J., and Henry, R.F.: Quantitative measurement of skin perfusion with Xenon-133, J. Nucl. Med. **21**:156, 1980.
8. Daniel, R.K., and Swartz, W.M.: Advances in microsurgery, Adv. Surg. II, 285, 1977.
9. Daniel, R.K., and Taylor, G.I.: Distant transfer of an island flap by microvascular anastomosis: a clinical technique, Plast. Reconstr. Surg. **52**:111, 1973.
10. Daniel, R.K., and Terzis, J.K.: Reconstructive microsurgery, Boston, 1977, Little, Brown & Co.
11. Erdi, A., et al.: Effect of low-dose subcutaneous heparin on whole-blood viscosity, Lancet **2**:342, Aug. 14, 1976.

12. Finseth, F., and Adelberg, M.G.: Prevention of skin flap necrosis by a course of treatment with vasodilator drugs, Plast. Reconstr. Surg. **61:**738, 1978.

13. Gallus, A., and Engel, G.: Heparin, The Society of Hospital Pharmacists of Australia, 1978.

14. Goldwyn, R.M., Lamb, D.L., and White, L.L.: An experimental study of large island flaps in dogs, Plast. Reconstr. Surg. **31:**528, 1963.

15. Goodman, L.S., and Gilman, A., editors: The pharmacological basis of therapeutics, ed. 5, New York, 1975, Macmillan, Inc.

16. Hayhurst, J.W., and O'Brien, B.M.: An experimental study of microvascular technique: patency rates and related factors, Br. J. Plast. Surg. **28:**128, 1975.

17. Hayhurst, J.W., O'Brien, B.M., Ishida, H., and Baxter, T.A.: Experimental digital replantation after prolonged cooling, Hand **6:**134, 1974.

18. Imai, Y., et al.: The role of the peripheral vasculature in changes in venous return caused by isoproterenol, norepinephrine and methoxamine in anesthetized dogs, Circ. Res. **43**(4):553, 1978.

19. Kety, S.S.: Measurement of regional circulation by the local clearance of radioactive sodium, Am. Heart J. **38:**321, 1947.

20. Kjellmer, I., Lindbjerg, I., Prerovsky, I., and Tonnesen, H.: The relation between blood flow in an isolated muscle measured with Xe-133 clearance and a direct recording technique, Acta Physiol. Scand. **69:**69, 1967.

21. Kleinert, H.E., et al.: Replantation utilizing microsurgery, Curr. Pract. Orthop. Surg. **7:**78, 1977.

22. Kolar, L., Wiedberdink, J., and Reneman, R.S.: Anticoagulation in microvascular surgery, Eur. Surg. Res. **5:**52, 1973.

23. Kostzews, R.M., and Jacobowitz, D.M.: Pharmacological actions of 6-hydroxydopamine, Pharmacol. Rev. **26**(3):199, 1974.

24. Mahadoo, T., Hebert, L., and Jaques, L.B.: Vascular sequestration of heparin, Thromb. Res. **12:**79, 1978.

25. O'Brien, B.M.: Replantation and reconstructive microvascular surgery, Ann. Roy. Col. Surg. Eng. **58:**87, 1976.

26. O'Brien, B.M.: Microvascular reconstructive surgery, Edinburgh, 1977, Churchill-Livingstone.

27. O'Brien, B.M., McLeod, A.M., and Morrison, W.A.: Microsurgery, Aust. N.Z. J. Surg. **47:**396, 1977.

28. Palmer, B.: Factors influencing the elimination rate of Xenon-133 injected intracutaneously: a study in rats, Scand. J. Plast. Reconstr. Surg. **6:**1, 1972.

29. Roizen, M.J., et al.: Effects of halothane on plasma catecholamines, Anesthesiology **41:**432, 1974.

30. Shimmel, J.S., Finseth, F.S., and Buncke, H.J.: Digital replantation: current technique and practice, Plast. Reconstr. Surg. (In Press.)

31. Shu, C.: Shear dependence of effective cell, volume as a determinant of blood viscosity, Science **168:**977, 1970.

32. Stahl, W.M.: Reconstruction of small arteries, Arch. Surg. **88:**384, 1964.

33. Stranc, M.F., and Stranc, W.E.: Tubed skin flaps. In Grabb, W.C., and Myers, M.B., editors: Skin flaps, Boston, 1975, Little, Brown & Co.

34. Thurston, J.B., Buncke, H.J., Chater, N.L., and Weinstein, P.R.: A scanning electron microscopy study of micro-arterial damage and repair, Plast. Reconstr. Surg. **57:**197, 1976.

Chapter 44

Improvement of tissue blood flow by vasodilator therapy with isoxsuprine: direct measurement by xenon washout

Frederick Finseth

Harry J. Buncke

Sir Harold Gillies once said that plastic surgery is a constant battle between beauty and the blood supply. This study is an effort to fortify the stance of the blood supply in this contest by the use of isoxsuprine.

The central control point for tissue circulation is the smooth muscle tone of vessels. Adjustments of this muscle tone control the resistance, the exchange, the capacitance, and the distribution functions of the peripheral circulation. Failure to adjust for excess smooth muscle tone spells defeat for the blood supply (and for beauty).

We have sought to control the adverse effects of excessive smooth muscle tone with the vasodilator drug isoxsuprine. Isoxsuprine increases survival in skin flaps in rats and dogs, in muscle flaps in the rabbit, and in myocutaneous flaps in the pig,[1,3-6] and isoxsuprine vasodilator therapy has been used clinically for salvage of the failing flap.[2]

Isoxsuprine is a beta-adrenergic receptor agonist-stimulator that also has a direct vascular smooth muscle relaxing effect. Its vasodilation effect is thought to result from both actions. Beta receptors of the smooth muscle of peripheral vasculature cause vasodilation. The principal sites of these receptors are precapillary smooth muscle and precapillary sphincters. These are the sites of control of the number of open capillaries, the capillary surface area, and capillary transport, as well as the sites of control of the *exchange function* of the circulation (in contrast to the *resistance function* of the arteriolar vascular smooth muscle, and yet distinct from the *capacitance function* of the post capillary and venular vascular smooth muscle). Thus the beta receptor is a logical target for obtaining an effect on the exchange function of the circulation.

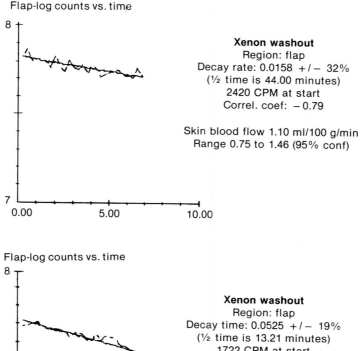

Fig. 44-1. Visual output from computer system, calculating tissue blood flow requirements from xenon washout. (Ohio Nuclear Model 410 gamma scintillation camera—Nuclear Medicine Computer System ADAC Clinical Data System).

XENON WASHOUT TECHNIQUE

Xenon washout is a technique for measuring capillary blood flow in tissue. We have sought to demonstrate the effect of isoxsuprine on blood flow to tissue in clinical circumstances by measuring capillary blood flow with the xenon washout technique. We have made these measurements in five patients with free microvascular tissue transfers, both before and after the administration of isoxsuprine.

The day after surgery, blood flow measurement was performed using the xenon washout technique. The patient was then given 10 mg of isoxsuprine intramuscularly. Two hours later the blood flow measurement was repeated. Measurements were taken in the free flap or injured tissue and in normal unoperated control skin elsewhere on the patient. Clinically stable patients without complications who could be transported safely were selected in consecutive order.

We injected 0.05 ml of normal saline with 50 μCi of dissolved xenon. Consecutive counts of radioactivity were made over 15-second intervals for a duration of 7 minutes. This information was fed into a computer that calculates the blood flow on the exponential rate of disappearance of the xenon radioactivity (Fig. 44-1).

1. 50 μCi xenon dissolved in 0.05 ml saline
2. Deep dermal injection
3. Consecutive radioactivity counts over 15-second intervals for 7-minute duration
4. Computer calculation of blood flow based on disappearance rate–washout of xenon

CASE REPORT
Patient I

The first patient had a burn injury of the right upper arm, elbow, and forearm; the hand was spared. His elbow was fixed at 60 degrees of flexion with no passive mobility. The extremity was essentially functionless because he had lost the ability to place his hand in useful positions. His left hand had also been severely burned, with loss of the digits and thumb; thus restoration of mobility to his right elbow was essential. Circumferential skin flap coverage of the elbow was needed to resurface the site for contracture release.

A free microvascular groin flap was anastomosed end to side to the brachial artery and a local vein (Fig. 44-2). On the first postoperative day blood flow measurements were made with the xenon washout technique before and 2 hours after administering a single dose. The blood flow acutely increased from 1.1 ml/100 g tissue/min to 3.6 ml/100 g/min (Fig. 44-3).

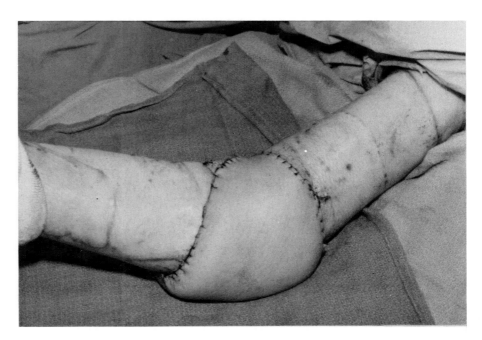

Fig. 44-2. Free microvascular groin flap to elbow.

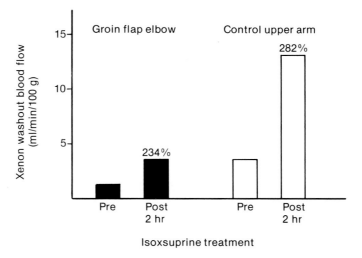

Fig. 44-3. Patient I. Bar graph representation of data.

Patient II

The second patient had a free microvascular groin flap for reconstruction of a web space following release of a thumb adduction contracture (Fig. 44-4). The blood flow increased from 2.3 ml/100 g/min to 3.3 ml/100 g/min, 2 hours after a single injection of 10 mg of isoxsuprine on the first postoperative day (Fig. 44-5).

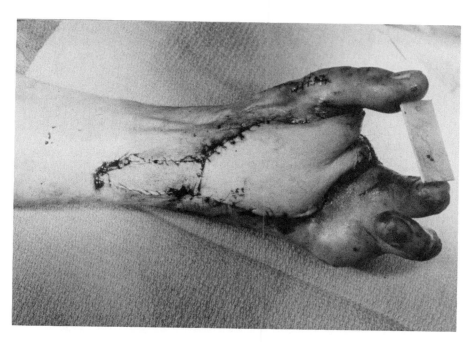

Fig. 44-4. Free microvascular groin flap to hand.

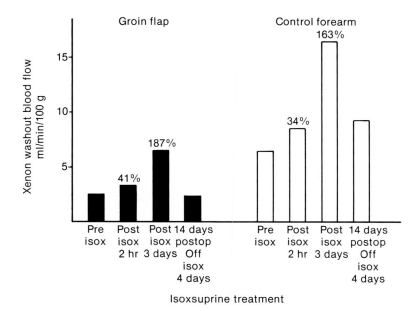

Fig. 44-5. Patient II. Bar graph representation of data.

Patient III

The third patient had a traumatic amputation of the dominant right thumb at the metacarpophalangeal joint level. A toe-to-hand thumb reconstruction was carried out (Fig. 44-6). On the first postoperative day blood flow increased from 4.6 ml/100 g/min to 9.6 ml/100 g/min, 2 hours after an injection of 10 mg of isoxsuprine (Fig. 44-7).

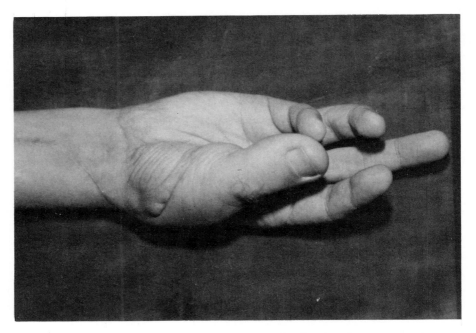

Fig. 44-6. Free microvascular great toe transfer for thumb reconstruction.

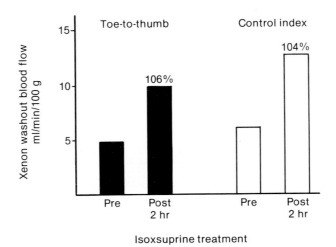

Fig. 44-7. Patient III. Bar graph representation of data.

Patient IV

The fourth patient had a large area of radionecrosis of the frontal bone from a recurrent brain tumor following a previous craniotomy and radiation therapy. Following debridement the wound consisted of a major defect with loss of skin, bone, and dura with exposure of the brain. The defect was repaired with a free latissimus dorsi muscle flap, anastomosing the vessels to the occipital artery and a local vein. The muscle flap was skin grafted. Again, on the first postoperative day, blood flow measurements were obtained and showed an increase from 1.1 ml/100 g/min to 2.9 ml/100 g/min, after a single injection of 10 mg of isoxsuprine (Fig. 44-8).

Patient V

The fifth patient had sustained a severe crush injury of the right wrist and hand for which he had undergone multiple operative procedures. He had a painful, relatively ischemic three-fingered hand with complete amputation of the thumb and index finger. An arteriogram showed obliteration of both the radial and ulnar arteries; the sole vascularization of the hand was from collateralization of the anterior interosseous artery, which reconstituted the superficial arch and common digital vessels. An attempt at revascularization by a vein bypass graft from the brachial artery to the superficial arch was unsuccessful. A trial was made of vasodilator therapy with isoxsuprine injections.

Six days after institution of this vasodilator regimen, repeat blood flow measurements were made. These demonstrated an increase of blood flow in the middle finger from 6.2 to 16.6 ml/100 g/min, in the ring finger from 2.6 to 11.0 ml/100 g/min, and in the small finger from 8.5 to 17.8 ml/100 g/min.

DISCUSSION

The blood flow to relatively ischemic tissue is promptly increased by administration of isoxsuprine; this increase can be maintained by the continued administration of isoxsuprine. The vasospasm and vasoconstriction that threaten a flap can be blocked, thus sustaining increased levels of blood flow and preventing necrosis in areas of marginal blood flow. Thromboses that result from a low-flow state at the anastomosis site might be averted by the increased flow rate provided by the action of isoxsuprine. Further, vascular spasm and its attending problems may be alleviated.

These findings suggest that (1) isoxsuprine has a positive effect on the cutaneous blood flow, (2) one focus of action of isoxsuprine is the precapillary sphincter, the regulatory point for capillary blood flow, and (3) the associated dilation of arteriovenous shunts does not physiologically "steal" blood from the capillary circulation.

SUMMARY

Our observations in five patients on whom objective measurements of blood flow were made by the xenon washout technique lead us to conclude that treatment with the vasodilator drug isoxsuprine substantially increased tissue blood flow.

REFERENCES

1. Acland, R.D.: Personal communication, 1980.
2. Finseth, F.: Clinical salvage of three failing skin flaps by treatment with a vasodilator drug, Plast. Reconstr. Surg. **63:**304, 1979.
3. Finseth, F., and Adelberg, M.G.: Prevention of skin flap necrosis by a course of treatment with vasodilator drugs, Plast. Reconstr. Surg. **61:**738, 1978.
4. Finseth, F., and Adelberg, M.G.: Experimental work with isoxsuprine for prevention of skin flap necrosis and for treatment of the failing flap, Plast. Reconstr. Surg. **63:**94, 1979.
5. Finseth, F., and Zimmermann, J.: Prevention of necrosis in island myocutaneous flaps in the pig by treatment with isoxsuprine, Plast. Reconstr. Surg. **64:** 536, 1979.
6. Finseth, F., Zimmermann, J., and Liggins, D.: Prevention of muscle necrosis in an experimental neurovascular island muscle flap by a vasodilator drug—isoxsuprine, Plast. Reconstr. Surg. **63:**774, 1979.

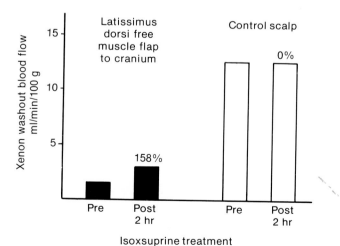

Fig. 44-8. Patient IV. Bar graph representation of data.

Index